# IMMUNOPATHOGENETIC
# MECHANISMS
# OF ARTHRITIS

# IMMUNOPATHO-GENETIC MECHANISMS OF ARTHRITIS

Edited by

## J. A. Goodacre
## and W. Carson Dick

*Department of Rheumatology*
*University of Newcastle upon Tyne*

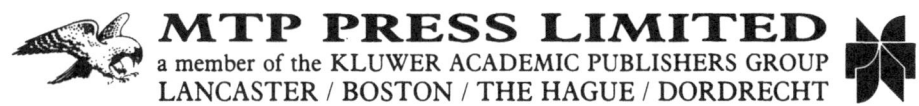
**MTP PRESS LIMITED**
a member of the KLUWER ACADEMIC PUBLISHERS GROUP
LANCASTER / BOSTON / THE HAGUE / DORDRECHT

Published in the UK and Europe by
MTP Press Limited
Falcon House
Lancaster, England

*British Library Cataloguing in Publication Data*

Immunopathogenetic mechanisms of arthritis.
   1. Arthritis    2. Immunogenetics
   I. Goodacre, J.    II. Dick, W. Carson
   616.7'220795      RC933

   ISBN-13: 978-94-010-7075-1     e-ISBN-13: 978-94-009-1293-9
   DOI: 10.1007/978-94-009-1293-9

Published in the USA by
MTP Press
A division of Kluwer Academic Publishers
101 Philip Drive
Norwell, MA 02061, USA

*Library of Congress Cataloging in Publication Data*

Immunopathogenetic mechanisms of arthritis.

   Includes bibliographies and index.
   1. Arthritis—Genetic aspects. 2. Immunopathology.
3. Immunogenetics. I. Goodacre, J. II. Dick, W.
Carson (William Carson) [DNLM: 1 Arthritis—immunology.
WE 344 1335]
RC933.144 1988    616.7'22079    87-33937

Typeset by Lasertext, Longford Trading Estate, Thomas Street, Stretford, Manchester

# CONTENTS

v

# List of contributors

**D. Alarcón-Segovia**
Department of Immunology and
  Rheumatology
Instituto Nacional de la Nutrición Salvador
  Zubirán
Vasco de Quiroga 15
Delegación Tlalpan
14000 Mexico, D. F.
Mexico

**A.C. Allison**
Department of Immunology
Institute of Biological Sciences
Syntex Research
3401 Hillview Avenue, Palo Alto
California 94303
USA

**J. Belch**
University Department of Medicine
Ninewells Hospital
Dundee DD1 9SY

**W. Carson Dick**
Department of Rheumatology
Royal Victoria Infirmary
Queen Victoria Road
Newcastle upon Tyne NE1 4LP

**A.R. Cross**
Department of Biochemistry
University of Bristol Medical School
University Walk
Bristol BS8 1TD

**G.W. Duff**
University of Edinburgh Department of
  Medicine
Rheumatic Diseases Unit
Northern General Hospital
Ferry Road
Edinburgh EH5 2DQ

**F.S. di Giovine**
University of Edinburgh Department of
  Medicine
Rheumatic Diseases Unit
Northern General Hospital
Ferry Road
Edinburgh EH5 2DQ

**J.A. Goodacre**
Department of Rheumatology
Royal Victoria Infirmary
Queen Victoria Road
Newcastle upon Tyne NE1 4LP

**I.D. Griffiths**
Department of Rheumatology
Royal Victoria Infirmary
Queen Victoria Road
Newcastle upon Tyne NE1 4LP

**O.T.G. Jones**
Department of Biochemistry
University of Bristol Medical School
University Walk
Bristol BS8 1TD

**L. Klareskog**
Department of Internal Medicine
Uppsala University
Uppsala University Hospital
751 85 Uppsala
Sweden

**S.C. Knight**
Division of Rheumatology
Medical Research Council Clinical Research
  Centre
Watford Road, Harrow
Middlesex HA1 3UJ

**J. Manson**
University of Edinburgh Department of
  Medicine
Rheumatic Diseases Unit
Northern General Hospital
Ferry Road
Edinburgh EH5 2DQ

**C.J.M. Melief**
Department of Immunology
The Netherlands Cancer Institute
Plesmanlaan 121
1066 CX Amsterdam
The Netherlands

**B. Pal**
Department of Rheumatology
Royal Victoria Infirmary
Queen Victoria Road
Newcastle upon Tyne NE1 4LP

**A.M. Solinger**
Department of Internal Medicine/Division
of Immunology
University of Cincinnati College of
Medicine
M.L. #563, 231 Bethesda Avenue
Cincinnati
Ohio 45267-0563
USA

**D.R. Stanworth**
Rheumatology and Allergy Research Unit
Department of Immunology
University of Birmingham Medical School
Vincent Drive
Birmingham B15 2TJ

**J.A. Symons**
University of Edinburgh Department of
Medicine
Rheumatic Diseases Unit
Northern General Hospital
Ferry Road
Edinburgh EH5 2DQ

**R.R.P. de Vries**
Department of Immunohaematology and
Bloodbank
University Hospital Leiden
Postbus 9600
2300 RE Leiden
The Netherlands

**H. Wigzell**
Department of Immunology
Karolinska Institutet
104 01 Stockholm
Sweden

**R.L. Wilder**
Arthritis and Rheumatism Branch
National Institute of Arthritis,
Musculoskeletal and Skin Diseases
National Institutes of Health
Bethesda, Maryland 20892
USA

# Preface

The fundamental problem facing scientists and clinicians in Rheumatology is that so little is known about the biology of joints. It is our view that a real interface between basic and clinical science offers the best chance of gaining a better understanding of arthritis and in this book we aim to provide a basis for such an interface. Each chapter provides a lucid account of the current literature, reflecting the eminence of each author in their own field. The contributors offer a variety of modern approaches to the study of inflammatory joint disease, illustrating some of the exciting opportunities for research which exist. We hope that those who share our view find these pages informative and stimulating.

*University of Newcastle upon Tyne, 1987.*　　　　　　　JOHN A. GOODACRE
W. CARSON DICK

# 1
# Polymorphonuclear leukocytes in acute inflammation

O. T. G. JONES and A. R. CROSS

## INTRODUCTION

The normal function of the professional phagocytes – polymorphonuclear leukocytes (PMN), monocytes, macrophages and eosinophils – is to protect the individual from microbial infection by seeking out and destroying the invading microbes. In order to perform this function effectively the phagocyte must move towards sites of infection, recognize, phagocytose, kill and digest the microbe and, if necessary, recruit other cells to assist. These phagocytic cells possess a membrane-bound enzyme system which can be activated to produce toxic oxygen radicals in response to a wide variety of stimuli. The purpose of this enzyme system is to destroy microbes, parasites or tumours by directing the radicals against the target cells. Whilst the beneficial effects of these oxygen radicals is well known, it has become clear that inappropriate production of oxygen radicals can have severe deleterious effects in diseases such as Behcet's disease, dermatitis herpetiformis, mucocutano-lymph node syndrome, rheumatoid arthritis, crystal-induced arthropathies, systemic lupus erythematosus, colitis ulcerosa, Crohn's disease, adult respiratory distress syndrome, reperfusion injury and carcinogenesis. In this chapter we shall concentrate on the properties of the oxygen radical generating system, its activation and the biological effects of its products.

## POLYMORPHONUCLEAR LEUKOCYTE FUNCTION

Phagocytes exhibit a number of discrete responses after exposure to a stimulus. The commonly measured responses are shown in Table 1.1.

Which particular combination of cellular responses is triggered may be both stimulus- and concentration-dependent; a PMN will respond to a low concentration of the chemotactic peptide N-formyl-Met-Leu-Phe (FMLP) by moving up a concentration gradient towards it (chemotaxis) but a higher concentration induces cellular production of superoxide. A large number of

1

**Table 1.1**   PMN responses to stimuli

---

Chemotaxis
Shape changes
Increased adhesiveness
Capping
Phagocytosis
Degranulation of specific and/or azurophilic (and/or tertiary?) granules
Secretion of lipoxygenase/cyclo-oxygenase products (e.g. leukotrienes and prostaglandins)
Superoxide production

---

substances have been found to stimulate PMN (Table 1.2).

This list contains examples of particulate stimuli (such as opsonized bacteria) and soluble stimuli (such as chemotactic peptides), both of which the PMN might normally be expected to encounter, and also substances such as the tumour promoter, phorbol myristate acetate (PMA), which the cells would not normally meet. In view of the large number of both stimuli and responses it is perhaps not surprising that a variety of mechanisms of signal transduction have been proposed to account for the cellular responses to the stimulus, these must explain both receptor-mediated and receptor-independent mechanisms of stimulation. In this review we will concentrate mainly on the mechanisms

**Table 1.2**   Substances known to stimulate PMN superoxide production

---

Opsonized particles and bacteria
Latex beads
Immune complexes
Complement fragments
Histamine-coated beads
Kallikrein
Crystals (e.g. urate, hydroxyapatite)

Fluoride ions
Lanthanum ions

Divalent cation ionophores (e.g. A23187)
Monovalent cation ionophores (e.g. valinomycin)

Phospholipase C
Phorbol myristate acetate
Fatty acids

Lectins
Cytochalasins

Membrane perturbing agents (e.g. SDS, digitonin)
DCCD (ATPase inhibitor)

Endotoxins

Chemotactic peptides (e.g. FMLP)
Leukocyte pyrogens
Platelet activating factor
Leukotrienes ($B_4$, $D_4$)
Platelet-derived growth factor
Bacterial lipopolysaccharide

Protease inhibitors

---

thought to be important in the activation of the superoxide generating oxidase of PMN, but firstly we should consider the nature of the superoxide generating oxidase itself.

## THE COMPOSITION OF THE SUPEROXIDE GENERATING SYSTEM OF PMN

The identification and characterization of the enzymic system responsible for the production of superoxide has been the subject of intense investigation in recent years. The 'increased respiration of phagocytosis' (the respiratory burst) had been reported by Baldridge and Gerard in 1933[1] and was thought to be a result of the stimulation of mitochondrial respiration necessary to provide the energy for phagocytosis. When the insensitivity of the increased oxygen uptake to inhibitors of mitochondrial respiration (cyanide and antimycin A) was described[2] attention was focussed on the nature of the enzyme responsible for the respiratory burst. Subsequently a variety of NADH-dependent soluble[3,4] or membrane-bound[5] oxidases and NADPH-dependent particulate[6,7] or NAD(P)H-dependent particulate enzymes[8,9] were described. In 1968 Paul and Sbarra[10] made direct measurements of hydrogen peroxide formation and in 1973 Babior and co-workers[11] established that superoxide was a major product of the NAD(P)H oxidase. It is now generally accepted that the enzyme is membrane-bound, exhibits a preference for NADPH ($K_m = 45\ \mu mol\ L^{-1}$) over NADH ($K_m = 450\ \mu mol\ L^{-1}$) and converts oxygen to its one electron reduced product, superoxide.

$$NADPH + 2O_2 \rightarrow NADP^+ + 2O_2^{-\cdot}$$

The enzyme activity is almost undetectable in resting (unstimulated) cells but increases enormously upon stimulation. In patients with the rare genetic disorder, chronic granulomatous disease (CGD), there is a predisposition to severe chronic recurrent infection, the neutrophils of these patients phagocytose normally but the respiratory burst is absent and NADPH oxidase activity (and radical production) is undetectable.

Much evidence suggests that the oxidase system is located on the plasma membrane of the PMN and becomes incorporated into the wall of the developing phagosome during phagocytosis. Briggs *et al.*[12] used a cytochemical method to locate superoxide production on the plasma membrane in the presence of a non-phagocytosable stimulus and inside the phagolysosome when a particulate stimulus was used. On subcellular fractionation NADPH oxidase activity was associated with the plasma membrane fraction[13,14]. Other evidence has come from the use of granule-depleted cytoplasts, which are virtually devoid of subcellular organelles but are capable of mounting a respiratory burst equivalent to that of the whole cell on the basis of membrane area[15,16].

Segal *et al.*[17] were the first to suggest that the oxidase was in fact a multicomponent electron transport chain and subsequently three redox components have been proposed, a flavin adenine dinucleotide (FAD) containing flavoprotein, a *b*-type cytochrome and ubiquinone.

3

## Flavoprotein

The oxidase was first proposed to be a flavoprotein by Babior and co-workers[18] who found that the addition of FAD to detergent extracts of oxidase-containing membranes restored activity lost in the presence of Triton X-100. The Triton solubilized enzyme had a dissociation constant for FAD of 61 nmol L$^{-1}$[119]. Other evidence for flavoprotein involvement has been obtained using the inhibitory effects of the flavin analogues 5-deaza-FAD and quinacrine[20-22]. The subcellular distribution of FAD is found to be very similar to the distribution of another proposed component of the oxidase, cytochrome $b_{-245}$[23] (see below). There are altered levels of FAD in PMN from patients with CGD[23-26]. Artificial reduction of the flavin by light in the presence of EDTA causes the reduction of the cytochrome $b_{-245}$ suggesting that the flavoprotein could be the reductase *in vivo*[23]. The redox potential of the flavoprotein has been determined ($E_{m7} = -280$ mV)[194].

## Cytochrome *b*

The presence of a novel cytochrome *b* in (equine) neutrophils was first reported by Hattori in 1961[27] and its involvement in the respiratory burst was proposed by Shinigawa *et al.* in 1966 in studies of rabbit PMN[28], on the basis of its oxidase-like properties (auto-oxidizability and the ability to bind carbon monoxide). Unfortunately these reports did not receive much attention until Segal and co-workers showed that the cytochrome was absent from some[17,29] but not all[30] patients with chronic granulomatous disease. The cytochrome was found to have a dual localization in both the plasma membrane and the specific granules, becoming incorporated into the phagolysosome during phagocytosis of latex beads[31,32]. Under anaerobic conditions the cytochrome became reduced on stimulation of the cells and was reoxidized by air[33]. It was not reduced in the cells of those CGD patients who did have the cytochrome[34]. Subsequent work has shown that the cytochrome *b*-negative form of the disease follows an X-linked form of inheritance and the cytochrome *b*-positive disease an autosomal form of inheritance[35]. *In vitro* complementation studies using monocytes from CGD patients elegantly confirmed these findings[36]. The gene for CGD codes for cytochrome $b_{-245}$[195,196].

Following the identification of the cytochrome b as a likely component of the superoxide generating system much work has been done to characterize it. The cytochrome has an extremely low oxidation-reduction potential ($-245$ mV)[37], lower than any other mammalian cytochrome *b* and sufficiently low to reduce oxygen to superoxide ($E_{m7} = -160$ mV)[38]. This unique property has proved invaluable in quantifying its concentration in cells containing other cytochromes and we have designated it cytochrome $b_{-245}$ (others have used the terminology cytochrome $b_{558}$). The cytochrome is present only in the other professional phagocytes: monocytes, macrophages and eosinophils[39]. Its synthesis is induced in a promyelocytic cell-line (HL-60), concomitant with the ability to produce superoxide, when the cells are induced to mature by dimethyl sulphoxide[40]. Cytochrome $b_{-245}$ forms a light-dissociable complex with carbon monoxide and although it has a relatively low affinity for this ligand ($K_m = 1.18\,\mathrm{mmol\,L^{-1}}$)[41], it does indicate the haem is sufficiently exposed to bind oxygen. Chemically reduced cytochrome $b_{-245}$ is reoxidized by oxygen very rapidly ($t\frac{1}{2} = 4.7\,\mathrm{ms}$)[41,42] which suggests that the cytochrome is the terminal component in the oxidase system. A number of groups have reported the purification of the cytochrome but with a wide range of reported molecular weights: a glycoprotein of 68–78 kDa[43]; 127 kDa[44]; 14, 12 and 11 kDa[45]; 32 kDa[46,47]. These discrepancies may be due to species differences and the anomalous behaviour on SDS-PAGE due to glycosylation and the extremely hydrophobic nature of the protein. Recent work suggests that the cytochrome is a heterodimer[197,198].

## Ubiquinone

In addition to the cytochrome and flavin components it has been suggested that quinone may be involved in the radical generating system[25,48–50], identified as ubiquinone-10[51,52]. It was claimed that quinone was not of mitochrondrial origin since phagolysosomal fractions isolated from neutrophils were enriched in ubiquinone. However, other subcellular fractionation studies have found only small quantities of ubiquinone and these have been associated only with the mitochrondrial fractions[53], furthermore, the ratio of cellular ubiquinone to cytochrome $c$ oxidase was 11.9:1 in the range typical for mitochondria (10.9–16.4:1)[54], and there was no enrichment of ubiquinone in phagolysosomes enriched in NADPH oxidase activity. Lutter et al.[16] also failed to detect ubiquinone in cytoplasts (which retain NADPH oxidase activity but are depleted in granules and organelles) and suggested that the large amounts of ubiquinone detected by others was a result of thrombocyte contamination. Bellavite et al.[55] were unable to detect ubiquinone in extracts of partially purified oxidase and concluded it was unlikely to be part of the oxidase. Final resolution of the controversy will probably require reconstitution studies. To date no other redox components have been implicated in the system and low temperature EPR studies have not detected any iron–sulphur or copper centres[37].

## ACTIVATION OF THE SUPEROXIDE GENERATING OXIDASE

A large number of signal-transduction mechanisms have been proposed to account for the activation of the oxidase by the diverse stimuli listed in Table 1.2. These include changes in the concentrations of cyclic nucleotides, altered intracellular concentrations of ions (particularly calcium), release of arachidonic acid and its metabolites, activation of protein kinases, limited proteolysis and membrane fusion. In the case of inflammatory stimuli the response of the cell is normally through a specific receptor-mediated event which leads to further intracellular signalling, finally arriving at a common pathway of activation. It is likely that those stimuli which do not have a specific receptor on the cell surface act at some later point on the activation pathway. One unexplained feature of receptor-mediated activation is the localized nature of the response; in the case of an opsonized zymosan particle or a non-phagocytosable surface

5

the formation of oxygen radicals takes place only in those areas of PMN membrane in contact with the particle and is not a generalized event[56,57] responses are also transient in the case of some stimuli[58,59].

## Ligand–receptor interaction

A number of receptors are present on the neutrophil plasma membrane (Table 1.3). The best characterized of these is the FMLP receptor and we will use this as an example of neutrophil receptor function.

There are approximately 40 000–60 000 FMLP receptors per cell (detected by labelling of cells with FML[$^3$H]P) of molecular weight of around 66 kDa. These receptors allow the PMN to respond in an adaptive way to discriminate differences in concentration from 1 nmol L$^{-1}$ to 50 $\mu$mol L$^{-1}$. This is achieved by altering the affinity of the available receptors through the involvement of GTP-binding proteins and receptor methylation. Low concentrations of stimulus cause chemotaxis, higher concentrations stimulate degranulation and superoxide production; these functions can be separated pharmacologically using aliphatic alcohols or polyene antibiotics (which alter membrane fluidity). In isolated PMN membranes two populations of receptors can be detected, low affinity ($K_d = 24.4$ nmol L$^{-1}$) and high affinity ($K_d = 0.53$ nmol L$^{-1}$)[69]. The high affinity receptors can be converted into the low affinity form by incubation of the membranes with a non-hydrolysable GTP analogue[69]. Snyderman et al.[70] have proposed the following scheme to account for these observations based on the model of the $\beta$-adrenergic receptor where the transduction of the receptor signal is via a guanine nucleotide-binding protein (N protein) which exhibits altered affinities for guanine nucleotides when bound to the ligand-receptor complex. Inhibition of these guanine nucleotide-binding proteins by cholera or pertussis toxins can inhibit or stimulate activation[71,72]. The model therefore describes not only the mechanism of receptor regulation but also the mechanism by which the binding of ligand to receptor transmits a signal to within the cell.

The nucleotide regulatory protein can transmit the signal intracellularly by altering an effector protein E, converting it to an active (or inactive state), E*, by phosphorylation or some conformation change. Possible effector proteins are enzymes such as phospholipases, protein kinases, methyl transferase, adenylate cyclase, etc.

**Table 1.3**  Human PMN receptors

| Stimulus | Reference |
|---|---|
| C5a (complement fragment) | 60 |
| C3b (stimulates phagocytosis not O$_2^-$ production) | 61 |
| FMLP | 62 |
| Fc component of IgG | 63 |
| Cell-derived chemotactic factor | 64 |
| Leukotriene B$_4$ (LTB$_4$) | 65 |
| Platelet activating factor (PAF) | 66 |
| Platelet-derived growth factor | 67 |

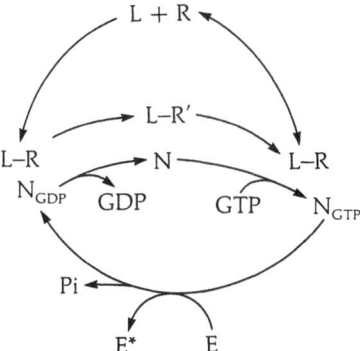

**Figure 1.1** In the model it is proposed that the affinity of the receptor is dependent on its association to the regulatory protein N which can bind guanine nucleotides. The transient high affinity state R' occurs when the receptor is bound to free N. (From Ref. 70)

Only a proportion of the receptors can be converted to the low affinity state by the addition of GTP. If cells are incubated with FMLP for 30 min, and washed to remove the stimulus, the number of high affinity receptors is increased markedly in a concentration-dependent manner. The high affinity receptors formed by pre-exposure to the stimulus are no longer susceptible to regulation by GTP, however. In these circumstances it is not known what alters the affinity of the receptors although it is known that their affinity can be altered by membrane fluidity. Yuli *et al.*[73] have shown, by the use of agents which alter membrane fluidity, that chemotaxis requires low doses of chemoattractants and is augmented by agents that increase the number of high affinity receptors, whereas superoxide production (and lysosomal enzyme release) is decreased when high affinity receptors predominate. Snyderman[70] has also suggested that methylation reactions may be involved in receptor regulation as well as being involved in the subsequent signal transduction.

## Intracellular second messengers

Following the interaction of the stimulus with the cell (either in a specific receptor-mediated fashion or otherwise), there follows the transmission of the signal through a pathway or set of pathways within the cell to a common intermediate, which in turn activates the oxidase itself.

## Cyclic nucleotides

Following stimulation with chemoattractants, immune complexes or iono-phores, two- or threefold increases in the levels of cAMP (but not cGMP) have been detected in PMN. The responses are rapid and precede the onset of $O_2^-$ production[74–76]. However, incubation of the cells with cAMP agonists did not promote the onset of the respiratory burst and in fact inhibited subsequent stimulus-induced $O_2^-$ formation. Thus cAMP seems to be involved in the inactivation rather than the activation process. Agonist-induced changes in cGMP levels do not appear to influence the respiratory burst[75,77].

## Membrane potential changes

Following stimulation of phagocytes very rapid changes of membrane potential, due to changes in ion flux, have been measured both directly (by the use of microelectrodes[78]) or by the use of fluorescent probes[79-81]. Changes have been measured in the fluxes of $H^+$, $Na^+$, $K^+$ and $Ca^{2+}$ which appear to be related to activation and indeed some ionophores have been shown to stimulate PMN[82,83]. Manipulation of the membrane potential by incubation of the cells in $Na^+$-free, high $K^+$ medium increased production of $O_2^-$ in response to FMLP[84]. However, in similar low $Na^+$, high $K^+$ medium, reduced responses to stimulation by immune complexes, zymosan or Con A were found[85,86]. Abnormal membrane depolarization has been described in some[87,88] but not all[89] patients with CGD. At the present time the relationship between membrane potential changes and the activation of the oxidase system is not clear; changes may arise from the electrogenic nature of the oxidase[199].

## Intracellular $Ca^{2+}$ and inositol phospholipid metabolism

There is evidence that extracellular $Ca^{2+}$ is involved in the activation of PMN by many stimuli. Activation of the oxidase by most stimuli is inhibited by the removal of extracellular calcium ions[90] whilst the calcium ionophores, A23187 and X357A can activate the respiratory burst directly[82,91] and certain stimuli cause increases in $Ca^{2+}$ uptake[92]. These studies suggest that for some stimuli the activation process is associated with an influx of extracellular $Ca^{2+}$; intracellular $Ca^{2+}$ might be involved with other regulatory mechanisms as in many other cell types. However, PMA and immune complexes can stimulate $O_2^-$ production in the absence of extracellular $Ca^{2+}$, whilst activation by other stimuli is diminished, but not abolished by EGTA[93] suggesting that intracellular $Ca^{2+}$ might be more important than $Ca^{2+}$ influx. Release of intracellular $Ca^{2+}$ following stimulation was demonstrated by Hoffstein[94] and the release has been shown to precede $O_2^-$ production[95]. Using the $Ca^{2+}$ activated photoprotein, obelin, Campbell and co-workers[96] have found that Con A, FMLP, complement and A23187 all caused rises in intracellular $Ca^{2+}$ which were necessary for activation of the respiratory burst. However, unopsonized latex beads were capable of inducing $O_2^-$ production even when intracellular $Ca^{2+}$ levels were prevented from rising by intracellular EGTA. The use of the fluorescent $Ca^{2+}$ probe, quin-2[97], has shown that whilst increases in intracellular $Ca^{2+}$, by release from intracellular stores, are of general importance to activation mechanisms in phagocytes, they are not sufficient in themselves to activate the respiratory burst[98], in agreement with the finding[99] that PMA does not increase intracellular $Ca^{2+}$. This does not explain the effect of calcium ionophores, however.

The mechanisms of intracellular $Ca^{2+}$ release have been recently reviewed by Berridge and Irvine[100]. It is thought that the release is mediated by

8

the activation of a phospholipase C which hydrolyses membrane bound phosphatidylinositol-4, 5-bisphosphate ($PIP_2$), to diacyl glycerol (DAG) and inositol-1,4,5-trisphosphate ($InsP_3$). $InsP_3$ from the membrane causes the release of $Ca^{2+}$ from intracellular stores. Increased breakdown of $PIP_2$, in response to stimuli, sufficient to cause intracellular $Ca^{2+}$ release has been measured by several groups[101–103].

## Protein kinase C

The finding that the binding site for phorbol esters within cells is the $Ca^{2+}$-activated, phospholipid-dependent, protein kinase C[104,105] has advanced understanding of cellular regulation. The link between this protein kinase and stimulus–response transduction was DAG (produced from $PIP_2$ breakdown) which dramatically increases its affinity for $Ca^{2+}$ thus activating kinase activity[106]. Activation of protein kinase C could modify many cellular functions by phosphorylation of other proteins. When protein kinase C is activated it is translocated from the cytosol to the plasma membrane[107–109], an effect stimulated by $Ca^{2+}$. A model has been proposed in which increases of intracellular $Ca^{2+}$ cause the translocation of protein kinase C to the membrane, prior to its activation by a second messenger, thus 'priming' the cell. This mechanism may explain the observation that incubation of PMN with low concentrations of chemoattractants[110] or other stimuli[111–113] potentiates activation of the cells by a second stimulus. This phenomenon of 'priming' has been further investigated by McPhail and colleagues[114], who showed that priming and activation could be clearly separated into two distinct events: low and high doses resulting in different intracellular responses. In a primed cell the lag period between exposure to the stimulus and the onset of the respiratory burst is reduced or absent and the rate of $O_2^-$ production is higher. In FMLP stimulation, removal of extracellular $Ca^{2+}$ with EGTA prevented oxidase activation but had no effect on its ability to prime for PMA. It was hypothesized that during priming protein kinase C was translocated to the plasma membrane where it was in the immediate vicinity of its substrate (some component of the $O_2^-$ generating system) – when the second (activating) signal arrives a more rapid and complete activation of the oxidase results.

Protein kinase C is the predominant protein kinase in neutrophils[115,116] and its substrates have been identified in neutrophil cytoplasts[117] where it phosphorylates a number of proteins. The phosphorylation of one of these proteins (molecular weight 46 kDa) paralleled the increase in $O_2^-$ production. Recently, Segal et al.[118] have shown that a polypeptide of similar molecular weight (44 kDa) is phosphorylated on stimulation of normal neutrophils or neutrophils from two patients with the X-linked form of CGD, but was not phosphorylated in neutrophils from four patients with the autosomal recessive form of the disease. It seems likely that this polypeptide is either a regulatory protein or part of the oxidase itself. Recently purified protein kinase C has been shown to activate $O_2^-$ production in a cell-free system[119]. However, protein kinase C may not be the whole answer to the activation process. Some

9

evidence from activation in cell-free systems suggests that phosphorylation is not essential for oxidase activation (see below), and three groups of workers have used different protein kinase C inhibitors to show that activation of the cells by FMLP or C5a is not inhibited[120–122]. Other recent reports[123] show that not all stimuli cause redistribution of protein kinase C or may even reverse membrane association[124].

### Activation of the oxidase in cell-free systems

Until recently it was impossible to activate the oxidase which forms $O_2^-$ in a cell-free system. Low levels of activation in broken-cell preparations treated with unsaturated fatty acids were reported independently by Bromberg and Pick (in guineapig macrophages)[125] and Heyneman and Vercauteren (in horse PMN)[126] in 1984. Shortly afterwards McPhail *et al.*[127] and Curnutte[128] reported arachidonate-dependent stimulation of $O_2^-$ production in cell-free sonicates of human PMN. High levels of $O_2^-$ production have now been achieved using the anionic detergents SDS and sodium dodecyl sulphonate in place of arachidonate[129]. In these cell-free systems there is a requirement for both a membrane fraction and a cytosolic fraction. The requirement for the cytosolic component is largely removed by pretreatment of the whole cell with low (sub-stimulatory) concentrations of PMA. It is not clear how detergents can activate the oxidase system, but there are a number of possibilities: an induced conformational change resulting in activation; removal of a membrane-associated inhibitory factor; alteration of the lipid environment around the oxidase allowing interaction with substrates or binding of activating factors; or finally a direct stimulation of protein kinase C.

### REACTIONS AND INTERACTIONS OF ACTIVATED OXYGEN SPECIES

The neutrophil NADPH oxidase produces $O_2^-$ on the outer face of the plasma membrane[11], which develops into the limiting membrane of the phagocytic vacuole, exposing target microorganisms to high local concentrations of the radical. There is also a substantial release of $O_2^-$ to the outside of the neutrophil during the respiratory burst, and this may contribute to tissue damage seen in inflammation and the activation of chemotactic factors[130]. $HO_2$ has a pK of 4.7 and is largely dissociated to $O_2^-$ at physiological pH, but the concentration of the protonated form of superoxide, which is much more reactive than $O_2^-$, is not negligible at the acid pH of the phagosome. $HO_2$ is also favoured by solution into a hydrophobic environment such as is found in biological membranes. Although superoxide is not a violent reagent it can act as a nucleophile in hydrophobic environments and can attack groups such as ester carbonyl groups present in phospholipids. Despite its relatively low reactivity in aqueous solution, $O_2^-$ can cause damage to a wide range of biological materials[131,132], including glutathione peroxidase which is an enzyme concerned in cellular defence against radical attack[133]. It can also act as a one-electron reductant, a property used in the common assay of

10

superoxide by following spectroscopically the reduction of added oxidized cytochrome $c$.

$$\text{cytochrome } c^{3+} + O_2^- \rightarrow \text{cytochrome } c^{2+} + O_2$$

Similarly $O_2^-$ can reduce tetrazolium salts to the blue formazans (the NBT test).

The main damaging biological effects of $O_2^-$ are believed to follow its dismutation to hydrogen peroxide ($H_2O_2$). This reaction is strongly pH-dependent, being favoured at acid pH, where there is a high concentration of protonated $O_2^-$ (i.e. $HO_2^-$). The uncatalysed reaction at pH 4.7 probably proceeds as shown below:

$$HO_2^- + O_2^- + H \rightarrow H_2O_2$$

At high pH, spontaneous dismutation is very slow. Superoxide reacts slowly with itself because two negatively charged species are involved:

$$O_2^- + O_2^- + 2H^+ \rightarrow H_2O_2$$

However this reaction is catalysed at neutral pH by superoxide dismutase, a metalloenzyme found in the cytosol (a Cu–Zn-protein) and in the mitochondria (a Mn-protein) of aerobic organisms[134].

$H_2O_2$ is not a radical and since its dissociation has a pK = 11.8 it is uncharged at physiological pH. Although poorly reactive in aqueous solution it can diffuse through membranes and give rise to toxic species remote from the site of its formation. The most reactive product derived *in vivo* from $H_2O_2$ is the hydroxyl radical, $OH$, formed in a transition metal-catalysed Haber-Weiss reaction. Iron is the metal commonly implicated in this reaction, although catalysis by copper and manganese ions may also be important biologically.

$$Fe^{3+} + O_2^- \rightarrow Fe^{2+} + O_2$$
$$Fe^{2+} + H_2O_2 \rightarrow Fe^{3+} + OH^- + OH$$

$OH$ reacts with great avidity with almost any compound containing hydrogen[135], including lipids, proteins, sugars and nucleotides. It is one of the most reactive species known in biology and so can travel a very limited distance from its site of formation; it is site-specific in that it reacts where formed. Examples of three types of reaction typical of $OH$ are shown below:

(1) *Hydrogen abstraction.* An example would be the reaction of a methylene group of a lipid.

$$R\text{-}CH_2\text{-}CH_2\text{-}R^1 + OH \rightarrow R\text{-}CH_2\text{-}CH\text{-}R^1 + H_2O$$

The lipid radical formed can react with oxygen to form a peroxy radical ($ROO$) and participate in a self-propagating chain of radical reactions causing extensive destruction of the lipids and membrane damage.

(2) *Addition reactions.* $OH$ can react with aromatic structures or with the purines and pyrimidines of nucleotides by addition, e.g.:

11

The radicals formed can then participate in further reactions, often involving oxygen, forming reactive products in a chain reaction.

(3)  *Electron transfer reactors.* The OH has a high oxidation–reduction potential and can act as an oxidant. A laboratory example of this type of reaction would be the oxidation of the ferrocyanide ion:

$$Fe(CN)_6^{4-} + OH \rightarrow Fe(CN)_6^{3-} + OH^-$$

or, more significant in biology, of chloride ion:

$$Cl^- + OH \rightarrow Cl + OH^-$$

Since iron in the Haber-Weiss reaction catalyses the formation of the very destructive OH radical from $H_2O_2$ and $O_2^-$, or from $H_2O_2$ itself, the availability of iron is important in the development of tissue damage from the radical attack[136] and in the microbicidal activity of the neutrophil[137]. Dissolved iron ions do not occur free in biological fluids; they are complexed to proteins, nucleic acids, phospholipids or to low molecular weight chelating molecules (such as ascorbate, citrate or ATP). The complexing of iron in haem proteins, where much of the body iron is found, is very tight and the same is true of ferric iron which is liganded to the specialised transport or storage proteins transferrin, lactoferrin and ferritin. It appears[138,139] that the iron complexes of molecules such as ATP or citrate can still catalyse the formation of OH but that iron in such haem complexes as myoglobin or haemoglobin is relatively inactive in this regard[137].

Specific granules of neutrophils are particularly rich in lactoferrin, which is stored in the granules in the iron-free form. Its role in the microbicidal and inflammatory activity of neutrophils is intriguing but still uncertain. It is released into the phagocytic vacuole as the granules fuse with the phagosomal membrane and passes to the exterior of the neutrophil before the developing phagocytic vacuole is sealed. Lactoferrin has a high affinity for iron in the ferric state (two atoms of ferric iron bound per mole) and its function may be protective, in complexing and preventing loosely bound iron from catalysing OH formation from $H_2O_2$. Partly iron-saturated lactoferrin does not catalyse lipid peroxidation and inhibits the catalytic function of added iron[140] while fully iron-saturated lactoferrin was found to be a poor catalyst of OH production[141] in a model system where $O_2^-$ was generated using xanthine oxidase. There have been reports[142] that the production of OH from superoxide produced by neutrophil NADPH oxidase was catalysed by iron-loaded lactoferrin. It is possible that conditions used for iron loading the lactoferrin are critical in its catalysis of OH production, or the iron may be released from its protected site in lactoferrin following reduction, by $O_2^-$, of bound $Fe^{3+}$ iron to the very much less tightly bound $Fe^{2+}$ form.

## Involvement of myeloperoxidase in the formation of toxic products from $H_2O_2$

Azurophil granules of human neutrophils are rich in the pale green haem-containing glycoprotein, myeloperoxidase. This is released into the phagocytic vacuole when target microbes of particles are ingested. Simultaneously, the respiratory burst is activated leading to local high concentrations of $O_2^-$ and $H_2O_2$ (formed by dismutation). Myeloperoxidase catalyses the oxidation of halogen ions, the most abundant of which is $Cl^-$ ($0.1\,mol\,L^{-1}$), which forms hypochlorite in the following reaction[143,144]:

$$H_2O_2 + Cl^- \xrightarrow{myeloperoxidase} OCl^- + H_2O$$

Some $OI^-$ may also be produced from $I^-$ although the low concentration of $I^-$ in human plasma ($0.1\,\mu mol\,L^{-1}$) suggests that its effects may not be important[145].

Hypochlorous acid is toxic to microorganisms and is important in the normal processes of killing infecting microorganisms. It can diffuse through the cell and react with amino groups to form chloramines, which persist as long-lived oxidants[146–148] and it can oxidize essential thiol groups of proteins to sulphoxide. Thus release of hypochlorite at an inflammatory site can directly cause tissue damage and also the activation of destructive neutral proteases (see later section on granule enzymes).

## Effects of active oxygen derivatives on DNA

It has become apparent that reactive oxygen intermediates produced by human neutrophils are capable of causing the malignant transformation of cells[149,150] which is noteworthy since carcinomas are frequently associated with some chronic inflammatory conditions, such as ulcerative colitis and chronic osteomyelitis. The activated oxygen species involved in producing transformation and DNA strand breaks[151] are yet to be established.

Oxidants are also known to affect the DNA repair enzyme polyadenosine diphosphate–ribose polymerase which ADP-ribosylates chromosomal proteins. The substrate for this enzyme is $NAD^+$, which is present in increased concentrations, as reduced pyridine nucleotides are oxidized in protection reactions against oxidative attack, and it is stimulated by DNA strand breaks produced by oxidative attack. The effect is cellular $NAD^+$ depletion[152] and perhaps modulation of gene expression.

## CELLULAR DEFENCE AGAINST ACTIVE OXYGEN ATTACK

Cells of all aerobic organisms, including neutrophils, contain metallo-enzymes called superoxide dismutases[153] which catalyse the conversion of $O_2^-$ to $H_2O_2$. They are located within the cytosol and mitochondria of mammalian cells and efficiently and rapidly scavenge $O_2^-$ radicals. The $H_2O_2$ which is produced is itself capable of giving rise to such toxic species as $OH^-$ and $OCl^-$ must also be removed if damage is to be minimized. This is the role of glutathione peroxidase, a cytosolic enzyme containing neither haem nor flavin but a selenium prosthetic group[154], which catalyses the following reaction:

$$2\,GSH + H_2O_2 \xrightarrow[peroxidase]{glutathione} GSSG + 2H_2O$$

13

Thus any $O_2^-$ or $H_2O_2$ which diffuses into the neutrophil cytosol from the phagosome can be converted to non-toxic products at the expense of reduced glutathione[155].

Reduced glutathione can be regenerated by the flavin enzyme glutathione disulphide reductase, which uses as electron donor NADPH supplied by the hexose monophosphate pathway. It is an enzyme with well defined crystal structure and mechanisms[156,157].

$$GSSG + NADPH + H^+ \xrightarrow[\text{reductase}]{\text{glutathione}} 2\ GSH + NADP^+$$

A variety of low molecular weight molecules help to protect cells against radical attack[131]. These include ascorbic acid, in the soluble phase of cells, and vitamin E in membranes. Both react with radicals to form stable products and thus quench radical reactions. Uric acid acts as an antioxidant in the plasma, and so does caeruloplasmin, a copper protein, which can accept electrons from $O_2^-$ and also act as a ferroxidase, to oxidise $Fe^{2+}$ to $Fe^{3+}$, thus inhibiting iron-dependent lipid peroxidation.

## THE GRANULES OF POLYMORPHONUCLEAR LEUKOCYTES

One of the most obvious morphological features of the human polymorpho-nuclear leukocyte is the abundance of membrane-limited granules in the cytoplasm; this striking characteristic has caused these cells to be classified as granulocytes, along with eosinophils and basophils. The granules are laid down early in the differentiation of neutrophils, the larger azurophil granules (or primary granules) appearing at the promyelocyte stage and the smaller specific granules (secondary granules) appearing in myelocytes[158]. In mature cells the specific granules are the most abundant. With the development of techniques of cell fractionation it has become apparent that there are sub-populations of granules differing slightly in density and enzyme content. In human neutrophils there is good evidence[159] for the presence of a third class of granule, sometimes given the name tertiary granule. The granules differ markedly in their contents and these differences are used in their classification. Azurophil granules are particularly rich in myeloperoxidase, a haem protein which gives the granules (and neutrophils) their characteristic pale green colour. An abundant marker protein for specific granules is lactoferrin, the iron-complexing protein, and for tertiary granules gelatinase is characteristic. A list of constituents of the granules of human neutrophils is given in Table 1.4: this catalogue, which is far from complete, is based in part on similar tabulations given by Gallin[160] and Baggiolini and Dewald[161].

Azurophil granules contain acid hydrolases typical of lysosomes, together with some constituents which are much more obviously concerned with microbicidal activity. In this latter group are found the antimicrobial cationic proteins[162] which include a chymotrypsin-like proteolytic protein, cathepsin G, which retains its antibacterial activity even after its chymotrypsin-like action has been abolished by heating or by treatment with diisopropylfluoro-phosphate[163,164]. Like most of the granule cationic proteins cathepsin G is rich in arginine. Another cationic protein, bacterial permeability increasing protein

14

**Table 1.4** Some characteristic constituents of the granule of human neutrophils

| Primary granules (azurophil granules) | Secondary granules (specific granules) | Tertiary granules |
|---|---|---|
| Neutral proteases:<br>  collagenase<br>  elastase<br>  cathepsin<br>  proteinase 3 | collagenase | gelatinase<br>proteinase 3 |
| Cathepsin B<br>Cathepsin D<br>$\beta$-Glucuronidase<br>$\beta$-Glycerophosphatase<br>$\alpha$-Mannosidase<br>N-acetyl-$\beta$-glucosaminidase<br>Ribonuclease (acid)<br>Deoxyribonuclease (acid) | receptors for FMLP<br>  and complement C3bi<br><br>cytochrome $b_{-245}$ | cathepsin B<br>cathepsin D<br>$\beta$-glucuronidase<br>$\beta$-glycerophosphatase<br>$\alpha$-mannosidase<br>N-acetyl-$\beta$-glucosaminidase |
| Lysozyme<br>Myeloperoxidase | lysozyme<br>vitamin B12-binding protein | |
| Antimicrobial<br>  cationic proteins | lactoferrin<br>complement activator | |

Modified from Gallim (1985)[160] and Baggiolini and Dewald (1984)[161]

(BPI) which has a molecular weight of 58 kDa (50 kDa in rabbit) is rich in lysine and represents 0.5% of the total protein of the human neutrophil[165]. This attaches to the negatively charged surface of bacteria and causes changes in the permeability of the outer membrane of the bacterial cell envelope to hydrophobic molecules, together with activation of enzymes which degrade outer membrane phospholipids and envelope peptidoglycans. The changes produced in the target organisms are subtle yet fatal. An arginine-rich protein of molecular weight 37 kDa, also present in azurophil granules[162], is bactericidal against a range of microbial species.

A group of arginine-rich low molecular weight peptides (six in the rabbit) called the defensins has also been characterized in human neutrophil azurophil granules[166-168]. These are peptides of 32–34 residues each containing three intramolecular disulphide bands with a common backbone sequence of eleven residues, which are bactericidal, fungicidal and anti-viral.

The contents of the neutrophil granules are emptied into the developing phagolysosome as target organisms or particles are engulfed by neutrophils and granules move towards the site of phagocytosis. Granule discharge takes place before the phagocytic vacuole is sealed[161,169,170] and so granule contents are released to the outside of the cell during phagocytosis as well as following the death of neutrophils. The specific granules fuse with the phagosome before the azurophil granules[171,172] and the tertiary granules appear to be highly responsive to stimuli, gelatinase being released from neutrophils even by stimuli that do not provoke a strong respiratory burst[159]. Indeed tertiary granules behave rather like secretory granules. Degranulation is promoted by soluble stimuli as well as phagocytic stimuli; phorbol[173] and concanavalin A[174] cause release of specific granule contents to the exterior.

Hydrolytic enzymes, particularly those proteases with neutral pH optima which are released to the exterior of neutrophils during phagocytosis, or after cell death, are likely to contribute to tissue damage in inflamed areas. Elastase is one of the main agents for neutrophil-mediated injury to endothelial cells[175] and for tissue destruction in pulmonary emphysema, chronic bronchitis, cystic fibrosis, adult respiratory distress syndrome (ARDS), atherosclerosis, arthritis, psoriasis and glomerulonephritis[176]. Elastase, a serine protease, optimally active around pH 7.0, degrades matrix macromolecules such as collagen, elastin, proteoglycans, fibrinogen and fibronectin as well as immunoglobins, complement and clotting factors. Several isoenzymes are present (at least three) differing in their carbohydrate content (varying from 18–20% carbohydrate). Activity is associated with the various sub-populations of primary granules[177].

Excessive loss of elastin in the lung may play a role in the pathogenesis of emphysema, and some of the products of the proteolytic activity of elastase are chemoattractants which draw more neutrophils to the inflammatory site. Elastase activity outside the phagosome is usually regulated by circulating inhibitors, including $\alpha$1-antitrypsin and $\alpha$2-macroglobin, or by locally produced inhibitors present in bronchial and cervical mucus and in seminal plasma[178]. The capacity of $\alpha$1-protease inhibitors to protect tissues from elastase damage is prevented by oxidative attack by the active oxygen species produced during the neutrophil respiratory burst[179]. These cause oxidation of methionine 358 at the active site of the inhibitor together with oxidation of up to three other methionine residues[180], causing the inhibitor to become ineffective[178,181]. Proteolysis of the inhibitor, perhaps by elastase itself acting on the oxidised form, also causes it to lose activity[180,182–185].

The products of the respiratory burst serve also to activate two other granule neutral proteinases important in the pathophysiology of connective tissue. Gelatinase, which attacks collagen, is synthesized and stored in granules in a latent form. On release from granules it is activated by products of the respiratory burst. Its activity after release from stimulated neutrophils is diminished if catalase is present to remove $H_2O_2$. The $H_2O_2$ appears to be required as a substrate of the myeloperoxidase/$Cl^-$ system for HOCl generation, since HOCl itself at around $50\,\mu mol\,L^{-1}$ could activate the gelatinase[186]. Neutrophil collagenase, which attacks interstitial collagen, is also activated by HOCl[187] and possibly directly by oxygen free radicals[188].

It is apparent that the products of the respiratory burst may contribute to inflammatory damage both directly, through attack on membrane lipids and on proteins, and indirectly through activation of lytic enzymes. The contributions of the granule proteins, myeloperoxidase and lactoferrin, to the formation of potentially inflammatory products has been discussed in an earlier section but it should be pointed out that the limiting membranes of human specific granules are particularly enriched in cytochrome $b_{-245}$, a component of NADPH oxidase[31], and this cytochrome is transported to the cytoplasmic membrane fraction as degranulation follows the respiratory burst[189–191]. Similarly the specific granule membrane contains receptors for FMLP and complement $C3bi$[192,193]. The addition to the plasma membrane of new membrane from specific granules may be important during the secretory process and in the maintenance of the respiratory burst.

16

# References

1. Baldridge, C.W. and Gerard, R.W. (1933). The extra respiration of phagocytosis. *Am. J. Physiol.*, **103**, 235–6
2. Sbarra, A.J. and Karnovsky, M.L. (1959). The biochemical basis of phagocytosis: metabolic changes during the ingestion of particles by polymorphonuclear leukocytes. *J. Biol. Chem.*, **234**, 1355–62
3. Baehner, R.L. and Karnovsky, M.L. (1968). Deficiency of reduced NADH oxidase in Chronic Granulomatous Disease. *Science*, **162**, 1277–9
4. Badwey, J.A. and Karnovsky, M.L. (1979). Production of superoxide and hydrogen peroxide by an NADH oxidase in Guineapig polymorphonuclear leukocytes: modulation by nucleotides and divalent cations. *J. Biol. Chem.*, **254**, 11530–7
5. Segal, A.W. and Peters, T.J. (1976). Characterization of the enzyme defect in Chronic Granulomatous Disease. *Lancet*, **i**, 1363–5
6. Patriarca, P., Cramer, R., Moncalvo, S., Rossi, F. and Romeo, D. (1971). Enzymatic basis of metabolic stimulation of leukocytes during phagocytosis: the role of activated NADPH oxidase. *Arch. Biochem. Biophys.*, **145**, 255–62
7. Hohn, D.C. and Lehrer, R.I. (1975). NADPH oxidase deficiency in X-linked Chronic Granulomatous Disease. *J. Clin. Invest.*, **55**, 707–13
8. Iyer, G. and Quastel, J.H. (1963). NADPH and NADH oxidation by Guineapig polymorphonuclear leukocytes. *Can. J. Biochem.*, **41**, 427–34
9. Curnutte, J.T., Kipnes, R.S. and Babior, B.M. (1975). Defect in pyridine nucleotide dependent superoxide production by a particulate fraction from granulocytes of patients with Chronic Granulomatous Disease. *N. Engl. J. Med.*, **293**, 628–32
10. Paul, B. and Sbarra, A.J. (1968). The role of the phagocyte in host-parasite interaction. xiii. The direct quantitative estimation of $H_2O_2$ in phagocytosing cells. *Biochim. Biophys. Acta*, **156**, 168–78
11. Babior, B.M., Kipnes, R.S. and Curnutte, J.T. (1973). Biological defence mechanisms: the production by leukocytes of superoxide, a potential bactericidal agent. *J. Clin. Invest.*, **152**, 741–4
12. Briggs, R.T., Drath, D.B., Karnovsky, M.L. and Karnovsky, M.J. (1975). Localization of NADH oxidase on the surface of human polymorphonuclear leukocytes by a new cytochemical method. *J. Cell Biol.*, **67**, 566–86
13. Dewald, B., Baggiolini, M., Curnutte, J.T. and Babior, B.M. (1979). Subcellular localization of the superoxide forming enzyme in human neutrophils. *J. Clin. Invest.*, **63**, 21–9
14. Yamaguchi, T., Sato, K., Shimada, K. and Kakinuma, K. (1982). Subcellular localization of a superoxide generating enzyme in Guinea pig polymorphonuclear leukocytes: fractionation of subcellular particles by using a Percoll density gradient. *J. Biochem.*, **91**, 31–6
15. Roos, D., Voetman, A.A. and Meerhof, L.J. (1983). Functional activity of enucleated human polymorphonuclear leukocytes. *J. Biol. Chem.*, **97**, 368–77
16. Lutter, R., van Zweiten, R., Weening, R.S., Hamers, M.N. and Roos, D. (1984). Cytochrome *b*, flavins and ubiquinone-50 in enucleated human neutrophils (polymorphonuclear leukocytes cytoplasts). *J. Biol. Chem.*, **259**, 9603–6
17. Segal, A.W., Jones, O.T.G., Webster, D. and Allison, A.C. (1978). Absence of a newly described cytochrome *b* from neutrophils of patients with Chronic Granulomatous Disease. *Lancet*, **ii**, 446–9
18. Babior, B.M. and Kipnes, R.S. (1977). Superoxide-forming enzyme from human neutrophils: evidence for flavin requirement. *Blood*, **50**, 517–24
19. Babior, B.M. and Peters, W.A. (1981). The superoxide producing enzyme from human neutrophils. *J. Biol. Chem.*, **256**, 2321–3
20. Light, D.R., Walsh, C., O'Callaghan, A., Goetzl, E.J. and Tauber, A.I. (1981). Characteristics of the cofactor requirements of the superoxide generating NADPH-oxidase of human polymorphonuclear leukocytes. *Biochemistry*, **20**, 1468–76
21. Wakeyama, H., Takeshigi, K. and Minikami, S. (1983). NADPH-dependent reduction of 2, 6-dichlorophenol indophenol by the phagocytic vesicles of pig polymorphonuclear leukocytes. *Biochem. J.*, **210**, 577–81
22. Bellavite, P., Cross, A.R., Serra, M.C., Davoli, A., Jones, O.T.G. and Rossi, F. (1983). The cytochrome *b* and flavin content and properties of the superoxide forming NADPH oxidase solubilized from activated neutrophils. *Biochim. Biophys. Acta*, **746**, 40–7

17

23. Cross, A.R., Jones, O.T.G., Garcia, R. and Segal, A.W. (1982). The association of FAD with the cytochrome $b_{-245}$ of human neutrophils. *Biochem. J.*, **208**, 759–63
24. Gabig, T.G. (1983). The NADPH-dependent superoxide-generating oxidase from human neutrophils: identification of a flavoprotein component that is deficient in a patient with Chronic Granulomatous Disease. *J. Biol. Chem.*, **258**, 6352–6
25. Gabig, T.G. and Lefker, B. (1984). Deficient flavoprotein component of the NADPH-dependent superoxide-generating oxidase in the neutrophils from three male patients with Chronic Granulomatous Disease. *J. Clin. Invest.*, **73**, 71–5
26. Ohno, Y., Buescher, E.S., Roberts, R. and Gallin, J.I. (1986). Re-evaluation of cytochrome *b* and FAD in neutrophils from patients with Chronic Granulomatous Disease with probable autosomal recessive inheritance of cytochrome *b* deficiency. *Blood*, **67**, 1132–8
27. Hattori, H. (1961). Studies on the labile, stable NADI oxidase and peroxidase staining reactions in the isolated particles of the horse granulocyte. *Nagoya J. Med. Sci.*, **23**, 362–78
28. Shinigawa, Y., Tanaka, C., Teraoka, A. and Shinigawa, Y. (1966). A new cytochrome in neutrophilic granules of rabbit leukocytes. *J. Biochem.*, **59**, 622–4
29. Segal, A.W. and Jones, O.T.G. (1978). Novel cytochrome b system in phagocytic vacuoles of human phagocytes. *Nature*, **276**, 515–17
30. Borregaard, N., Johansen, K.S., Taudorff, E. and Wandall, J.H. (1979). Cytochrome *b* is present in neutrophils from patients with Chronic Granulomatous Disease. *Lancet*, **i**, 949–51
31. Segal, A.W. and Jones, O.T.G. (1979). The subcellular distribution and some properties of the cytochrome *b* component of the microbicidal oxidase system of human neutrophils. *Biochem. J.*, **182**, 181–8
32. Segal, A.W. and Jones, O.T.G. (1980). Rapid incorporation of the human neutrophil plasma membrane cytochrome b into phagocytic vacuoles. *Biochem. Biophys. Res. Commun.*, **92**, 710–15
33. Segal, A.W. and Jones, O.T.G. (1979). Reduction and subsequent oxidation of a cytochrome *b* of human neutrophils after stimulation with phorbol myristate acetate. *Biochem. Biophys. Res. Commun.*, **88**, 130–4
34. Segal, A.W. and Jones, O.T.G. (1980). Absence of cytochrome *b* reduction in stimulated neutrophils from both female and male patients with Chronic Granulomatous Disease. *FEBS. Lett.*, **110**, 111–14
35. Segal, A.W., Cross, A.R., Borregaard, N., Valerius, N.H., Soothill, J.F. and Jones, O.T.G. (1983). Absence of cytochrome $b_{-245}$ in Chronic Granulomatous Disease. A multicentre European evaluation of its incidence and relevance. *N. Engl. J. Med.*, **308**, 245–51
36. Hamers, M.N., de Boer, M., Meerhof, L.J., Weening, R.S. and Roos, D. (1984). Complementation in monocyte hybrids revealing genetic heterogeneity in Chronic Granulomatous Disease. *Nature*, **307**, 553–5
37. Cross, A.R., Jones, O.T.G., Harper, A.M. and Segal, A.W. (1981). Oxidation–reduction properties of the cytochrome *b* found in the plasma membrane fraction of human neutrophils. A possible oxidase in the respiratory burst. *Biochem. J.*, **194**, 599–606
38. Wood, P.M. (1974). The redox potential of the system oxygen–superoxide. *FEBS. Lett.*, **44**, 22–4
39. Segal, A.W., Garcia, F., Goldstone, A.H., Cross, A.R. and Jones, O.T.G. (1981). Cytochrome $b_{-245}$ of neutrophils is also present in human monocytes, macrophages and eosinophils. *Biochem. J.*, **196**, 363–7
40. Roberts, P.J., Cross, A.R., Jones, O.T.G. and Segal, A.W. (1982). Development of cytochrome $b_{-245}$ and an active oxidase system in association with maturation of a human promyelocytic (HL-60) cell-line. *J. Cell. Biol.*, **95**, 720–6
41. Cross, A.R., Higson, F.K., Jones, O.T.G., Harper, A.M. and Segal, A.W. (1982). The enzymatic reduction and kinetics of oxidation of the cytochrome $b_{-245}$ of neutrophils. *Biochem. J.*, **204**, 479–85
42. Cross, A.R., Parkinson, J.F. and Jones, O.T.G. (1985). Mechanism of superoxide-producing oxidase of neutrophils: $O_2$ is necessary for the fast reduction of cytochrome $b_{-245}$ by NADPH. *Biochem. J.*, **226**, 881–4
43. Harper, A.M., Dunne, M.J. and Segal, A.W. (1984). Purification of cytochrome $b_{-245}$ from human neutrophils. *Biochem. J.*, **219**, 519–27

44. Lutter, R., van Schaik, M.L.J., van Zweiten, R., Wever, R., Hamers, M.N. and Roos, D. (1985). Purification and partial characterization of the b-type cytochrome from human polymorphonuclear leukocytes. *J. Biol. Chem.*, **260**, 2237−44
45. Pember, S.O., Heyl, B.L., Kinkade, J.M. and Lambeth, J.D. (1984). Cytochrome $b_{558}$ from (bovine) granulocytes. Partial purification from Triton X-114 extracts and properties of the isolated cytochrome. *J. Biol. Chem.*, **259**, 10590−5
46. Serra, M.C., Bellavite, P., Davoli, A., Bannister, J.V. and Rossi, F. (1984). Isolation from neutrophil membranes of a complex containing active NADPH oxidase and cytochrome $b_{-245}$. *Biochim. Biophys. Acta*, **788**, 138−46
47. Bellavite, P., Papini, E., Zeni, L., Della Bianca, V. and Rossi, F. (1985). Studies on the nature and activation of superoxide-forming NADPH-oxidase of leukocytes: identification of a phosphorylated component of the active enzyme. *Free Rad. Res. Commun.*, **1**, 11−29
48. Millard, J.A., Gerard, K.W. and Schneider, D.L. (1979). The isolation from rat peritoneal leukocytes of plasma membrane enriched in alkaline phosphatase and b-type cytochrome. *Biochem. Biophys. Res. Commun.*, **90**, 312−19
49. Crawford, D.R. and Schneider, D.L. (1981). Evidence that a quinone may be required for the production of superoxide and hydrogen peroxide in neutrophils. *Biochem. Biophys. Res. Commun.*, **99**, 1277−86
50. Sloan, E.P., Crawford, D.R. and Schneider, D.L. (1981). Isolation of plasma membrane from human neutrophils and determination of cytochrome b and quinone content. *J. Exp. Med.*, **153**, 1316−28
51. Crawford, D.R. and Schneider, D.L. (1982). Identification of ubiquinone-50 in human neutrophils and its role in microbicidal events. *J. Biol. Chem.*, **257**, 6662−8
52. Cunningham, C.C., DeChatelet, L.R., Spach, P.I., Parce, J.W., Thomas, M.J., Lees, C.J. and Shirley, P.S. (1982). Identification and quantification of electron transport components in human polymorphonuclear leukocytes. *Biochim. Biophys. Acta*, **682**, 430−5
53. Cross, A.R., Jones, O.T.G., Garcia, R. and Segal, A.W. (1983). The subcellular localization of ubiquinone in human neutrophils. *Biochem. J.*, **216**, 765−8
54. Szarkowska, L. and Klingenberg, M. (1963). On the role of ubiquinone in mitochondria. Spectrophotometric and chemical measurements of its redox reactions. *Biochem. Z.*, **338**, 674−8
55. Bellavite, P., Jones, O.T.G., Cross, A.R., Papini, E. and Rossi, F. (1984). Composition of partially purified NADPH oxidase from pig neutrophils. *Biochem. J.*, **223**, 639−48
56. Ohno, Y-I., Hirai, K-I., Kanoh, T., Uchino, H. and Ogawa, K. (1982). Subcellular localization of hydrogen peroxide production in human neutrophils stimulated with particles and an effect of cytochalasin B on the cells. *Blood*, **60**, 253−60
57. Vissers, M.C.M., Day, W.A. and Winterbourn, C.C. (1985). Neutrophils adherent to a non-phagocytosable surface (glomerular basement membrane) produce oxidants only at the site of attachment. *Blood*, **66**, 161−6
58. Goldstein, I.M., Roos, D., Kaplan, H.B. and Weissmann, G. (1975). Complement and immunoglobulins stimulate superoxide production by human leukocytes independently of phagocytosis. *J. Clin. Invest.*, **56**, 1155−63
59. Becker, E.L., Sigman, M. and Oliver, J.M. (1979). Superoxide production induced in rabbit polymorphonuclear leukocytes by synthetic chemotactic peptides and A23187. The nature of the receptor and the requirement for calcium. *Am. J. Pathol.*, **95**, 81−6
60. Chenoweth, D.E. and Hugli, T.E. (1978). Demonstration of specific C5a receptor on intact human polymorphonuclear phagocytes. *Proc. Natl. Acad. Sci. USA*, **75**, 3943−7
61. Wright, S.D. and Siverstein, S.C. (1983). Receptors for C3b and C3bi promote phagocytosis but not the release of toxic oxygen from human phagocytes. *J. Exp. Med.*, **158**, 2016−23
62. Williams, L.T., Snyderman, R., Pike, M.C. and Lefkovitz, R.J. (1977). Specific receptor sites for chemotactic peptides on human polymorphonuclear leukocytes. *Proc. Natl. Acad. Sci. USA*, **74**, 1204−8
63. Lobuglio, A.F., Cotran, R.S. and Jandl, J.H. (1967). Red cells coated with Immunoglobulin G: binding and sphering by mononuclear cells in man. *Science*, **158**, 1582−5
64. Spilberg, I. and Mehta, J. (1979). Specific neutrophil receptor for cell-derived growth factor. *J. Clin. Invest.*, **63**, 85−8
65. Goldman, D.W. and Goetzl, E.J. (1982). Specific binding of leukotriene $B_4$ to receptors on human polymorphonuclear leukocytes. *J. Immunol.*, **129**, 1600−4

66. Goetzl, E.J., Derian, C.K., Tauber, A.I. and Valone, F.H. (1980). Novel effects of 1-O-Hexadecyl-2-acyl-SN-glycerophosphorylcholine mediators on human leukocyte function: delineation of the specific roles of the acyl substituents. *Biochem. Biophys. Res. Commun.*, **94**, 881–88

67. Tzeng, D.Y., Deuel, T.F., Huang, J.S., Senior, R.M., Boxer, L.A. and Baehner, R.L. (1984). Platelet-derived growth factor promotes polymorphonuclear leukocytes activation. *Blood*, **64**, 1123–8

68. Sklar, L.A., Jesaitis, A.J. and Painter, R.G. (1984). The neutrophil N-formyl peptide receptor: dynamics of ligand–receptor interactions and their relationships to cellular responses. *Contemp. Top. Immunobiol.*, **14**, 29–82

69. Koo, C., Lefkowitz, R.J. and Snyderman, R. (1982). The oligopeptide chemotactic factor receptor on human polymorphonuclear leukocytes membranes exists in two affinity states. *Fed. Proc.*, **41**, 272

70. Snyderman, R., Pike, M.C., Edge, S. and Lane, B.C. (1984). A chemoattractant receptor on macrophages exists in two affinity states regulated by guanine nucleotides. *J. Cell Biol.*, **98**, 444–8

71. Satoh, M., Nanri, H., Takeshige, K. and Minikami, S. (1985). Pertussis toxin inhibits intracellular pH changes in human neutrophils stimulated by FMLP. *Biochem. Biophys. Res. Commun.*, **131**, 64–9

72. Okamura, N., Uchida, M., Ohtsuka, T., Kawanishi, M. and Ishibashi, S. (1985). Diverse involvement of $N_1$ protein in superoxide anion production in polymorphonuclear leukocytes depending on the type of membrane stimulants. *Biochem. Biophys. Res. Commun.*, **130**, 939–44

73. Yuli, I., Tomonaga, A. and Snyderman, R. (1982). Chemoattractant receptor functions in human polymorphonuclear leukocytes are divergently altered by membrane fluidizers. *Proc. Natl. Acad. Sci. USA*, **79**, 5906–10

74. Herlin, T., Petersen, C.S. and Esmann, V. (1978). The role of calcium and cAMP in regulation of glycogen metabolism in phagocytosing human polymorphonuclear leukocytes. *Biochim. Biophys. Acta*, **542**, 63–76

75. Simchowitz, L., Fischbein, L.C., Spilberg, I. and Atkinson, J.P. (1980). Induction of a transient elevation in intracellular levels of adenosine-3',5'-cyclic monophosphate by chemotactic factors: an early event in human neutrophil activation. *J. Immunol.*, **124**, 1482–1491

76. Smolen, J.E., Korchak, H.M. and Weissman, G. (1980). Increased levels of cAMP in human polymorphonuclear leukocytes after surface stimulation. *J. Clin. Invest.*, **65**, 1077–85

77. Nakagawara, A. and Minikami, S. (1975). Generation of superoxide anions by leukocytes treated with cytochalasin E. *Biochem. Biophys. Res. Commun.*, **64**, 760–7

78. Gallin, E.K. and Gallin, J.I. (1977). Interactions of chemotactic factors with human macrophages: induction of membrane potential changes. *J. Cell. Biol.*, **75**, 277–89

79. Utsumi, K., Sugiyama, K., Miyahara, M., Naito, M., Awai, M. and Inoue, M. (1977). The effect of concanavalin A on membrane potential of polymorphonuclear leukocytes monitored by fluorescent dye. *Cell Struct. Func.*, **2**, 203–9

80. Seligmann, B.E., Gallin, E.K., Martin, D.L., Shain, W. and Gallin, J.I. (1980). Interaction of chemotactic factors with human polymorphonuclear leukocytes: studies using a membrane potential-sensitive cyanine dye. *J. Membr. Biol.*, **52**, 257–72

81. Simchowitz, L. (1985). Chemotactic factor-induced activation of sodium/proton exchange in human neutrophils. *J. Biol. Chem.*, **260**, 13248–55

82. Romeo, D., Zabucchi, G., Miani, N. and Rossi, F. (1975). Ion movement across leukocyte plasma membrane and excitation of their metabolism. *Nature*, **253**, 542–4

83. Zabucchi, G., Soranzo, M.R., Rossi, F. and Romeo, D. (1975). Exocytosis in human polymorphonuclear leukocytes induced by A23187 and calcium. *FEBS. Lett.*, **54**, 44–8

84. Della Bianca, V., Bellavite, P., De Togni, P., Fumarulo, R. and Rossi, F. (1983). Studies on stimulus response coupling in human neutrophils: role of monovalent cations in the respiratory and secretory response to fMLP. *Biochim. Biophys. Acta*, **755**, 497–505

85. Miles, P.R., Bowman, L. and Castranova, V. (1981). Transmembrane potential changes during phagocytosis in rat alveolar macrophages. *J. Cell Physiol.*, **106**, 109–17

86. Korchak, H.M. and Weissmann, G. (1980). Stimulus response coupling in the human neutrophil: transmembrane potential and the role of extracellular sodium. *Biochim. Biophys. Acta*, **601**, 180–94

87. Whitin, J.C., Chapman, C.E., Simons, E.R., Chovaniec, M.E. and Cohen, H.J. (1980). Correlation between membrane potential changes and superoxide production in human granulocytes stimulated with phorbol myristate acetate: evidence for defective activation in Chronic Granulomatous Disease. *J. Biol. Chem.*, **255**, 1874–8

88. Seligmann, B.E. and Gallin, J.I. (1980). Use of lipophilic probes of membrane potential to assess human neutrophil activation: abnormality in Chronic Granulomatous Disease. *J. Clin. Invest.*, **66**, 493–503

89. Lew, P.D., Southwick, F.S., Stossel, T.P., Whitin, J.C., Simons, E.R. and Cohen, H.J. (1981). A variant of Chronic Granulomatous Disease: deficient oxidative metabolism due to a low affinity NADPH oxidase. *N. Engl. J. Med.*, **305**, 1329–33

90. Cohen, H.J. and Chovaniec, M.E. (1978). Superoxide production by digitonin-stimulated guineapig granulocytes. The effects of NEM, divalent cations and glycolytic and mitochondrial inhibitors on the activation of the superoxide generating system. *J. Clin. Invest.*, **61**, 1088–96

91. Schell-Frederick, E. (1974). Stimulation of the oxidative metabolism of polymorphonuclear leukocytes by the calcium ionophore A12187. *FEBS Lett.*, **48**, 37–40

92. Naccache, P.H., Volpi, M., Showell, H.J., Becker, E.L. and Sha'afi, R.I. (1979). Transport of sodium, potassium and calcium across rabbit polymorphonuclear leukocytes membranes. Effect of chemotactic factor. *Science*, **203**, 461–3

93. Smolen, J.E., Korchak, H.M. and Weissmann, G. (1981). The roles of extracellular and intracellular calcium in lysosomal enzyme release and superoxide generation by human neutrophils. *Biochim. Biophys. Acta*, **677**, 512–20

94. Hoffstein, S.T. (1979). Ultrastructural demonstration of calcium loss from local regions of the plasma membrane of surface stimulated human granulocytes. *J. Immunol.*, **123**, 1395–402

95. Smolen, J.E. and Weissmann, G. (1982). The effect of various stimuli and calcium antagonists on the fluorescence response of chlorotetracycline-loaded human neutrophils. *Biochem. Biophys. Acta*, **720**, 172–80

96. Campbell, A.K. and Hallett, M.B. (1983). Measurement of intracellular calcium ions and oxygen radicals in polymorphonuclear leukocyte-erythrocyte 'ghost' hybrids. *J. Physiol.*, **338**, 537–50

97. Tsien, R.Y. (1981). A non-disruptive technique for loading calcium buffers and indicators into cells. *Nature*, **290**, 527–8

98. Korchak, H.M., Vienne, K., Rutherford, L.E. and Weissmann, G. (1984). Stimulus–response coupling in the human neutrophil: temporal analysis of changes in cytosolic calcium and calcium efflux. *Fed. Proc.*, **43**, 2749–54

99. Lagast, H., Pozzan, T., Lew, P.D. and Waldvogel, F.A. (1983). PMA stimulates the plasma membrane calcium pump of human and guineapig neutrophils without raising cytosolic free calcium. *Clin. Res.*, **31**, 410–18

100. Berridge, M.J. and Irvine, R.F. (1984). Inositol triphosphate, a novel second messenger in cellular signal transduction. *Nature*, **312**, 315–21

101. Volpi, M., Yassin, R., Naccache, P.H. and Sha'afi, R.I. (1983). Chemotactic factor causes rapid decrease in phosphatidyl-4,5-bisphosphate and phosphatidylinositol-4-monophosphate in rabbit neutrophils. *Biochem. Biophys. Res. Commun.*, **112**, 957–64

102. Dougherty, R.W., Godfrey, P.P., Hoyle, P.C., Putney, J.W. and Freer, R.J. (1984). Secretagogue-induced phosphoinositide metabolism in human leukocytes. *Biochem. J.*, **222**, 307–14

103. Cockroft, S., Barrowman, M.M. and Gomperts, B.D. (1985). Breakdown and synthesis of polyphosphoinositides in FMLP stimulated neutrophils. *FEBS Lett.*, **181**, 259–63

104. Castagna, M., Takai, Y., Kaibuchi, K., Sano, K., Kikkawa, U. and Nishizuka, Y. (1982). Direct activation of calcium-activated, phospholipid-dependent protein kinase by tumour-promoting phorbol esters. *J. Biol. Chem.*, **257**, 7847–51

105. Neidel, J.E., Kuhn, L.J. and Vandenbark, G.R. (1983). Phorbol diester receptor co-purifies with protein kinase C. *Proc. Natl. Acad. Sci. USA*, **80**, 36–40

106. Kishimoto, A., Takai, Y., Mori, T., Kikkawa, U. and Nishizuka, Y. (1980). Activation of calcium and phospholipid dependent protein kinase by diacyl glycerol, its possible relationship to phosphatidyl inositol turnover. *J. Biol. Chem.*, **255**, 2273–6

107. Kraft, A.S., Anderson, W.B., Cooper, H.L. and Sands, J.J. (1982). Decrease in cytosolic calcium/phospholipid dependent protein kinase activity following phorbol ester treatment of EL4 thymoma cells. *J. Biol. Chem.*, **257**, 13193–6

108. Wolf, M., LeVine, H., May, W.S., Cuatrecasas, P. and Sayhoun, N. (1985). A model for intracellular translocation of protein kinase C involving synergism between calcium and phorbol esters. Nature, 317, 546–9
109. May, W.S., Sayhoun, N., Wolf, M. and Cuatrecasas, P. (1985). Role of intracellular calcium mobilization in the regulation of protein kinase C-mediated membrane processes. Nature, 317, 549–51
110. Van Epps, D.E. and Garcia, M.L. (1980). Enhancement of neutrophil function as a result of prior exposure to chemotactic factor. J. Clin. Invest., 66, 167–75
111. Badwey, J.A., Curnutte, J.T., Berde, C.B. and Karnovsky, M.L. (1982). Cytochalasin E diminishes the lag phase in the release of superoxide by human neutrophils. Biochem. Biophys. Res. Commun., 106, 170–4
112. Bender, J.G., McPhail, L.C. and Van Epps, D.E. (1983). Exposure of human neutrophils to chemotactic factors potentiates activation of the respiratory burst. J. Immunol., 130, 2316–23
113. Guthrie, L.A., McPhail, L.C., Henson, P.M. and Johnston, R.B. (1984). Priming of neutrophils for enhanced release of oxygen metabolites by bacterial lipopolysaccharide (endotoxin): evidence for increased activity of the superoxide-forming enzyme. J. Exp. Med., 160, 1656–71
114. McPhail, L.C. and Snyderman, R. (1984). Mechanisms of regulating the respiratory burst in leukocytes. Contemp. Top. Immunobiol., 14, 247–81
115. Minakucha, R., Takai, Y., Yu, B. and Nishizuka, Y. (1981). Widespread occurrence of calcium activated phospholipid-dependent protein kinase in mammalian tissues. J. Biochem., 89, 1651–4
116. Helfman, D.M., Appelbaum, B.D., Vogler, W.R. and Kuo, J.F. (1983). Phospholipid-sensitive calcium-dependent protein kinase and its substrates in human neutrophils. Biochem. Biophys. Res. Commun., 111, 847–53
117. Gennaro, R., Florio, C. and Romeo, D. (1985). Activation of protein kinase C in neutrophil cytoplasts: localization of protein substrates and possible relationships with stimulus response coupling. FEBS Lett., 180, 185–90
118. Segal, A.W., Heyworth, P.G., Cockcroft, S. and Barrowman, M.M. (1985). Stimulated neutrophils from patients with autosomal recessive Chronic Granulomatous Disease fail to phosphorylate a $M_r$ 44 000 protein. Nature, 316, 547–9
119. Cox, J.A., Jeng, A.Y., Sharkey, N.A., Blumberg, P.M. and Tauber, A.I. (1985). Activation of the human neutrophil nicotinamide adenine dinucleotide phosphate (NADPH)-oxidase by protein kinase C. J. Clin. Invest., 76, 1932–8
120. Cooke, E. and Hallett, M.B. (1985). The role of C-kinase in the physiological activation of the neutrophil oxidase: evidence from using pharmacological manipulation of C-kinase activity in whole cells. Biochem. J., 232, 323–7
121. Naccache, P.H., Molski, M.M. and Sha'afi, R.I. (1985). Polymyxin B inhibits phorbol 12-myristate 13-acetate but not chemotactic factor induced effects in rabbit neutrophils. FEBS Lett., 193, 227–30
122. Gerard, C., McPhail, L.C., Marfat, A., Stimler-Ferard, N.P., Bass, D.A. and McCall, C.E. (1986). Role of protein kinases in stimulation of human polymorphonuclear leukocytes oxidative metabolism by various agonists: differential effects of a novel protein kinase inhibitor. J. Clin. Invest., 77, 61–5
123. Nishihira, J., McPhail, L.C. and O'Flaherty, J.T. (1986). Stimulus-dependent mobilization of protein kinase C. Biochem. Biophys. Res. Commun., 134, 587–94
124. Costa-Casnellie, M.R., Segel, G.B. and Lichtman, M.A. (1985). Concanavalin A and phorbol ester cause opposite subcellular redistribution of protein kinase C. Biochem. Biophys. Res. Commun., 133, 1139–44
125. Bromberg, Y. and Pick, E. (1984). Unsaturated fatty acids stimulate NADPH-dependent superoxide production by a cell-free system derived from macrophages. Cell Immunol., 88, 213–21
126. Heyneman, R.A. and Vercauteren, R.E. (1984). Activation of an NADPH oxidase from horse polymorphonuclear leukocytes in a cell-free system. J. Leuk. Biol., 36, 751–9
127. McPhail, L.C., Clayton, C.C. and Snyderman, R. (1984). Evidence that activation of human neutrophil NADPH oxidase involves association of a cytosolic factor with membrane components. Clin. Res., 32, 315A

128. Curnutte, J.T., Badwey, J.A., Robinson, J.M., Karnovsky, M.J. and Karnovsky, M.L. (1984). Studies of the mechanism of superoxide release from human neutrophils stimulated with arachidonate. *J. Biol. Chem.*, **259**, 11851–7
129. Bromberg, Y. and Pick, E. (1985). Activation of NADPH dependent superoxide production in a cell-free system by SDS. *J. Biol. Chem.*, **260**, 13539–45
130. Petrone, W.F., English, D.K., Wong, K. and McCord, J.M. (1980). Free radicals and inflammation: superoxide-dependent activation of a neutrophil chemotactic factor in plasma. *Proc. Natl. Acad. Sci. USA*, **77**, 1159–63
131. Halliwell, B. and Gutteridge, J.M.C. (1985). The importance of free radicals and catalytic metal ions in human diseases. *Mol. Aspects Med.*, **8**, 89–193
132. Halliwell, B. and Gutteridge, J.M.C. (1985). *Free Radicals in Biology and Medicine*. (Oxford: Clarendon Press)
133. Blum, J. and Fridovich, I. (1985). Inactivation of glutathione peroxidase by superoxide radicals. *Arch. Biochem. Biophys.*, **240**, 500–8
134. Fridovich, I. (1978). Superoxide radicals, superoxide dismutases and the aerobic lifestyle. *Photochem. Photobiol.*, **28**, 733–40
135. Anbar, M. and Neta, P. (1967). A compilation of specific bimolecular rate constants for the reactions of hydrated electrons, hydrogen atoms and hydroxyl radicals with inorganic and organic compounds in aqueous solution. *Int. J. Appl. Radiat. Isot.* **18**, 495–523
136. Blake, D.R., Gallagher, P.J., Potter, A.P., Bell, M.J. and Bacon, P.A. (1984). The effect of synovial iron on the progression of rheumatic disease. *Arthr. Rheum.*, **27**, 495–501
137. Halliwell, B. and Gutteridge, J.M.C. (1986). Oxygen free radicals and iron in relation to biology and medicine: some problems and concepts. *Arch. Biochem. Biophys.*, **246**, 501–14
138. Flitter, W., Rowley, D.A. and Halliwell, B. (1983). Superoxide-dependent formation of hydroxyl radicals in the presence of iron salts. *FEBS Lett.*, **158**, 310–12
139. Floyd, R.A. (1983). Direct demonstration that ferrous ion complexes of di- and triphosphate nucleotides catalyse hydroxyl free radical formation from hydrogen peroxide. *Arch. Biochem. Biophys.*, **225**, 263–70
140. Gutteridge, J.M.C., Patterson, S.K., Segal, A.W. and Halliwell, B. (1981). Inhibition of lipid peroxidation by the iron binding protein. *Biochem. J.*, **199**, 259–61
141. Winterbourn, C.C. (1983). Lactoferrin catalysed hydroxyl radical production. *Biochem. J.*, **210**, 15–19
142. Bannister, J.V., Bellavite, P., Davioli, A., Thornalley, P.J. and Rossi, F. (1982). The generation of hydroxyl radicals following superoxide production by neutrophil NADPH oxidase. *FEBS Lett.*, **150**, 300–2
143. Klebanof, S.J. (1967). Iodination of bacteria: A bactericidal mechanism. *J. Exp. Med.*, **126**, 1068–78
144. McRipley, R.J. and Sbarra, A.J. (1967). Role of the phagocyte in host–parasite interactions. XII. Hydrogen peroxide-myeloperoxidase bactericidal systems in the phagocyte. *J. Bacteriol.*, **94**, 1425–30
145. Thomas, E.L. and Fishman, M. (1986). Oxidation of chloride and thiocyanate by isolated leukocytes. *J. Biol. Chem.*, **261**, 9694–701
146. Weiss, S.J., Lampert, M.B. and Test, S.T. (1983). Long-lived oxidants generated by human neutrophils: characterisation and bioactivity. *Science*, **222**, 625–8
147. Thomas, E.L., Grisham, M.B. and Jefferson, M.M. (1983). Myeloperoxidase-dependent effect of amines on functions of isolated neutrophils. *J. Clin. Invest.*, **72**, 441–54
148. Grisham, M.B., Jefferson, M.M., Melton, D.F. and Thomas, E.L. (1984). Chlorination of endogenous amines by isolated neutrophils. *J. Biol. Chem.*, **254**, 4022–6
149. Weitzman, S.A., Weitberg, A.B. and Stossel, T.P. (1985). Phagocytes as carcinogens: malignant transformation produced by human neutrophils. *Science*, **227**, 1231–3
150. Cerutti, P.A. (1985). Pro-oxidant states and tumour promotion. *Science*, **227**, 375–81
151. Lesko, S.A., Lorentzen, R.J. and Tso, P.O.P. (1980). Role of superoxide in deoxyribonucleic acid strand scission. *Biochemistry*, **19**, 3023–8
152. Schraufstatter, I.U., Hinshaw, D.B., Hyslop, P.A., Spragg, R.G. and Cochrane, C.G. (1986). Oxidant injury of cells. DNA strand breaks activate polyadenosine diphosphate-ribose polymerase and leads to depletion of nicotinamide adenine dinucleotide. *J. Clin. Invest.*, **77**, 1312–20

153. Fridovich, I. (1986). Superoxide dismutases. In Meister, A. (ed.) *Advances in Enzymology*, **58**, 61–97. (New York: John Wiley & Sons)

154. Epp, O., Ladenstein, R. and Wendel, A. (1983). The refined structure of the selenoenzyme glutathione peroxidase at 0.2 nm resolution. *Eur. J. Biochem.*, **133**, 51–69

155. Reed, P.W. (1969). Glutathione and hexose monophosphate shunt in phagocytosing and hydrogen peroxide treated rat leukocytes. *J. Biol. Chem.*, **244**, 2459–64

156. Schirmer, R.H. and Schultz, G.E. (1983). Flavoproteins of known three dimensional structure. In *Collog. Mosbach.*, **34** *Biological Oxidations*. pp. 93–113. (Berlin: Springer Verlag)

157. Schultz, G.E., Schirmer, R.H. and Pau, E.F. (1982). FAD-binding site of glutathione reductase. *J. Mol. Biol.*, **160**, 249–64

158. Bainton, D.F., Ullyot, J.L. and Farquhar, M.G. (1971). The development of neutrophilic polymorphonuclear leukocytes in human bone marrow. Origin and content of azurophil and specific granules. *J. Exp. Med.*, **134**, 907–34

159. Dewald, B., Bretz, U. and Baggiolini, M. (1982). Release in gelatinase from a novel secretory compartment of neutrophils. *J. Clin. Invest.*, **70**, 518–25

160. Gallin, J.I. (1985). Neutrophil specific granule deficiency. *Annu. Rev. Med.*, **36**, 263–74

161. Baggiolini, M. and Dewald, B. (1984). Exocytosis by neutrophils. *Contemporary Topics in Immunology*, **14**, 221–46

162. Spitznagel, J.K. (1984). Non-oxidative antimicrobial reactions of leukocytes. *Contemporary Topics in Immunology*, **14**, 283–343

163. Odeberg, H. and Olsson, I. (1976). Mechanism for the microbicidal activity of cationic proteins of human granulocytes. *Infect. Immun.*, **14**, 1269–75

164. Thorne, K.J.I., Oliver, R.C. and Barrett, A.J. (1976). Lysis and killing of bacteria by lysosomal proteinases. *Infect. Immun.*, **14**, 555–63

165. Elsbach, P. and Weiss, J. (1985). Oxygen dependent and oxygen independent mechanisms of microbicidal activity of neutrophils. *J. Immunol. Lett.*, **11**, 159–63

166. Selsted, M.E., Brown, D.M., De Lange, R.J., Harwig, S.S.L. and Lehrer, R.I. (1985). Primary structures of six antimicrobial peptides of rabbit peritoneal neutrophils. *J. Biol. Chem.*, **260**, 4579–84

167. Selsted, M.E., Harwig, S.S.L., Ganz, T., Schilling, J.W. and Lehrer, R.I. (1985). Primary structures of three human neutrophil defensins. *J. Clin. Invest.*, **76**, 1436–9

168. Ganz, T., Selsted, M.E., Szklarek, D., Harwig, S.S.L., Daher, K., Bainton, D.F. and Lehrer, R.I. (1985). Defensins: Natural peptide antibiotics of human neutrophils. *J. Clin. Invest.*, **76**, 1427–35

169. Weissmann, G., Zurier, R.B. and Hoffstein, S. (1972). Leukocytic proteases and the immunologic release of lysosomal enzymes. *Am. J. Pathol.*, **68**, 539–64

170. Hawkins, D. (1972). Neutrophilic leukocytes in immunological reactions. Evidence for selective release of lysosomal constituents. *J. Immunol.*, **108**, 310–17

171. Bainton, D.F. (1973). Sequential degranulation of two types of polymorphonuclear leukocyte granules during phagocytosis of microorganisms. *J. Cell Biol.*, **58**, 249–64

172. Estensen, R.D., White, J.G. and Holmes, B. (1974). Specific degranulation of human polymorphonuclear leukocytes. *Nature*, **248**, 347–8

173. Wright, D.G. and Gallin, J.I. (1977). A functional separation of human neutrophil granules: generation of C5a by a specific granule product and inactivation of C5a by azurophil granule products. *J. Immunol.*, **119**, 1068–76

174. Hoffstein, S., Soberman, R., Goldstein, I. and Weissman, G. (1976). Concanavalin A induces microtubule assembly and specific granule discharge in human polymorphonuclear leukocytes. *J. Cell Biol.*, **68**, 781–7

175. Smedly, L.A., Tonnesen, M.G., Sandhaus, R.A., Haslett, C., Guthrie, L.A., Johnston, R.B., Henson, P.M. and Worthen, G.S. (1986). Neutrophil mediated injury to endothelial cells. Enhancement by endotoxin and essential role of neutrophil elastase. *J. Clin. Invest.*, **77**, 1233–43

176. Janoff, A. (1985). Elastase in tissue injury. *Annu. Rev. Med.*, **36**, 207–16

177. Garcia, R.C., Peterson, C.G.B., Segal, A.W. and Venge, P. (1985). Elastase in the different primary granules of the human neutrophil. *Biochem. Biophys. Res. Commun.*, **132**, 1130–6

178. Travis, J. and Salvesen, G.S. (1983). Human plasma proteinase inhibitors. *Annu. Rev. Biochem.*, **52**, 655–709

179. Carp, H. and Janoff, A. (1980). Phagocyte-derived oxidants suppress the inhibitory capacity of α1-proteinase inhibitor *in vitro*. *J. Clin. Invest.*, **66**, 987–95
180. Ossanna, P.J., Test, S.T., Matheson, N.R., Regiani, S. and Weiss, S.J. (1986). Oxidative regulation of neutrophil elastase–α1-proteinase inhibitor interactions. *J. Clin. Invest.*, **77**, 1939–51
181. Clark, R.A., Stone, P.J., Hag, A.E., Calore, J.D. and Franzblau, C. (1981). Myeloperoxidase-catalysed inactivation of α-1-protease inhibitor by human neutrophils. *J. Biol. Chem.*, **256**, 3348–53
182. McGuire, W.W., Spragg, R.G., Cohen, A.B. and Cochrane, C.G. (1982). Studies on the pathogenesis of the adult respiratory distress syndrome. *J. Clin. Invest.*, **69**, 543–53
183. Cochrane, C.G., Spragg, R.G. and Revak, S.D. (1983). Pathogenesis of the adult respiratory distress syndrome: evidence of oxidant activity in bronchoalveolar lavage fluid. *J. Clin. Invest.*, **71**, 754–61
184. Stockley, R.A. and Afford, S.C. (1984). Qualitative studies of lung lavage α-1-proteinase inhibitor. *Hoppe-Seyler's Z. Physiol. Chem.*, **365**, 503–10
185. Stockley, R.A. and Afford, S.C. (1984). The effect of leukocyte elastase on the immunoelectrophoretic behaviour of α-1-antitrypsin. *Clin. Sci.*, **66**, 217–24
186. Peppin, G.J. and Weiss, S.J. (1986). Activation of the endogenous metalloproteinase, gelatinase, by triggered human neutrophils. *Proc. Natl. Acad. Sci. USA*, **83**, 4322–6
187. Weiss, S.J., Peppin, G.J., Ortiz, X., Ragdale, J. and Test, S.T. (1985). Oxidative autoactivation of latent collagenase by human neutrophils. *Science*, **227**, 747–9
188. Burkhardt, H., Schwingel, M., Menninger, H., Macartney, H.W. and Tschesche, H. (1986). Oxygen radicals as effectors of cartilage destruction. Direct degradative effect on matrix components and indirect action via activation of latent collagenase from polymorphonuclear leukocytes. *Arthr. Rheum.*, **29**, 379–87
189. Garcia, R.C. and Segal, A.W. (1984). Changes in the subcellular distribution of the cytochrome $b_{-245}$ on stimulation of human neutrophils. *Biochem. J.*, **219**, 233–42
190. Borregaard, N. and Tauber, A.I. (1984). Subcellular localisation of the human neutrophil NADPH oxidase. *J. Biol. Chem.*, **259**, 47–52
191. Ohno, Y., Seligman, B.E. and Gallin, J.I. (1985). Cytochrome *b* translocation to human neutrophil plasma membranes and superoxide release. *J. Biol. Chem.*, **260**, 2409–14
192. Gallin, J.I. and Seligman, B.E. (1984). Mobilisation and adaptation of human neutrophil chemoattractant FMLP receptors. *Fed. Proc.*, **43**, 2732–6
193. O'Shea, J., Seligman, B.E., Gallin, J.I., Chusel, T., Berger, M. and Brown, E. (1984). Distinct modulation of complement receptors on human neutrophils. *Fed. Proc.*, **43**, 1505
194. Kakinuma, K., Kaneda, M., Chiba, T. and Ohnishi, T. (1986). Electron spin resonance studies on a flavoprotein in neutrophil plasma membranes: redox potentials of the flavin and its participation in NADPH oxidase. *J. Biol. Chem.*, **261**, 9426–32
195. Dinauer, M.C., Orkin, S.H., Brown, R., Jesaitis, A.J. and Parkos, C.A. (1987). The glycoprotein encoded by the X-linked chronic granulomatous disease locus is a component of the neutrophil cytochrome *b* complex. *Nature*, **327**, 717–20
196. Teahan, C., Rowe, P., Parker, P., Totty, N. and Segal, A.W. (1987). The X-linked chronic granulomatous disease gene codes for the β-chain of cytochrome $b_{-245}$. *Nature*, **327**, 720–1
197. Segal, A.W. (1987). Absence of proteins from neutrophils in X-linked CGD: evidence for a subunit structure of cytochrome $b_{-245}$. *Nature*, **326**, 88–91
198. Parkos, C.A., Allen, R.A., Cochrane, C.G. and Jesaitis, A.J. (1987). A new method of purification of b-cytochrome from the plasma membrane of human granulocytes yields two polypeptides of $M_r = 91,000$ and $M_r = 22,000$. *J. Clin. Invest.*, **80**, 732–41
199. Henderson, L.M., Chappell, J.B. and Jones, O.T.G. (1987). The superoxide-generating NADPH oxidase of human neutrophils is electrogenic and associated with a $H^+$ channel. *Biochem. J.*, **246**, 325–9

# 2
# The role of eicosanoids in inflammation

J. BELCH

## INTRODUCTION

Inflammation is a process which occurs in tissues following sublethal injury through different causes, either mechanical, chemical or biological. These various stimuli are followed by production, release and local accumulation/ diffusion of a number of biologically active substances: the inflammatory mediators. Each of these has some role in initiating or modulating the inflammatory process. In most instances, inflammation may be regarded as a physiological response leading to tissue repair. It is evident, however, that such a basic and important process has to be regulated carefully. Mechanisms originally designed for host defence may themselves cause disease if the initiating stimulus cannot be eliminated. These mechanisms are highly complex and interrelated. This should be emphasized because, although the connection between eicosanoids and inflammation is becoming obvious, and their importance is likely to increase, they are merely one feature of a very complex process.

## EICOSANOIDS

In the biological systems for the regulation of various cell functions, the essential fatty acids (EFAs) have unique roles as precursor molecules for potent inflammatory mediators with far-reaching effects: the prostaglandins (PGs) and leukotrienes (LTs). Structurally, the first PGs described had the well-known 'hairpin' confirmation with a cyclopentane ring between the two chains. However, later on, compounds such as prostacyclin (PGI$_2$) with a double-ring structure; thromboxane A$_2$ (TXA$_2$) with an oxane ring; and the LTs with the straight-chain conformation combined with amino acids, led to the suggestion that the generic name 'eicosanoids' be used to encompass all the metabolic products of EFAs.

26

Descriptions of the fatty acid content of natural products and foods demonstrated that seed material was generally a rich source of linoleic acid, whereas the lipid of green leafy vegetables contained γ-linolenic acid[1]. The derivation of PGs and LTs from these EFAs is illustrated in Figure 2.1. Thus dihomo-γ-linolenic (DGLA) leads to the formation of the 1 series (monoenoic) PGs; arachidonic acid (AA) to the 2 series (bisenoic); and eicosapentanoic (EPA) to the 3 series (trisenoic) PGs. The series of LT also alters depending on the precursor EFA. The most studied EFA is AA, the precursor of the 2 series PGs and the 4 series LTs. This is because AA is the commonest dietary EFA. Recently, however, the other series of PGs and LTs have been receiving attention and the recent advances in this area have been included in this chapter.

## PROSTAGLANDINS

Prostaglandins, discovered independently by von Euler[2] and Goldblatt[3] in the 1930s have progressed from being an uncharacterized biological substance of a lipid nature into an extensive family of compounds derived from polyunsaturated fatty acids, mainly AA. They are synthesized and released by almost every tissue in the body and participate in many different biological functions. Of the many areas in which the functions of PGs have been studied, a substantial degree of understanding has been brought to the participation of PGs in the development of the signs and symptoms of inflammation.

### Metabolism of arachidonic acid

Oxidative metabolism of AA within the cell occurs via two major enzyme pathways (Figure 2.2): the first is via a lipoxygenase enzyme leading to the formation of the LTs, the second is via a cyclo-oxygenase enzyme system.

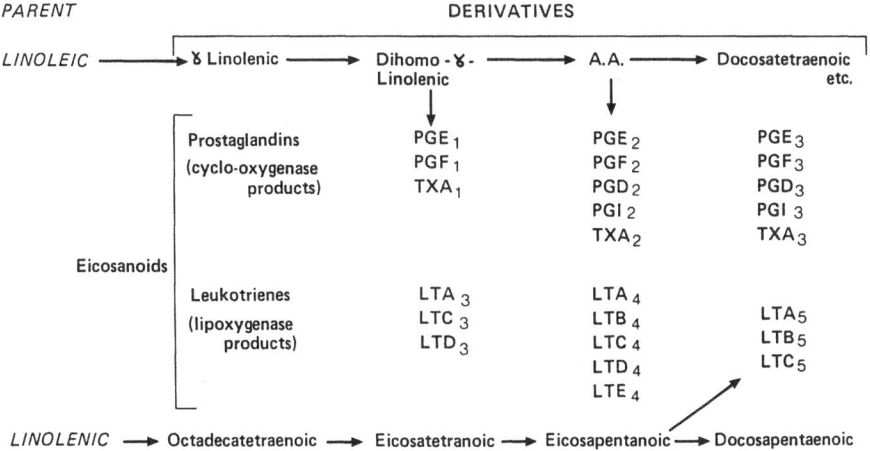

**Figure 2.1** Derivation of prostaglandins (PGs) and leukotrienes (LTs) from essential fatty acids

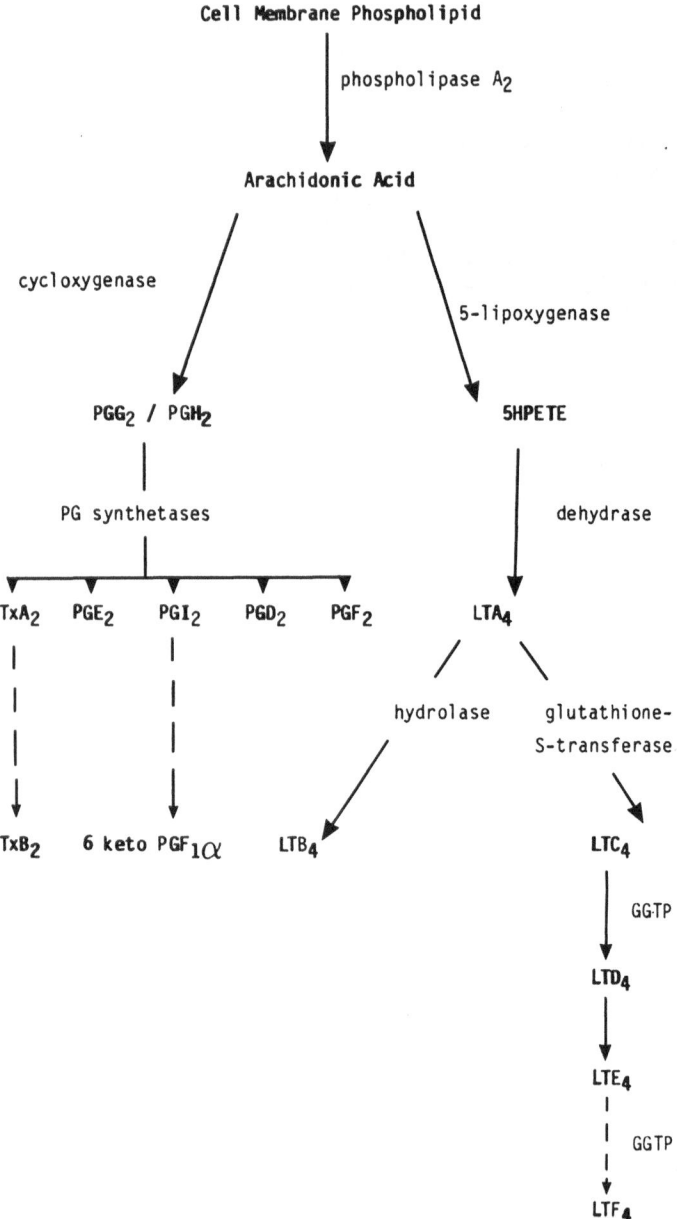

**Figure 2.2** Metabolism of arachidonic acid. PG = prostaglandin; LT = leukotriene; Tx = thromboxane; 5HPETE = 5-hydroperoxyeicosatetranoic acid; GGTP = glutamyl transpeptidase

AA, via the action of cyclo-oxygenase, forms biologically active short-lived intermediaries – the endoperoxides $PGG_2$ and $PGH_2$. From these, via the action of various synthetase enzymes, a range of metabolic transformations leads to the formation of the stable PGs, $PGE_2$, $D_2$, $F_{2\alpha}$ and $A_2$, and the unstable short-lived $PGI_2$ and $TXA_2$ which are rapidly converted into stable and inert 6 keto-$PGF_{1\alpha}$ and $TXB_2$, respectively.

## Sources of prostaglandins

Since the early 1960s, many workers have demonstrated the presence of PGs in a wide variety of inflammatory exudates, ranging from joint effusions to intra-ocular inflammatory exudate[4]. However, the source of these PGs remained unknown until experiments in the early 1970s showed that polymorphonuclear leukocytes (PMNs) when stimulated generated E-type PGs[5]. Later experiments demonstrated that macrophages and possibly lymphocytes were also capable of generating PGs[6]. The spleen has also been implicated recently[7]. Currently, although all the major immuno-inflammatory cell types appear able to generate products of arachidonic acid metabolism, the macrophage seems to be the most important, with the glass-adherent monocyte producing PGs in the peripheral blood[8]. The type and amount of PG produced depends on the cell type, the stimulus applied and the sex of the individual studied[9].

## Biological actions

The inflammatory properties of the cyclo-oxygenase products can, for ease of discussion, be logically divided into three sections:
The development of the cardinal signs of inflammation
The effect on PMNs
The effect on lymphocytes.

*The cardinal signs of inflammation*
These are summarized in Table 2.1. The vascular changes which are the hallmark of inflammation are hyperaemia and increased vascular permeability; this produces redness and oedema. Arteriolar relaxation causes the tissues to become engorged with blood. Microvascular blood flow is initially increased but subsequently slows until, in some vessels, there may be stasis which causes clotting if prolonged. Some of the most convincing evidence that PGs are involved in inflammation is based on their potent action on vascular smooth muscle (Table 2.1). Vasodilatation is caused by the release into the tissues of $PGI_2$, $E_1$, $E_2$ and $D_2$. The effects of these compounds are, however, antagonized to a certain degree by the vasoconstrictor activities of the endoperoxides, and $PGF_{2\alpha}$ and $TXA_2$. It has been suggested that this vasoconstrictor effect of $TXA_2$, in combination with its platelet aggregating effect, may help to prevent haemorrhage in inflammation[10].

While only weakly active in producing oedema, the endoperoxides and $PGI_2$, $E_2$ and $F_{2\alpha}$ contribute synergistically to the swelling caused by bradykinin and histamine[11].

29

**Table 2.1**  Prostaglandins and the cardinal signs of inflammation

| Cardinal sign | Prostaglandin involvement |
|---|---|
| Rubor (redness) | Some PGs are potent vasodilators |
| Tumor (oedema) | Most PGs augment oedema induced by other agents – this may simply reflect vasodilatation |
| Dolor (pain) | Most PGs induce hyperalgesia and pain due to synergy with histamine and bradykinin |
| Calor (heat) | AA metabolites induce fever; NSAIs are antipyretic; ?fever caused by unknown cyclo-oxygenase product |
| Functio laesia (loss of function) | Potent effects on movement and function of inflammatory cells (PMNs, lymphocytes, macrophages, platelets) |

The role of AA metabolites in the provocation of pain is very complex. In various experiments, Ferreira[12] has found that AA *per se* provokes overt pain. In contrast, the PG endoperoxides provoke only modest hyperalgesia[13]. $PGI_2$ causes hyperalgesia which becomes overt pain upon addition of bradykinin and histamine[14]. The $PGI_2$-invoked hyperalgesia is shortlived, in contrast to the long-lived hyperalgesia of $PGE_1$ and $E_2$. These PGEs also act synergistically with bradykinin and histamine. Indeed, most of the oxidative products of AA appear to potentiate pain induced by bradykinin and histamine, rather than being themselves the cause. The analgesic effect of non-steroidal inflammatory agents (NSAIs) (see Figure 2.3 later) would, however, suggest that the hyperalgesic action of PGs may be important in the sensation of pain in human diseases. However, such experiments could easily be interpreted as suggesting that currently unidentified cyclo-oxygenase products may be the mediators of such pain.

The role of PGs in fever is unclear at the present time. Whereas AA itself can provoke fever, the known stable PG derivatives by themselves are not pyrogenic[15]. Although $PGE_1$ is a potent pyretic agent when injected into the cerebral ventricles, it appears that this effect may be due to secondary release of interleukin 1 rather than a direct effect[16]. Again, the antipyretic effects of the NSAIs question this hypothesis or suggest the existence of other fever-inducing but as yet undiscovered cyclo-oxygenase products.

The fifth cardinal sign of inflammation is loss of function. The PG-mediated inhibition of cellular activity during inflammation has been well documented and probably relates to alterations in cellular cyclic AMP (cAMP). This is further discussed in the context of the effects of PGs on PMNs and lymphocytes but includes also an inhibition of both fibroblast growth and IgE-induced histamine release from basophils[17].

*Effect of prostaglandins on PMNs*

PGs have been shown to affect both PMN movement and PMN release of lysosomal enzymes. Since the earliest response to injury is usually the influx of PMNs, the chemotactic activity of AA derivatives has attracted considerable attention. AA itself is chemotactic[14] and this activity is significantly enhanced when the lipid is exposed to ultraviolet light. This suggests that oxidative products of AA do have potent chemotactic effects. However, although $TXA_2$ is chemotactic for mouse PMNs, it does not affect human leukocytes[18]. The stimulatory effects of the other PGs on human cells have been rather weak, and are also species dependent. Furthermore, inhibition of PG production does not correlate with reduction in leukocyte migration[19]. It is likely, therefore, that the oxidative products of AA responsible for stimulating chemotaxis are the leukotrienes and this effect will be discussed later.

In contrast to the pro-inflammatory effects of PGs described previously, their actions on tissue components appear to be mostly inhibitory. It has therefore been suggested that the endogenous PGs have a negative feedback role in chronic inflammation, initially aiding development of the cardinal signs of inflammation followed by a later suppressant effect. Many reports have demonstrated that an increase in intracellular cAMP, resulting from the actions of certain PGs, modulates the PMN in a general inhibitory way[14]. Since 1971 it has been appreciated that some of the stable PGs added to human PMNs inhibit the release of lysosomal hydrolases[20]. As these effects can be mimicked if the cells are treated with exogenous cAMP, it was thought that the PGs mediate their inhibitory response in this way. Indeed, it has now been shown that their inhibitory capacity is directly proportional to the increase in PMN cAMP[21]. Furthermore, $PGI_2$ is a most potent cyclase stimulator and has been shown to prevent PMN chemotaxis. $PGI_2$ also inhibits the margination and adherence of leukocytes in the blood vessels[22]. It is of interest that total leukocyte numbers are most elevated when $PGI_2$ production is lowest, suggesting that $PGI_2$ may suppress PMN accumulation in acute inflammation. In contrast, $PGF_{2\alpha}$ raises cyclic guanosine monophosphate (cGMP) and may enhance chemokinesis[14].

*Effect of prostaglandins on lymphocytes*
There is considerable evidence to suggest that PGs may influence T-cell activity such as the response to mitogens or antigens, production of lymphokines and possible suppressor or helper functions. As with the PMN, the effect of the PGEs and $PGI_2$ is in general inhibitory. The finding that macrophages are important in producing PGs is of particular interest, in view of the potential modulation of T-cell proliferation and lymphokine generation, effects which are associated with increased levels of cAMP. Exogenously added $PGE_2$ and $PGI_2$ inhibit both *in vitro* functions of lymphocytes[23] and *in vivo* responses mediated by lymphocytes[24]. PGEs and $PGI_2$ inhibit lymphocyte proliferation, generation of lymphokines and T lymphocyte mediated cytotoxicity. Goodwin and Webb[25] also detected an enhancement of suppressor T-cell activity. It should be noted, however, that conflicting results have been published in the literature which has led to some confusion in this area. These opposing results may reflect differences in dose. Very low concentrations of PGEs appear to enhance mitogenesis, but high doses inhibit the response. A PGE bell-shaped dose response curve has been previously reported with other cells such as the platelet.

PGD₂ and PGA₂ are, however, less inhibitory of lymphocyte function than PGs of the E or I group, and PGs of the F series have been shown to activate lymphocytes[26]; this is thought to be due to their ability to increase cGMP levels.

Our knowledge of the PG-mediated regulation of B lymphocyte function is still very poor, with many apparent contradictions in the literature. Human B lymphocytes will secrete immunoglobulins when stimulated with the B-cell activator such as pokeweed mitogen (PWM). Some experiments indicate that high-dose PGEs will inhibit generation of IgG and IgM antibodies, while at lower doses E-type PGs may stimulate the response[27]. The high-dose studies have been criticized because the concentration of PGs used are not 'physiological'. However, it should be remembered that PGs are autocoids; they are produced locally in very high concentrations (as reflected by the concentrations in inflammatory exudates) and responses by lymphocytes to PG concentrations of $10^{-6}$ to $10^{-8}$ mol $L^{-1}$ perhaps do reflect those occurring *in vivo*. These high doses of $PGE_1$ will suppress sheep red blood cell haemagglutinin responses, suggesting an inhibition of the appearance of antibody-forming cells and treatment *in vivo* with $PGE_1$ has been reported to enhance the survival time of murine homographs through depletion of B-cells[27].

In general, therefore, the initial pro-inflammatory effects of the PGs are balanced by their later, mostly inhibitory effects on tissue components.

## INTERACTION OF PGs WITH OTHER MEDIATORS OF INFLAMMATION

Synergism between PGs and other substances was first reported by Goldblatt in 1935[3] who showed that there was synergism between adrenalin and PGs in producing smooth muscle contractions. In later experiments, PGs were shown to sensitize smooth muscle to the contractile effects of vasopressin, oxytocin and histamine. However, we still do not know how important these interactions are on smooth muscle *in vivo*. Interactions between PGs and other substances have more recently been observed in the intact animal; these are believed to be important in the context of the inflammatory response.

### Histamine and bradykinin

In some early experiments on the effects of PGs on human skin, it was noted that some, notably $PGE_1$ and $PGE_2$, were able to potentiate pain induced by histamine and bradykinin[12]. More recently, $PGI_2$ has been found to be an important potentiator of the pain response[10]. Histamine and bradykinin increase venular permeability to macromolecules. Addition of PGs, which themselves produce little oedema, result in a marked potentiation of the responses to histamine and bradykinin[28]. This relates predominantly to the PGs ability to promote vasodilatation and it is of interest that other vasodilators, e.g. vasoactive intestinal peptide (VIP) can also act synergistically with histamine and bradykinin[29].

32

## Complement-derived peptides

Injection of certain bacteria, yeasts or immune complexes, results in local oedema which can be suppressed by inhibitors of PG synthesis. This supports the hypothesis that two endogenous mediators act synergistically to induce oedema formation. As neither antihistamines nor kinin inhibitors inhibited the oedema response, investigation was begun to identify the permeability-increasing mediator. This was identified as the cleavage produce C5a of the fifth component of complement[30]. Histamine and bradykinin act directly on venular endothelial cells to cause leakage; however C5a has a different mechanism of action. It has been shown that increased permeability cannot be induced by C5a in animals depleted of circulating PMNs, but that responses to histamine and bradykinin are unchanged[31]. Thus responses to C5a appear to depend on an interaction by endothelial cells and the circulating neutrophils and the addition of PG augments this effect. Furthermore, C3 fragments have been shown to enhance PG release from monocytes in culture[32].

## Oxygen radicals

Cells such as PMNs can consume large quantities of oxygen when phagocytosing particles. This oxygen is transformed into oxidising substances such as superoxide ($O_2^-$). Superoxide helps in the killing and digestion of phagocytosed material. However, if produced in excess, oxidising substances may leak from the cell and contribute to the surrounding inflammatory reaction. The superoxide anion forms a hydroxyl radical (OH) with hydrogen peroxide ($H_2O_2$). This is thought to be the main factor in oxygen-centred inflammatory mechanisms. Oxygen radicals are produced by the AA pathway, especially during the conversion of $PGG_2$ to $PGH_2$ by the enzyme hydroperoxidase[33]. Thus, any stimulus which activates PG production will also augment the production of free radicals. In turn the oxidative products of free radical reactions, lipid peroxides, are necessary at low level to activate $PGH_2$ synthetase and are thus important promoters of the conversion of AA to the PGs. Furthermore, peroxides are important influences in determining whether $PGI_2$ or $TXA_2$ production will predominate. High peroxide levels will selectively enhance $TXA_2$ production by their ability to inactivate $PGI_2$ synthetase.

We have recently, however, shown that $PGE_1$ is a free radical scavenger[34] and this again supports the hypothesis that PGs are initially pro-inflammatory, allowing increased free radical production with later anti-inflammatory free radical scavenging effects.

## Interleukin-1

Interleukin-1 (IL-1) is an important cytokine with effects on a wide variety of target tissues. Some of these effects include induction of fever, lymphocyte proliferation, the acute phase response and muscle catabolism. In addition, IL-1 has been shown to stimulate $PGE_2$[35] and $PGI_2$[36] synthesis; in this way IL-1 contributes to the production of the PGs. Recent evidence[37] suggests that these products of the cyclo-oxygenase pathway then down-regulate the further production of IL-1. This implies a feedback regulation of IL-1 by prostaglandins demonstrating the classic characteristic of a hormone in inducing its own inhibitor. This autoregulatory effect of PGs on IL-1 production is supported by the finding of Boraschi *et al.*[38] showing that $\gamma$-interferon can augment macrophage IL-1 production by suppressing $PGE_2$ release.

## Platelets

Several PGs have profound effects on platelet responses. The PG products that induce aggregation and release of platelet products are the endoperoxides ($PGG_2$ and $PGH_2$) and $TXA_2$. Others inhibit platelet responses, e.g. $PGD_2$, $PGE_1$, $E_2$ and $PGI_2$. As with the PMN, these platelet activating or inhibitory properties are dependent on the PGs ability to decrease or increase cAMP. The importance of the platelet in thrombosis has been known for many years; however, more recently, it has become apparent that some of the platelet release products are important in the inflammatory process.

Serotonin is released from the dense granules of the platelet and can have profound effects on vascular tone and permeability. In addition, serotonin is a fibrogenic agent and may therefore affect the connective tissue composition at sites of chronic inflammation[39].

It has been known for some years that platelets also contain acid hydrolases. Studies have shown that these lysosomal enzymes are found in part of the platelet $\alpha$-granule fraction; however, the roles of these enzymes in inflammation remain to be fully determined. The ability of the acid hydrolases to attack connective tissue is presumably severely limited by the buffering action of the surrounding plasma. Likewise, the neutral proteinases would be affected by plasma inhibitors such as $\alpha$1-antitrypsin and $\alpha$2-macroglobulin. It is likely that such enzymes could only be effective in the immediate pericullular environment. They may therefore play a role in promoting further platelet secretion, but are unlikely to make a major contribution to the degradation of connective tissue.

Platelet-derived growth factor (PDGF) promotes proliferation of smooth muscle cells. It is also thought to degranulate mast cells and be leukotactic. Platelet activating factor (PAF) is a phospholipid product of platelets and white cells and is released in response to various stimuli. It is a potent activator of platelet activation, but additionally may play an important role as a mediator of inflammation and allergy. Intravenous PAF causes profound thrombocytopenia, vascular permeability and later anaphylactic shock. It is likely that it mediates these effects by $TXA_2$ and LT production[40]. The platelet itself is a potent producer of $TXA_2$. Over 99% of the PG endoperoxides formed by platelet cyclo-oxygenase are directed along the thromboxane synthetase pathway. The resultant $TXA_2$ production will modify both platelet aggregation and the inflammatory process, as previously described. Thus the

PGs with anti-platelet effects would diminish the inflammatory response by preventing platelet release, whereas those that aggregate platelets such as $PGG_2$, $PGH_2$ and $TXA_2$ would augment it.

## PROSTAGLANDINS AND PATHOLOGICAL INFLAMMATION

In the preceding pages we have seen that the PGs have a role in the general inflammatory process. However, what evidence do we have regarding their involvement in pathological inflammation? Certainly, authors have reported elevated PG levels in synovial fluid taken from patients with rheumatoid arthritis (RA)[4] and culture of RA synovial tissue has also demonstrated increased PG production[41]. However, as we have seen, although elevated levels would initially augment the development of the cardinal signs of inflammation, they should also, by their later suppressant effects on cellular function, aid in the termination of the process. It has been proposed that a breakdown in this down-regulatory pathway could lead to the development of chronic inflammation. A disorder of PG regulation has been suggested as being relevant in RA[42] and multiple sclerosis[43], where a breakdown in PG suppression could lead to an overactive immune response.

We have shown that PGs infused therapeutically produce an initial gratifying response in the Raynaud's phenomenon associated with systemic sclerosis (SS)[44]. This is followed by the development of resistance to the effects of the PGs. Later work has shown that tachyphylaxis, manifest by a decrease in numbers of cell PG receptor sites, has occurred[45]. It may be that excess PGs produced during the initial phase of inflammation allow the development of cellular resistance to the later suppressant effects of PGs. In support of this theory are the findings that lymphocytes[46] and endothelial cells[47] from patients with SS are resistant to the effects of $PGE_1$, and we have found similar results with SS platelets using $PGI_2$[48]. The introduction of a higher dose of PG, such as is infused pharmacologically, would then suppress cellular function. This could explain the apparent paradox that, despite findings of high levels of PGEs in adjuvant arthritis, infusions of $PGE_1$ appear to prevent and suppress this arthritis[49].

In immunologically related diseases, manipulation of AA metabolism could therefore have a wider spectrum than mere inhibition by NSAIs of the pro-inflammatory aspects of PGs.

## LEUKOTRIENES

The series of biologically active derivatives of AA was recently extended by the discovery of a new group of compounds, the leukotrienes. These LTs have pronounced biological effects which are related to immediate hypersensitivity responses and inflammation. They have only recently been characterized chemically but their role in allergic reactions was noted many years ago. In the 1930s a substance was detected in the lung extracellular fluid that was clearly not one of the mediators liberated from mast cell granules, but that caused a long-lasting and profound constriction of the airways[50].

35

It later became known as slow reacting substance of anaphylaxis (SRS-A) which has recently been shown to consist of a mixture of substances. They are thio-ethers; fatty acids linked by a sulphur atom to one or more amino acids. Their chemical structure was delineated by Samuelsson et al. in 1979[51], who named them leukotrienes because they were made by leukocytes and had three conjugated double bonds in their parent molecule.

## Metabolism of arachidonic acid

The PGs and LTs share a common origin, that is AA. In the case of the LTs, this branch is initiated by the 5-lipoxygenase enzyme (Figure 2.2). AA is converted into 5-hydroperoxyeicosatetranoic acid (5HPETE) which is modified to become $LTA_4$ (the subscript 4 indicates that there are four double bonds). $LTA_4$ is converted by the enzymatic addition of water into $LTB_4$, or by the addition of glutathione into $LTC_4$. The tripeptide glutathione consists of a chain of amino acids cysteine, glycine and glutamic acid. When glutamic acid is removed, $LTC_4$ is transformed into $D_4$ and the loss of glycine from $D_4$ leads to the formation of $E_4$. We now know that a mixture of $C_4$, $D_4$ and $E_4$ constitutes SRS-A.

It should be noted that, in cellular systems, $LTA_4$ can also be hydrolysed non-enzymatically to form 6-*trans*-$LTB_4$ and 12-epi-6-*trans*-$LTB_4$. The stereochemistry of $LTB_4$ is of particular biological importance, as both the non-enzymatic hydrolysis products and stereochemically dissimilar *synthetic* $LTB_4$ have considerably reduced biological activity[52]. Furthermore, other enzymes apart from 5-lipoxygenase, such as 12-lipoxygenase and 15-lipoxygenase are active in this system leading to the formation of compounds which might also be important to the inflammatory process. Also, as with the PGs, it is not only the essential fatty acid AA which leads to the formation of LTs. Other C20 fatty acids can also be metabolized to LTs, e.g. eicosatetranoic acid to the series 5 LTs[53] (Figure 2.1). These LTs have similar biological profiles to those of the 4 series but in general tend to differ in potency of effect. Use can be made of this therapeutically to modify inflammation by alteration in dietary fatty acids and this is discussed later.

Depending on the cell type and availability of enzymes, AA is converted to whichever LT is required. A variety of stimuli can thus be converted into a multitude of compounds, which can regulate or mediate various cell functions. For ease of discussion, $LTB_4$ with its specific effects on white blood cells will be dealt with first, then $LTC_4$, $D_4$ and $E_4$ with their effects predominantly on smooth muscle.

## $LTB_4$

$LTB_4$ was purified and characterized initially as a product of human neutrophils[51]. Since then other cells have been shown to generate $LTB_4$ after incubation with stimuli such as calcium ionophore, the chemotactant N-formyl-Met-Leu-Phe (FMLP), opsonized zymosan, complement fragments and AA. Much of the *in vitro* data comes from cells stimulated by A23187, the calcium ionophore[52]. This is a non-physiological stimulus, and of more interest are the records of $LTB_4$ generation following more physiological stimuli, e.g. lymphokines and complement fragment C5a. Other cells have been reported as producing $LTB_4$ (macrophages, eosinophils, T lymphocytes, basophils and also erythrocytes and keratinocytes) so that although PMNs are the major source it appears that $LTB_4$ can be generated from a large number of different cell types.

The production of $LTB_4$ can be decreased by agents that increase cellular cAMP levels[53]. This may be of some importance to the regulation of metabolism as $LTB_4$ can also stimulate the formation of cAMP[52], providing a possible negative feedback inhibition of $LTB_4$ production. In any case, $LTB_4$ is rapidly de-activated, mainly by its conversion to the more polar and less active 20-carboxy derivatives[52].

The actions of $LTB_4$ are listed in Table 2.2. PMNs present the first line of defence against foreign and pathogenic stimuli. As such they have to perform several functions including the detection of, movement towards and accumulation at sites of injury or infection. This phenomenon is termed chemotaxis. Once at the site of infection (aggregation) the PMN phagocytoses the offending particles. Following this there is a discharge of various lysosomes which promote the destruction of the engulfed particle. The most potent and certainly the best documented effects of $LTB_4$ are those on the above behaviour and function of leukocytes.

$LTB_4$ has been shown to stimulate chemokinesis (random movement) of PMNs and it is a potent chemotactic and aggregating agent[54]. Furthermore, its potency is thought to be equivalent to that of the established cytotoxin C5a and the synthetic peptide FMLP[52]. In addition it also stimulates release of PMN lysosomal enzymes. The doses required, however, are considerably higher than those used to effect chemokinesis or aggregation, and it is much less potent that FMLP as a degranulating agent[54].

Recently $LTB_4$ has been implicated in eosinophil chemotaxis and release of peroxidase. $LTB_4$ will enhance the expression of complement receptors[55] which might be linked to the ability of $LTB_4$ to increase the complement-dependent killing of *Schistosoma mansonii*.

An essential component of the inflammatory response is the adhesion of PMN to the endothelial lining of blood vessels. $LTB_4$ effectively stimulates PMN adhesion to endothelial cell surfaces, and possibly to smooth muscle and dermal fibroblasts.

**Table 2.2**  Biological actions of the leukotrienes

| Actions of $LTB_4$ | Actions of $LTC_4$, $D_4$, $E_4$ |
| --- | --- |
| Stimulation of leukocyte functions<br>    chemokinesis<br>    chemotaxis<br>    adherence<br>    aggregation<br>    degranulation | Smooth muscle contraction<br><br>Leakage from venules<br><br>Small airways constriction |
| Enhanced expression of C3b receptors | |
| Suppression of lymphocytes | |

In addition to its potent actions on PMNs, $LTB_4$ in common with the PGs may be a possible mediator of lymphocyte responses. A number of workers[56] have suggested that LTs inhibit lymphocyte activities *in vitro*, e.g. the lymphocyte response to mitogen. In contrast other studies, examining the effect of drug-induced lipoxygenase inhibition, suggest the opposite[52]. However, the inhibitor drugs employed were not specific for $LTB_4$ and therefore the effects seen may have been due to removal of other lipoxygenase products. As yet, therefore, $LTB_4$ cannot be ascribed any definite role in modulating lymphocyte behaviour.

$LTB_4$ effects upon smooth muscle are not nearly so potent as those of other LTs. The weak contraction of smooth muscle tissue seen *in vitro* is thought to be due to $LTB_4$-induced $TXA_2$ release[57], as it is blocked by cyclo-oxygenase inhibition. Further interaction of $LTB_4$ with the products of the cyclo-oxygenase enzyme is seen with $PGE_2$. If $PGE_2$ or $LTB_4$ are injected individually into the skin, the vascular permeability does not change. However, if given together, there is a significant increase in plasma exudation[54].

## $LTC_4$, $LTD_4$ and $LTE_4$

It is now thought that human SRS-A consists mainly of $LTD_4$, but also some $LTC_4$. It is, however, important to be aware that there is a marked species difference in LT production, e.g. rat SRS-A contains $E_4$ in addition to $C_4$ and $D_4$[58]. All of the cysteine-containing LTs have been found in a variety of cell systems and the stimuli for production are similar to those reported for $LTB_4$, e.g. calcium ionophore A23187. We have seen that $LTC_4$ is metabolized to $D_4$ and thus to $E_4$. It has recently been found that $E_4$ can be converted to $F_4$. As this results in loss of biological activity, it probably represents part of the pathway for metabolism and degradation of the LTs.

The actions of these LTs are listed in Table 2.2. One of their most potent effects is their action on smooth muscle preparations. The standard assay for SRS-A was constriction of guineapig ileum, and in this muscle preparation $C_4$, $D_4$ and $E_4$ are thousands of times more potent than histamine[53]. This smooth muscle effect is best recognized in the airways where LTs have been shown to produce bronchoconstriction both directly and via release of $TXA_2$[59].

The bronchoconstrictor properties of these LTs are well recognized but their role in the development of inflammation is not so clear. In particular $C_4$ and $D_4$ lack significant chemotactic activity[60]. The circulatory system, however, and in particular the microvascular bed is an area where LTs might have important mediator functions. An increase in vessel permeability allows exudation of plasma into the extravascular space. This contributes to the swelling and oedema of inflamed tissues and allows transport of other inflammatory mediators to the active site. $LTC_4$, $D_4$ and $E_4$ promote such a plasma exudation from post-capillary venules, again at much lower concentra-tions than required for histamine[61]. This effect appears to be caused by a direct action on the endothelial lining as it occurs quickly and does not require release of histamine, PGs or the presence of PMNs. In contrast, that produced by $LTB_4$ occurs later, requires adherent PMNs and possible interaction with $PGs^{54}$.

A further contribution to tissue damage may occur as a result of the smooth muscle constriction. The LTs $C_4$ and $D_4$ are potent vasoconstrictors, in particular affecting the coronary, cerebral and uterine vessels[62]. However, species difference makes overall analysis of the numerous studies difficult. It is likely, however, that LTs will be relevant in the pathological constriction seen in vascular beds following immunological reactions.

## INTERACTIONS OF LEUKOTRIENES WITH OTHER MEDIATORS OF INFLAMMATION

As with the PGs, interactions between LTs and other substances have been observed and it has been suggested that this interaction and mediator synergism are important phenomena in inflammation.

### Cyclo-oxygenase products

The effects of the cyclo-oxygenase and lipoxygenase products are interrelated. Synergism occurs between leukotrienes and the vasodilatory PGs, causing plasma leakage, and may be important in the formation of oedema. Interestingly, $LTC_4$ stimulates release of $PGE_2$ and $PGI_2^{63}$. This will lead to an increase in plasma exudate, but also leads to an increase in cAMP. cAMP has been shown to decrease $LTB_4$ production[53]; thus there is the potential for feedback regulation of $LTB_4$-generation at an inflammatory site.

As discussed, PGs are known to act synergistically with C5a to produce oedema[30]. The ability of $LTB_4$ to enhance the expression of complement receptors on human neutrophils may increase this effect[55]. There is also some evidence that $LTB_4$ enhances the effects of bradykinin and thus further oedema formation[64].

It is also of interest that $LTB_4$ may produce hyperalgesia. However, Levine et al.[65] have shown that the $LTB_4$-induced hyperalgesia is not mediated via PG release but is dependent on PMN activation and localization at the site of inflammation.

### Oxygen radicals

Recently we have shown[66] that LTs can stimulate superoxide anion production, the order of activity being $D_4 > C_4 > B_4$. In turn, Henderson and Klebanoff[67] have shown that LTs can be inactivated by the hydroxyl ion. Thus free radical production may modulate LT activity and vice versa.

39

## Interleukin-1

Inhibition of LT production has been shown to decrease IL-1 production[68], a finding which we confirmed using the lipoxygenase inhibitor BW755C (Wellcome Research)[69]. In contrast, the cyclo-oxygenase inhibitor indomethacin had no effect. When LTB$_4$ was added directly to a pro-monocytic cell line (U937) we detected an increase in production of IL-1 (thymocyte activation assay).

## Platelets

The metabolism of exogenous AA by leukocytes is enhanced by the addition of platelets. Maclouf et al.[70] have recently demonstrated that the 12-HPETE derived from platelet AA activates the 5-lipoxygenase enzyme of leukocytes. This will lead to increased LT production, in particular LTB$_4$. Although inflammation can proceed in the absence of circulating platelets[71] the interaction described suggests that platelets may be involved in the initiation or amplification of LT-modulated inflammation. Gorman et al.[72] have shown that PAF can stimulate PMNs to synthesize LTB$_4$. Furthermore, PAF has been shown to mediate its action on the pulmonary circulation by increasing production of lipoxygenase products.

## LEUKOTRIENES AND PATHOLOGICAL INFLAMMATION

Theoretically, therefore, it is possible that LTs play a part in the production of inflammation. However, little work has so far been carried out to support a hypothesis that excess LT production contributes to excess pathological inflammation. One reason for this is that methodological and other problems have been associated with LT measurement in biological samples. Recently, high pressure liquid chromatography (HPLC) and radioimmunoassay have both been used with some success. Klickstein et al.[73], using HPLC, detected excess lipoxygenase products in the synovial fluid of RA patients and patients with spondylitis, as compared to osteoarthritic controls. Davidson et al.[74] have supported these data with the finding of detectable levels of LTB$_4$ by HPLC in rheumatoid synovial fluid; these levels subsequently fell after disease-modifying therapy. However, these findings do not clarify whether LTB$_4$ causes an increase in synovial fluid cell count (via its chemotactic effect) or whether the increased cell count (brought on by some other stimuli) releases greater quantities of LTB$_4$. The usual question is raised as to cause or consequence regarding inflammatory mediators.

In a recent study of RA patients, we have shown that the RA PMNs produced more LTB$_4$ when stimulated with calcium ionophore, than did age and sex-matched controls[75]. As mentioned earlier, it has been suggested that patients receiving cyclo-oxygenase inhibitors respond by diverting substrate to the lipoxygenase pathway. We compared patients on NSAIs to those off NSAI therapy, and could detect no significant difference in LTB$_4$ production from PMNs. Both groups showed elevated LTB$_4$ levels. Family studies are now under way to investigate whether this increase in production is genetically linked. Assay of the 5-lipoxygenase enzyme in family groups might also prove interesting.

It seems likely that increased PMN production of leukotrienes and increased levels of LTs in biological fluids will be detected in many inflammatory states. Whether these LTs are cause or consequence of excess inflammation is unknown. It is interesting to speculate, however, that no matter if the excess LTs are a primary or secondary effect, their removal via inhibition of synthesis may allow improvement in the clinical symptoms of inflammatory diseases.

## THERAPEUTIC MANIPULATION OF THE ARACHIDONIC ACID PATHWAY

The finding of increased PG and LT levels in inflammatory exudates suggests that inhibition of their synthesis might ameliorate the signs and symptoms of inflammation. Inhibition of both PG and LT formation is possible at a number of sites in the AA cascade and this is illustrated in Figure 2.3.

### Cyclo-oxygenase inhibitors

The finding in 1971 that drugs such as indomethacin and aspirin are selective inhibitors of PG synthesis[76] led Vane to propose that this was the mechanism of their therapeutic and toxic effects. The decrease in $PGE_2$ and $PGI_2$ accounts for the reduction in erythema, oedema and hyperalgesia seen with these drugs. Furthermore, the PGs synergize with other inflammatory mediators so that their removal will reduce the effectiveness of bradykinin, histamine, free radicals, complement-derived peptides, etc.

Prostaglandin production is not normally increased unless there is tissue damage, and this explains why cyclo-oxygenase inhibitors are not analgesic or antipyretic in the absence of inflammation. A large number of NSAIs inhibit PG synthesis, and there is a good correlation between their potency in decreasing the cardinal signs of inflammation and in reducing PG formation[77].

The toxicity of these drugs, however, is also related to their potency as PG inhibitors. NSAIs have the common property of causing gastrointestinal irritation, which can lead to peptic ulceration and haemorrhage. When a group of drugs with diverse chemical structures share the same therapeutic and toxic effects, it suggests that the same mechanism of action underlies both processes. The recognition of this led to the suggestion that PG production in the gastric mucosa was a protective mechanism and that removal of PGs leads to injury[76]. $PGI_2$ and $E_2$ are produced in the gastric mucosa and are potent mucosal vasodilators. Removal of this vasodilatory effect via NSAI administration could lead to areas of local ischaemia within the gastric mucosa which would be susceptible to attack by acid or pepsins. The inhibition of gastric cyclo-oxygenase by NSAI correlates closely with the ulcerogenicity of these drugs[78].

Some NSAIs have been associated with renal tubular necrosis. Vasodilator

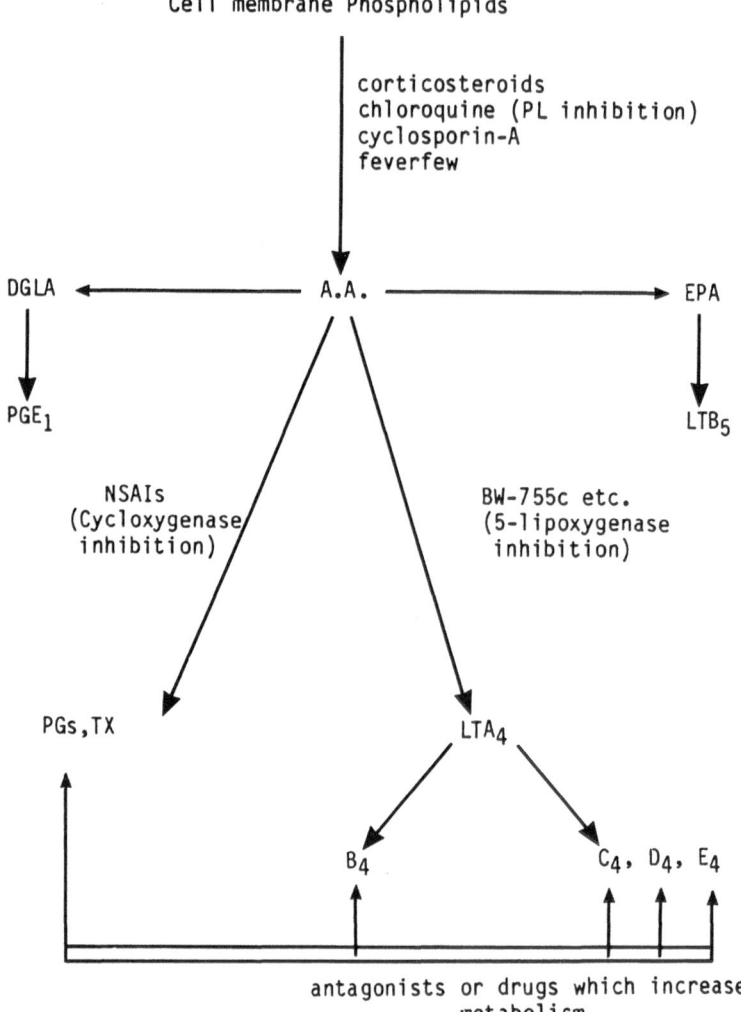

**Figure 2.3** Therapeutic approaches to arachidonic acid (AA) metabolism. PG = prostaglandin; LT = leukotriene; TX = thromboxane; PL = phospholipase; EPA = eicosapentanoic acid; DGLA = dihomo-γ-linolenic acid; NSAI = non-steroidal anti-inflammatory agent

PGs maintain blood flow and glomerular filtration rate in diseases where renal function is impaired. It is possible that cyclo-oxygenase inhibition might be detrimental in these patients. $PGF_{2\alpha}$ and $PGE_2$ are potent contractors of uterine smooth muscle and are mediators of parturition and labour. Manufacturers advise special precautions in the use of aspirin-like drugs in normal pregnancy. PG inhibition may also cause premature closure of the foetal ductus in late pregnancy.

There has been renewed interest recently in evaluation of non-acetylated salicylate preparations in the treatment of RA. Among these salicylsalicylic acid (salsalate) has gained increasing support. Although technically classified as an NSAI, salsalate does not share the propensity to inhibit PG synthesis. Its efficacy derives from its behaviour as a pro-drug of salicylic acid – the active part of all salicylate formulations – and this may lead to reduction in gastrointestinal side-effects following oral administration[79].

Apart from the toxicity of NSAIs, there have been reports suggesting that inhibition of cyclo-oxygenase diverts substrate AA to form more lipoxygenase productions. This possible increase in LT production may explain why these drugs can give good symptomatic relief but do little to ameliorate the underlying process of the disease. Analgesia and decreased oedema would result from decreasing PG levels, but increased LT production would allow the more chronic PMN-mediated components of inflammation to proceed unchecked. Although we have not confirmed this in our own group of RA patients[75], more work is required in this area.

## 5-Lipoxygenase inhibitors

Although there are fairly specific inhibitors of cyclo-oxygenase, there are few compounds known to selectively inhibit only the 5-lipoxygenase enzyme. However, as inhibition of PG production alone may lead to substrate diversion and increased LT formation, it is a reasonable hypothesis that a selective lipoxygenase inhibitor would augment the PG-mediated components of inflammation. Inhibitors of both pathways are likely to have significant clinical advantages over selective single enzyme inhibitors.

Most recent published work relates to BW755c (Wellcome Research Laboratories). This pyrazoline derivative is a dual inhibitor of both the cyclo-oxygenase and lipoxygenase enzymes[80]. It has been shown to decrease oedema, PG concentrations and leukocyte numbers in inflammatory exudates, and has a similar profile of anti-inflammatory activity to dexamethasone. However, despite these encouraging results, it should be stressed that BW755c is an experimental compound and most of the reported work has been carried out either in vitro or in animal models of inflammation.

Other potential lipoxygenase inhibitors are nor-dihydroguaiaretic acid (NDGA), propyl gallate, some aromatic disulphites, flavinoids such as rutin and quercetin, and ETYA, an acetylenic analogue of AA[52]. As with BW755c, however, these compounds are in the early stage of development.

Benoxaprofen is a weak cyclo-oxygenase inhibitor and it has been suggested that benoxaprofen also decreases 5-lipoxygenase activity. Salmon et al.[81] suggest however that this lipoxygenase inhibition is only an in vitro phenomenon and they have demonstrated that LTB$_4$ levels are not reduced by the drug in exudate obtained from an animal model of inflammation. It is possible, therefore, that the toxic effects of benoxaprofen, which led to its withdrawal, cannot be attributed to inhibition of the 5-lipoxygenase enzyme.

Colchicine has also been suggested as a dual inhibitor in vitro[82] – in vivo work is awaited to assess the relevance of these findings. Stenson and Lobos[83] reported that sulphasalazine, in addition to PG inhibition, decreased the

43

synthesis of 5HETE by human neutrophils. We have recently investigated its effect on rat basophil leukaemia cells (unpublished observations). We measured production of $LTC_4$ by HPLC after calcium ionophore stimulation and have found decreased production of the LT after addition of the drug. The metabolite 5-amino-salicylate appears to be the most active against LT generation.

The lack of specificity of lipoxygenase inhibitors may cause problems, thus compounds with the ability to block the conversion of $LTA_4$ to $B_4$ or specific $LTB_4$ antagonists may be more useful (Figure 2.3).


## Phospholipase inhibitors

The inhibition of AA release from phospholipid would result in reduced formation of both cyclo-oxygenase and lipoxygenase products (Figure 2.3). It might be expected that such dual inhibition might be more clinically effective than the inhibition of only one or other pathway. NSAIs are, in general, very weak phospholipase (PL) inhibitors. However other drugs, notably the corticosteroids, do act at this level.

In order to understand the mechanism of action of PL inhibitors, it is important to review some of the basic properties of these enzymes. $PLA_1$ and $PLA_2$ are a heterologous group of enzymes distributed throughout the body. They can be classified into membrane-bound or soluble forms. There seems to be a population of $PLA_2$ enzymes in cell membranes, which are accessible from outside the cell. This is suggested by the fact that very high molecular weight proteins are capable of blocking AA release from membranes when present in the medium surrounding the cell. In common with PLA, PLC is found in most cells. However, while there do not appear to be any membrane-associated forms of the enzyme its soluble form is usually located in lysosomes. Because AA is usually esterified to the $\beta$ position, $PLA_2$ inhibition has a greater effect on its metabolism.

The glucocorticoids in particular are known to interfere with the production of eicosanoids. It was noted that, although they had no direct action on the eicosanoid generating enzymes *in vitro*, they could suppress the production of eicosanoids by intact cells. It is now known that they act by inducing the synthesis and/or release of proteins that possess anti-$PLA_2$ properties, macrocortin and lipomodulin[84]. The relative novelty of these compounds, however, has meant that data concerning their precise mechanisms of action are, as yet, unavailable.

Other drugs used in the treatment of RA may also affect $PLA_2$. Chloroquine and cyclosporin A will decrease PG production and their effects are thought to be due to $PLA_2$ inhibition[85]. Feverfew extract, a compound favoured by those with an interest in 'alternative medicine', has also been shown to decrease $PLA_2$ activity.

It is of interest that mepacrine and chlorpromazine decrease both $PLA_2$ and PLC activity. Propranolol inhibits PLC only as does the glucocorticoid-induced inhibitor of $PLA_2$[86]. Thus corticosteroids affect both $PLA_2$ and PLC in an inhibitory fashion. The side effects of these potent drugs are, however, legion and this precludes their use in all but the most severely affected patients.

## Manipulation of dietary essential fatty acids

Stimulation of cells involved in immune reactions results in mobilization of fatty acids from phospholipid pools for the synthesis of various PGs and LTs. Depending upon the availability of the EFA, determined largely by dietary constituents, biosynthesis may be directed in favour of a particular PG or LT type. Thus, a diet rich in AA leads to the formation of the 2 series PGs and the 4 series LTs with the pro-inflammatory effects as earlier described. The ingestion of a rich diet in evening primrose oil (EPO) will elevate levels of dihomo-γ-linolenic acid (DGLA), which will result in an increase in production of the monoenoic PGs, e.g. $PGE_1$. DGLA cannot itself be converted to LTs but can form a 15-hydroxyl derivative that blocks transformation of AA to LTs[87]. Dietary DGLA may therefore act as a competitive inhibitor of 2 series PGs and 4 series LTs and thus suppress inflammation (Figure 2.1).

Recent studies have shown that the chemotaxis of rat PMNs is impaired by such a diet[88]. In addition we have found that $MRL_1$ mice, who develop a spontaneous autoimmune arthritis, have a significant amelioration in the development of proteinuria and other vasculitic manifestations, with pro-longation of lifespan, when given an EPO-rich diet[89].

We have recently completed a double-blind placebo controlled study of EPO (12 capsules per day) in RA patients[80]. Initial results suggest that in a high proportion of the treated patients the dosage of NSAI can be reduced or even stopped. When placebo capsules were substituted after one year on active treatment the patients relapsed over a 3-month period. Early analysis of the results, however, show no effect on C-reactive protein and erythrocyte sedimentation rates, suggesting that EPO does not have a 'second line' effect. It is likely, therefore, as most clinicians suspect, that the aetiopathogenic mechanism of RA does not lie in over-production of AA products, and their inhibition may result in improved symptoms but not in decreased disease activity.

High dietary levels of another EFA, eicosapentanoic acid (EPA) would provide a substrate for production of PGs of the 3 series and LTs of the 5 series. Prescott[91] has shown that the potency of $LTB_5$ in inducing PMN aggregation is 10% of the potency of $LTB_4$. Kremer et al.[92] investigated the effect of a diet rich in EPA on the clinical manifestation of RA. Although the results suggested a benefit in the 17 treated patients when compared to the 20 controls, the improvement was not dramatically better than that seen in the placebo group. Furthermore, a 12-week study period will be too short to evaluate any long-term effects. We have looked at patients receiving a mixture of EPA and EPO for one year[90]; again, a decrease in NSAI dosage was observed without exacerbation of RA symptoms. A flare in disease activity was produced when placebo capsules were substituted. It is not clear, however, whether the benefits obtained were due to the EPO or the EPA; further long-term studies are therefore required.

45

## Direct prostaglandin treatment

It should be remembered that the late effects of the PGs are to decrease the activation of inflammatory cells such as platelets, PMNs and lymphocytes. We have hypothesized a disorder of PG regulation as being important in RA where a breakdown in PG suppression could lead to continuation of the inflammatory response.

Work with patients suffering from systemic sclerosis has shown that *pharmacological* doses of $PGE_1$ and $I_2$ reintroduce the suppressant effect on inflammatory cells[44,46]. However, despite the fact that adjuvant arthritis can be ameliorated by infusion of $PGE_1$[49], no work has yet been carried out in patients with RA. We have infused $PGI_2$ into RA patients with vasculitic leg ulcers (unpublished observation) and have witnessed healing and improved joint symptoms. However, such results could easily be explained by the hospitalization and subsequent bed rest during the infusions. The effect of direct PG therapy on inflammatory joint disease can only be assessed by double-blind controlled studies.

In conclusion, arachidonic acid is a source of inflammatory mediators. It is possible that the development of inhibitors of both PGs and LTs could lead to the discovery of important new drugs for the treatment of RA. A combined cyclo-oxygenase and lipoxygenase inhibitor should have similar properties to the anti-inflammatory steroids. There is evidence that compounds like BW755c do not enhance the development of bacterial infection, and it is possible that such compounds will have steroid-like therapeutic activity but be free from steroid-related toxicity. Furthermore, the effect of dietary manipulation of this system should be further evaluated.

So far, however, studies suggest that such therapeutic manoeuvres may decrease the inflammatory symptoms but without altering the disease activity itself. Many mediators are involved in inflammation and it is likely that the AA metabolites are only one part of this complicated process.

### References

1. Crawford, M.A. (1983). Background to essential fatty acids and their prostanoid derivatives. *Br. Med. Bull.*, **6**, 210−13
2. von Euler, U.S. (1934). On the specific vasodilatory and plain muscle stimulating substance from accessory genital glands in man and certain animals (prostaglandin and vestiglandin). *Arch. Exp. Pathol. Pharmacol.*, **175**, 78−84
3. Goldblatt, M.W. (1934). Properties of human seminal plasma. *J. Physiol.*, **84**, 208−18
4. Trang, L.E., Granstrom, E. and Lovgren, O. (1977). Levels of prostaglandins $F_{2\alpha}$ and thromboxane $B_2$ in joint fluid in rheumatoid arthritis. *Scand. J. Rheumatol.*, **6**, 151−4
5. Zurier, R.B. (1975). The potential role of prostaglandins in skeletal and muscle disorders. *Ann. Clin. Lab. Sci.*, **5**, 276−81
6. Parker, C.W. (1980). Editorial comments: modulation of lymphoid cell function and allergic responses. *Adv. Cyclic Nucleotide Res.*, **12**, 181−5
7. Osheroff, P.L. and Webb, D.R. (1978). Stimulation of splenic prostaglandin level by DNP protein antigens. *Cell. Immunol.*, **38**, 319−27
8. Editorial (1981). Prostaglandins and immunity. *Lancet*, **ii**, 24−5
9. Du, J.T., Vennos, E., Ramey, E. and Ramwell, P.W. (1984). Sex differences in arachidonate cyclo-oxygenase products in elicited rat peritoneal macrophages. *Biochem. Biophys.* **794**, 256−60

10. Higgs, G.A., Palmer, R.M.J., Eakins, K.E. and Moncada, S. (1984). Arachidonic acid metabolism as a source of inflammatory mediators and its inhibition as a mechanism of action for anti-inflammatory drugs. *Mol. Aspects Med.*, **4**, 275–301

11. Winkelstein, A. and Kelley, V.E. (1980). The effects of PGE₁ on lymphocytes in NZB/NZN mice. *Clin. Immunol. Immunopathol.*, **17**, 212–8

12. Ferreira, S.H. (1972). Prostaglandins, aspirin-like drugs and analgesia. *Nature (N. Biol.)*, **240**, 200–3

13. Willis, A.L. and Cornelsen, M. (1973). Repeated injection of prostaglandin E₂ in rat paws induces chronic swelling and a marked decrease in pain threshold. *Prostaglandins*, **3**, 353–7

14. Weissmann, G., Smolen, J.E. and Korchak, H. (1980). Prostaglandins and inflammation: Receptor/cyclase coupling as an explanation of why PGEs and PGI₂ inhibit functions of inflammatory cells. In Samuelsson, B., Ramwell, P.W. and Paoletti, R. (eds. ) *Advances in Prostaglandin and Thromboxane Research.* pp. 1637–53. (New York: Raven Press)

15. Cranston, W.I. (1979). Central mechanisms of fever. *Fed. Proc.*, **38**, 49–51

16. Feldberg, W. and Milton, A.S. (1979). Prostaglandins and body temperature. In Vane, J.R. and Ferreira, S.H. (eds.) *Inflammation.* pp. 617–56. (Berlin: Springer Verlag)

17. Orange, R.P., Austen, W.G. and Austen, K.F. (1971). Immunological release of histamine and slow reactive substance of anaphylaxis from the lung. I. Modulation by agents influencing cellular levels of cyclic AMP. *J. Exp. Med.*, **134**, 136–148

18. Kitchen, E.A., Boot, J.R. and Dawson, W. (1978). Chemotactic activity of thromboxane B₂, prostaglandins and their metabolites for polymorphonuclear leukocytes. *Prostaglandins*, **16**, 239–42

19. Walker, J.R., Smith, M.J.H. and Ford-Hutchinson, A.N. (1976). Anti-inflammatory drugs, prostaglandins and leukocyte migration. *Agents Actions*, **6**, 602–9

20. Weissmann, G., Dukor, P. and Zurier, R.B. (1971). Effect of cyclic AMP on release of lysosomal enzymes from phagocytes. *Nature*, **231**, 131–5

21. Oropeza-Rendon, R.L., Speth, V., Hillier, G., Weber, K. and Fischer, H. (1979). Prostaglandin E₁ reversibly induces morphological changes in macrophages and inhibits phagocytosis. *Exp. Cell Res.*, **119**, 365–70

22. Boxer, L.A., Allen, J.M., Schmidt, M., Yocher, M. and Baehner, R.L. (1980). Inhibition of polymorphonuclear leukocyte adherence by prostacyclin. *J. Lab. Clin. Med.*, **95**, 672–8

23. Smith, J.W., Steiner, A.L. and Parker, C.W. (1971). Human lymphocytic metabolism. Effects of cyclic and noncyclic nucleotides on stimulation by phytohemagglutinin. *J. Clin. Invest.*, **50**, 442–448

24. Quagliata, F., Lawrence, V.J.W., Phillips, A. and Quagliata, J.M. (1973). Prostaglandin E₁ as a regulator of lymphocyte function. Selective action on B lymphocytes and synergy with procarbazine in depression of immune responses. *Cell. Immunol.*, **6**, 457–65

25. Goodwin, J.S. and Webb, D.R. (1981). Studies on the cyclic AMP response to prostaglandin in human lymphocytes. In Goodwin, J.S. (ed.) *Suppressor Cells in Human Disease.* pp. 99–135. (New York and Basle: Dekker)

26. Diamantstein, T. and Ulmer, A. (1975). The antagonistic action of cyclic GMP and cyclic AMP on proliferation of B and T lymphocytes. *Immunology*, **28**, 113–19

27. Starte, N.D. and Panayi, G.S. (1984). Prostaglandin regulation of B-lymphocyte function. *Immunol. Today*, **5**, 175–8

28. Basran, G.S., Morley, J., Paul, W. and Turner-Warwick, M. (1982). Evidence in man of synergistic interaction between putative mediators of acute inflammation and asthma. *Lancet*, **i**, 935–7

29. Williams, T.J. (1982). Vasoactive intestinal polypeptide is more potent than prostaglandin E₂ as a vasodilator and oedema potentiator in rabbit skin. *Br. J. Pharmacol.*, **77**, 505–9

30. Williams, T.J. and Jose, P.J. (1981). Mediation of increased vascular permeability after complement activation. Histamine-independent action of rabbit C5a. *J. Exp. Med.*, **153**, 136–53

31. Wedmore, C.V. and Williams, T.J. (1981). Control of vascular permeability by poly-morphonuclear leukocytes in inflammation. *Nature*, **289**, 646–50

32. Rutherford, B. and Schenkein, H.A. (1983). C3 cleavage products stimulate release of prostaglandins by human mononuclear phagocytes *in vitro. J. Immunol.*, **130**, 874–7

33. Warso, M.A. and Lands, W.E.M. (1983). Lipid peroxidation in relation to prostacyclin and thromboxane physiology and pathophysiology. *Br. Med. Bull.*, **39**, 277–80

34. Belch, J.J.F., Chopra, M., Smith, E., Forbes, C.D. and Sturrock, R.D. Prostaglandin $E_1$ is a free radical scavenger. (Submitted for publication)
35. Kunkel, S.L. and Chensue, S.W. (1985). Arachidonic acid metabolites regulate interleukin-1 production. *Biochem. Biophys. Res. Commun.*, **128**, 892–7
36. Belch, J.J.F., Shapiro, D., Shenkin, A. and Sturrock, R.D. (1986). Prostacyclin production from vascular endothelium is enhanced by Interleukin-1. In *Marker Proteins in Inflammation.* Vol. 3. pp. 41–42. (Berlin: W. de Gruyter)
37. Kunkel, S.L., Chensue, S.W. and Phan, S.H. (1986). Prostaglandins as endogenous mediators of interleukin-1 production. *J. Immunol.*, **136**, 186–92
38. Boraschi, D., Censini, S. and Tagliabue, A. (1984). Interferon-gamma reduces macrophage-suppressive activity by inhibiting prostaglandin $E_2$ release and inducing interleukin-1 production. *J. Immunol.*, **133**, 764–8
39. Dorsch, C.A. and Killmayer, J. (1983). The effect of native and single stranded DNA on the platelet release reaction: Enhancement of aggregated IgG-induced serotonin release. *Arthr. Rheum.*, **26**, 179–85
40. Young, J.M., Maloney, P.J., Shizu, N.J. and Jeffrey, S.C. (1985). Pharmacological investigation of the mechanisms of platelet-activating factor induced mortality in the mouse. *Prostaglandins*, **30**, 545–57
41. Peitila, P., Moilanen, E., Seppala, E., Nissila, M., Lepisto, P., Laiteinen, O. and Vapaatalo, H. (1984). Differences in the production of arachidonic acid metabolites between healthy and rheumatic synovial fibroblasts. *Scand. J. Rheumatol.*, **13**, 243–6
42. Morley, J. (1974). Prostaglandins and lymphokines in arthritis. *Prostaglandins*, **8**, 315–25
43. Kirby, P.J., Morley, J., Ponsford, J.R. and McDonald, W.I. (1976). Defective PGE reactivity in leucocytes of multiple sclerosis patients. *Prostaglandins*, **11**, 621–30
44. Belch, J.J.F., Newman, P., Drury, J.R., McKenzie, F., Leiberman, P., Capell, H.A., Forbes, C.D. and Prentice, C.R.M. (1983). Intermittent prostacyclin infusions in patients with Raynaud's syndrome: a double blind trial. *Lancet*, **i**, 313–15
45. Belch, J.J.F., Madhok, R., Shaw, B., Leiberman, P., Forbes, C.D. and Sturrock, R.D. (1985). Double-blind trial of CL115, 347, a transdermally absorbed prostaglandin $E_2$ analogue, in treatment for Raynaud's phenomenon. *Lancet*, **i**, 1130–3
46. Inoshita, T., Whiteside, T.L., Rodman, G.P. and Taylor, F.H. (1981). Abnormalities of T-lymphocyte subsets in patients with progressive systemic sclerosis. *J. Lab. Clin. Med.*, **97**, 265–70
47. Whicker, J.T., Martin, M.F.R. and Dieppe, P.A. (1980). Absence of prostaglandin stimulated increase in acute phase proteins in systemic sclerosis. *Lancet*, **i**, 1187–8
48. Belch, J.J.F., O'Dowd, A., Forbes, C.D. and Sturrock, R.D. (1985). Platelet sensitivity to a prostacyclin analogue in systemic sclerosis. *Br. J. Rheumatol.*, **24**, 346–50
49. Bouta, I.L., Parnham, M.J. and van Vleit, L. (1978). Combination of theophylline and prostaglandin $E_1$ as inhibitors of the adjuvant-induced arthritis syndrome of rats. *Ann. Rheum. Dis.*, **37**, 212–17
50. Feldberg, W., Kellaway, C.H. (1938). Liberation of histamine and formation of a lecithin-like substance by cobra venom. *J. Physiol.*, **94**, 187–226
51. Samuelsson, I., Borgeat, P., Hammarstrom, S. and Murphy, R.C. (1979). Introduction of a nomenclature: Leucotrienes. *Prostaglandins*, **17**, 785–7
52. Bray, M.A. (1983). The pharmacology and pathophysiology of leukotriene $B_4$. *Br. Med. Bull.*, **39**, 249–54
53. Piper, P.J. (1983). Pharmacology of leukotrienes. *Br. Med. Bull.*, **39**, 255–9
54. Smith, M.J.H. (1982). Biological activities of leukotriene $B_4$ (Isomer III). In Samuelsson, B. and Paoletti, R. (eds.) *Advances in Prostaglandin, Thromboxane and Leukotriene Research.* Vol. 9, pp. 283–92. (New York: Raven Press)
55. Nagy, L., Lee, T.H., Goetzl, E.J., Pickett, W.C. and Kay, A.B. (1982). Complement receptor enhancement and chemotaxis of human neutrophils and eosinophils by leukotrienes and other lipoxygenase products. *Clin. Exp. Immunol.*, **47**, 541–7
56. Aldigier, J.C., Gualde, N., Mexmain, S., Chable-Rabinovitch, H., Matinaud, M.H. and Rigaud, M. (1984). Immunosuppression induced *in vivo* by 15-hydroxyeicosatetranoic acid (15HETE). *Prostaglandin Leukotriene Med.*, **13**, 99–107
57. Piper, P.J., Samhoun, M.N. (1982). Stimulation of arachidonic acid metabolism and generation of thromboxane $A_2$ by leukotrienes $B_4$, $C_4$, and $D_4$ in guinea-pig lung in vitro. *Br. J. Pharmacol.*, **77**, 267–75

58. Ohnishi, H., Kosuzume, H., Kitamura, Y., Yamaguchi, K., Nobuhara, M. and Suzuki, Y. (1980). Structure of slow reacting substance of anaphylaxis (SRS-A). *Prostaglandins*, **20**, 655–66

59. Austen, K.F., Corey, E.J., Drazen, J.M., Leitch, A.G. (1983). The effect of indomethacin on the contractile response of the guinea-pig lung parenchymal strip to leukotrienes $B_4$, $C_4$, $D_4$ and $E_4$. *Br. J. Pharmacol.*, **80**, 47–53

60. Goetzl, E.J., Goldman, D.W., Naccache, P.H., Sha'afi, R.I. and Pickett, W. (1982). Mediation of leukocyte components of inflammatory reactions by lipoxygenase products of arachidonic acid. In Samuelsson, B. and Paoletti, R. (eds.) *Advances in Prostaglandin, Thromboxane and Leukotriene Research*. Vol. 9, pp. 273–82. (New York: Raven Press)

61. Samuelsson, B. (1983). Leukotrienes: mediators of immediate hyper-sensitivity reactions and inflammation. *Science*, **220**, 568–75

62. Tagari, P., Boullin, D.J., Du Boulay, G.H. and Aitken, V. (1983). Vaso-constrictor and vasodilatory effects of leukotriene D4 and FPL 55712 on human and rat cerebral arteries. In Samuelsson, B. and Paoletti, R. (eds.) *Advances in Prostaglandin, Thromboxane and Leukotriene Research*. Vol. 12, pp. 357–64. (New York: Raven Press)

63. Gimbrone, M.A., Brock, A.F. and Schafer, A.I. (1984). Leukotriene $B_4$ stimulates polymorphonuclear leukocyte adhesion to cultured vascular endothelial cells. *J. Clin. Invest.*, **74**, 1552–5

64. Higgs, G.A., Palmer, R.M.J., Eakins, K.E. and Moncada, S. (1981). Arachidonic acid metabolism as a source of inflammatory mediators and its inhibition as a mechanism of action for anti-inflammatory drugs. *Mol. Aspects Med.*, **4**, 275–301

65. Levine, J.D., Lau, W., Kwiat, G. and Goetzl, E.J. (1984). Leukotriene $B_4$ produces hyperalgesia that is dependent on polymorphonuclear leukocytes. *Science*, **225**, 743–5

66. Chopra, M., Belch, J.J.F., Brown, D.H., Sturrock, R.D. and Smith, W.E. (1985). The action of leukotrienes in a free radical generating system. In Higgs, G.A. and Williams, T.J. (eds.) *Inflammatory Mediators*. pp. 240–1. (London: Macmillan)

67. Henderson, W.R., Klebanoff, S.J. (1983). Leukotriene production and inactivation by normal, chronic granulomatous disease and myeloperoxidase-deficient neutrophils. *J. Biol. Chem.*, **258**, 13522–7

68. Dinarello, C.A., Bishai, I., Rosenwasser, L.J. and Coceani, F. (1984). The influence of lipoxygenase inhibitors on the *in vitro* production of human leukocytic pyrogen and lymphocyte activating factor (Interleukin-1). *Int. J. Immunopharmacol.*, **6**, 43–50

69. Shapiro, D., Belch, J.J.F., Sturrock, R.D. and Shenkin, A. (1986). Effects of drugs altering arachidonic acid metabolism on production of interleukin-1 by monocyte-like cells. *Proc. Nutr. Soc.*, **45**, 31–2

70. Maclouf, J., Fruteau de Laclos, B. and Borgeat, P. (1982). Stimulation of leukotriene biosynthesis in human blood leukocytes by platelet-derived 12-hydroxyeicosatetraenoic acid. *Proc. Natl. Acad. Sci. USA*, **79**, 6042–6

71. Ubatuba, F.B., Harvey, E.A. and Ferreria, S.H. (1975). Are platelets important in inflammation? *Agents Actions*, **5**, 31–4

72. Gorman, R.R., Morton, D.R., Hopkins, N.K. and Lin, A.H. (1983). Acetyl glyceryl ether phosphorylcholine stimulates $LTB_4$ synthesis and cAMP accumulation in human polymorphonuclear leukocytes. In Samuelsson, B. and Paoletti, R. (eds.) *Advances in Prostaglandin, Thromboxane and Leukotriene Research*. Vol. 12, pp. 57–63. (New York: Raven Press)

73. Klickstein, L.B., Shapleigh, C., Goetzl, E.J. (1980). Lipoxygenation of arachidonic acid as a source of polymorphonuclear leukocyte chemotactic factors in synovial fluid and tissue in rheumatoid arthritis and spondyloarthritis. *J. Clin. Invest.*, **66**, 1166–70

74. Davidson, E.M., Rae, S.A. and Smith, M.J.H. (1983). Leukotriene $B_4$, a mediator of inflammation present in synovial fluid in rheumatoid arthritis. *Ann. Rheum. Dis.*, **42**, 677–9

75. Belch, J.J.F., O'Dowd, A., Ansell, D. and Sturrock, R.D. (1986). Leukotriene $B_4$ ($LTB_4$) production in patients with rheumatoid arthritis. Presented at British Society for Rheumatology Annual General Meeting, November 19–21, London

76. Vane, J.R. (1971). Inhibition of prostaglandin synthesis as a mechanism of action for the aspirin-like drugs. *Nature*, **231**, 232–5

77. Higgs, G.A., Harvey, E.A., Ferreira, S.H. and Vane, J.R. (1976). The effects of anti-inflammatory drugs on the production of prostaglandins *in vivo*. In Samuelsson, B. and

Paoletti, R. (eds.) *Advances in Prostaglandin and Thromboxane Research*. Vol. 1, pp. 105–10. (New York: Raven Press)

78. Whittle, B.J.R., Higgs, G.A., Eakins, K.E., Moncada, S. and Vane, J.R. (1980). Selective inhibition of prostaglandin production in inflammatory exudates and gastric mucosa. *Nature*, **284**, 271–3

79. Singleton, P.T. (1980). Salsalate: its role in the management of Rheumatic Disease. *Clin. Ther.*, **3**, 80–102

80. Higgs, G.A. and Flower, R.J. (1981). Anti-inflammatory drugs and the inhibition of arachidonate lipoxygenase. In Piper, P.J. (ed.) *SRS-A and Leukotrienes*. pp. 197–207. (London: Wiley & Sons)

81. Salmon, J.A., Tilling, L.C. and Moncada, S. (1984). Benoxaprofen does not inhibit formation of leukotriene $B_4$ in a model of acute inflammation. *Biochem. Pharmacol.*, **33**, 2930–2

82. Editorial (1983). Colchicine effect in gout may be due to leukotriene inhibition. *Hosp. Pract.*, **18**, 186–93

83. Stenson, W.F. and Lobos, E. (1982). Sulphasalazine inhibits the synthesis of chemotactic lipids by neutrophils. *J. Clin. Invest.*, **69**, 494–7

84. Fuller, W.R., Kelsey, C.R., Cole, P.J., Dollery, C.T. and MacDermot, J. (1984). Dexamethasone inhibits the production of thromboxane $B_2$ and leukotriene $B_4$ by human alveolar and peritoneal macrophages in culture. *Clin. Sci.*, **67**, 653–6

85. Fan, T.P.D. and Lewis, G.P. (1985). Mechanism of cyclosporin A induced inhibition of prostacyclin synthesis by macrophages. *Prostaglandins*, **30**, 735–48

86. Chan, L-Y. and Tai, H-H. (1982). Resolution into two different forms and study of the properties of phosphatidylinositol-specific phospholipase C from human platelet cytosol. *Biochim. Biophys. Acta*, **713**, 344–51

87. Voorlees, J.J. (1983). Leukotrienes and other lipoxygenase products in the pathogenesis and therapy of psoriasis and other dermatoses. *Arch. Dermatol.*, **119**, 541–7

88. Kunkel, S.L., Ogawa, H., Ward, P.A. and Zurier, R.B. (1982). Suppression of chronic inflammation by evening primrose oil. *Prog. Lipid Res.*, **20**, 885–8

89. Godfrey, D., Belch, J.J.F., Watson, J., Sturrock, R.D. and Stimpson, W. (1986). Manipulation of essential fatty acid intake in $MRL_1$ mice: effect on disease manifestations. *Prog. Lipid Res.* (In press)

90. Belch, J.J.F., Ansell, D., Madhok, R. and Sturrock, R.D. (1986). The effect of evening primrose oil (EPO) and EPO/fish oil combination on rheumatoid arthritis: a double blind study. Presented at the British Society of Rheumatology Annual General Meeting, November 19–21, London

92. Prescott, S.M. (1984). The effect of eicosapentanoic acid on leukotriene $B_4$ production by human neutrophils. *J. Biol. Chem.*, **259**, 7615–21

92. Kremer, J.M., Biganoette, J., Michalek, A.V., Timchalk, M.A., Lininger, L., Rynes, I.R., Huych, C., Zieminski, J. and Bartholomew, L.E. (1985). Effects of manipulation of dietary fatty acids on clinical manifestations of rheumatoid arthritis. *Lancet*, **i**, 184–7

# 3
# Immunogenetics: HLA and arthritis

R. R. P. DE VRIES

## INTRODUCTION: THE IMMUNOGENETIC APPROACH TO ARTHRITIS

To develop arthritis one needs a trigger and an immune system. Everybody has an immune system but luckily only few of us suffer from clinically relevant arthritis. The easiest explanation for arthritis being an exception rather than the rule would be that in most cases the trigger is absent. If an infection with an arthritogenic pathogen were obligatory for arthritis then such an infection might be a rare event. However, in most instances of arthritis there is no evidence for such an easy explanation.

Although everybody has an immune system, which in the vast majority of individuals seems to function normally, it has become clear during the last two decades that subtle differences do exist between individuals and may be clinically relevant. These differences may be genetically determined and the discipline in which this discovery was made is called immunogenetics.

Immunogenetics is by definition younger than immunology and genetics though it is actually 87 years old. It was born as the ABO blood groups and its only immunological aspect was that the alleles of this blood group system and those of other genetic polymorphisms discovered later in this century were identified by immunological methods. Because several blood group antigens appeared to be transplantation antigens, immunology became not only a tool but also a subject of study for immunogeneticists. This led to a specialization in immunogenetics which will be the subject of this chapter: the study of genetically determined differences in immune reactivity and the resulting differences in disease susceptibility or severity.

Thus far the major contribution from immunogenetics to a better understanding of the pathogenesis of arthritis has been the definition of genetic markers for susceptibility to certain types of arthritis; the human major histocompatibility complex (the HLA system) has notably provided such genetic markers. These markers have offered insight into the mode of inheritance, led to subdivision into apparently genetically heterogeneous

51

entities and demonstrated a common genetic factor for certain types of arthritis. To a very limited extent such genetic markers may be applied to the management of individual patients: as a diagnostic aid, to predict prognosis or reaction to therapy and for genetic counselling. However, the major challenge for immunogeneticists is to clarify the mechanism of the association between a genetic marker (e.g. HLA-B27) and a certain type of arthritis (e.g. ankylosing spondylitis). In this chapter I will confine myself to the associations between HLA-markers and arthritis and to one hypothesis, namely the so-called 'immune response gene hypothesis'.

Immune response genes (Ir-genes) are polymorphic genes that code for differences in immune reactivity between individuals[1]. An important aspect of Ir-genes is that they may be studied in healthy individuals thus providing a probe to study mechanisms conferring susceptibility to immunologically mediated disease which is similar to the way in which the study of immunodeficient individuals has led to a better insight into how the immune system prevents disease.

The ultimate goal of this immunogenetic approach to several diseases, and to arthritis in particular, is to unravel the following chain of events (Table 3.1).

(1) Polymorphic Ir-genes contain the genetic information for:

(2) Qualitative or quantitative differences in expression of Ir-gene products, which:

(3) Lead to differences in immune reactivity towards certain antigens between individuals, which in turn:

(4) Lead to differential susceptibility to or severity of certain types of arthritis.

Although one can also apply this immunogenetic approach to non-specific immune reactivity, I will confine myself to antigen-specific immune responses. The main reason for doing this is that my discussion is restricted to the most extensivey studied Ir-genes, namely the Ir-genes linked to the major histocompatibility complex (MHC) which code for antigen-specific differences in immune reactivity[1]. This immediately leads to a problem which was mentioned at the start of this introduction: in most cases of arthritis we do not know the inciting antigen. This paradox will be an essential part of my discussion and I will try to demonstrate that the above-mentioned immunogenetic approach may offer leads for identifying antigens responsible for the triggering and/or perpetuation of arthritis.

**Table 3.1** The immunogenetic approach to arthritis

| 1. Ir-gene | : | A or B |
|---|---|---|
| 2. Ir-gene product | : | a or b |
| 3. Ir to antigen x | : | appropriate or inappropriate |
| 4. Result | : | no arthritis or arthritis |

## HLA CLASS I AND II MOLECULES AND IMMUNE RESPONSE REGULATION

The HLA system[2,3] is the major histocompatibility complex of man. It is situated on the short arm of chromosome 6. As shown in Figure 3.1 it comprises two different types of very polymorphic genes, namely class I and class II genes. Between the class I and class II genes several genes coding for factors of the complement system (C2, C4 and factor B) are situated, as well as the gene coding for the steroid hormone 21-hydroxylase. These genes are neither structurally nor functionally related to the HLA class I and II genes and therefore I consider them as not belonging to the HLA system. This does not mean that notably the polymorphic complement genes may not be relevant for differential susceptibility to arthritis. However I will not include them in the present discussion which will focus on the HLA class I and II genes. Several class I-like genes have recently been discovered, which are situated telomeric from the class I genes. The function of the products of these class I-like genes is unknown and they will also remain outside the scope of this chapter. There are three functional class I genes (A, B and C) and at least three sets of class II genes coding for these class II products (DP, DQ and DR). Except for DP, these genes are all situated so close to each other (recombination frequency less than 2%) that they are usually inherited together or as a so-called haplotype.

A unique feature of the HLA system is its extreme polymorphism: it is by far the most polymorphic genetic system known in man. This implies that

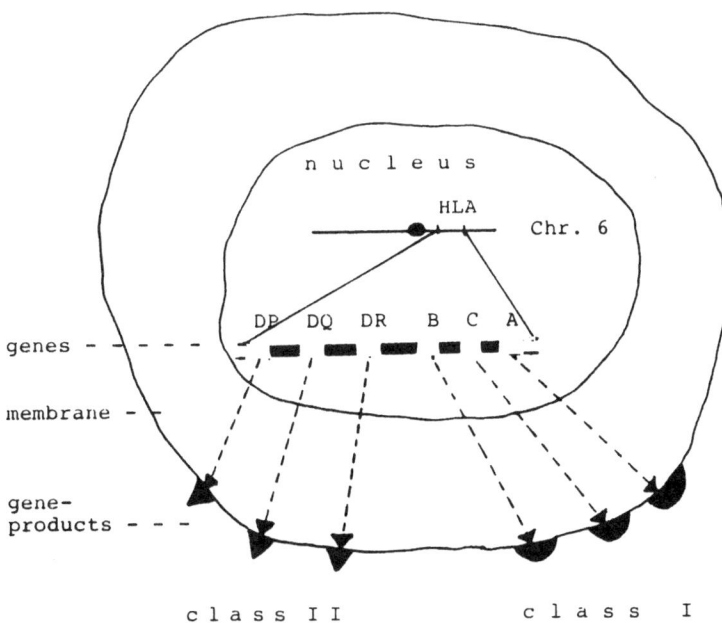

**Figure 3.1** The HLA system

most individuals will have a unique set of HLA class I and II alleles, unless they are genetically closely related. Apart from the fact that this extreme polymorphism provides us with a powerful tool for genetic studies, it is probably also essential for the function of the system as will be discussed later. The theoretically virtually infinite number of combinations is restricted to some degree because of the fact that so-called linkage disequilibria exist: certain combinations of alleles of different loci occur more (or less) often than predicted from their respective gene frequencies. These linkage disequilibria may be (or have been) functionally important as will also be discussed later. Moreover, they have practical relevance for the demonstration of disease susceptibility genes because products of genes linked to a particular disease susceptibility genes may serve as genetic markers.

The products of HLA class I genes (A, B and C) are glycoproteins which constitute the so-called heavy chain (molecular weight 44 kDa) of class I molecules. This heavy chain is a transmembrane protein produced by and present on the membrane of virtually all nucleated cells. Non-covalently attached to the heavy chain is $\beta_2$-microglobulin ($\beta_2$m) which has a molecular weight of 12 kDa and is coded by a non-polymorphic gene situated on chromosome 15. The extracellular part of the class I heavy chain consists of three immunoglobulin-like domains and $\beta_2$m is attached to the domain closest to the cell membrane*. The polymorphism of the HLA class I genes is mainly expressed by the two outer domains of the heavy chain.

HLA class II molecules are also found on the cell membrane, but usually only on cells belonging to the immune system. They show a particularly strong expression on specialized antigen presenting cells such as dendritic and Langerhans cells, and are also present on (most) B-cells macrophages (to a variable degree) and activated T-cells. They consist of two non-covalently associated glycoprotein chains, which are called $\alpha$ and $\beta$. In this case both chains have two domains, both penetrate the cell wall and both are coded by HLA genes. Thus the three class II molecules officially recognized today[6], namely DP, DQ and DR each consist of an $\alpha$- and $\beta$-chain which are both coded by a separate HLA class II gene: $DP_\alpha$ and $DP_\beta$, $DQ_\alpha$ and $DQ_\beta$, and $DR_\alpha$ and $DR_\beta$., respectively. The situation is however more complicated. For instance, there are usually two $DR_\beta$ genes per haplotype which code for two different DR molecules ($DR_{\alpha\beta I}$ and $DR_{\alpha\beta III}$). The polymorphism of the class II genes, like that of the class I genes, is mainly expressed on the outer domains of the molecule.

An important function of both class I and class II HLA molecules is the presentation of antigens to T-cells. In contrast to B-cells, T-cells are only activated by antigen when this is presented on the membrane of a cell by a

---

*It is interesting that the domain to which $\beta_2$m is bound shows marked homology with $\beta_2$m, the domains of class II molecules adjacent to the cell membrane (see below), the constant domains of immunoglobulin molecules and the constant domains of other members of the so-called 'immunoglobulin superfamily' such as the T-cell receptor for antigen. This indicates a common evolutionary origin and suggests that this conserved domain structure is functionally important[4].

(self-) HLA class I or II molecule. These molecules also select the type of T-cells that will respond to a given antigen. Usually CD4 positive T-cells respond to antigens presented by class II molecules and CD8 positive cells to antigens presented by class I molecules. Because the best defined T-cell subset involved in the regulation of the immune response, the helper T-cell, is CD4 positive, class II molecules have a central role in the regulation of the immune response. Because regulatory T-cells recognize antigen presented by HLA class II molecules, it is easy to envisage that the physiological restriction of HLA class II molecules to antigen presenting cells (B-cells and activated T-cells) has a function in focusing the immune response. However, the details of the actual interactions involved are still far from clear. Cytotoxic T-cells usually have the CD8 phenotype and kill cells with specific antigens presented on their surface by class I molecules, but CD4-positive T-cells may also be cytotoxic and will usually kill cells carrying specific antigen and class II molecules. Thus, both class I and class II molecules are involved in the effector phase of the cellular immune response. Because every nucleated cell carries at least class I molecules on its surface it is capable of presenting, for example, virus or tumour antigens to cytotoxic T-cells and is thus lysed by cytotoxic T-cells.

Not only qualitative differences (class I *versus* class II), but also quantitative differences in expression of HLA molecules play an important regulatory role in the immune response[6]: the magnitude of the T-cell response is a direct function of the concentrations of antigens and MHC molecules on the surface of the antigen presenting cell[7].

Thus the regulation of the expression of HLA class I and II molecules plays an important regulatory role in the immune response. To put it simply: they have to be present and/or upregulated where T-cell action is needed and absent or down-regulated where that is inappropriate. Several molecules regulating this expression have been identified: interferons give a positive signal for both class I and II expression, whereas class II expression is specifically upregulated by $\gamma$-interferon and tumour necrosis factor (G.F. Botazzo, personal communication) and down-regulated by, for example, E class prostaglandins and $\alpha$-fetoprotein[6]. Moreover it has been observed that class II expression, which is usually restricted to cells belonging to the immune system, may be induced on virtually all cells in pathological conditions[8]. Such so-called 'aberrant' class II expression has been observed on non-lymphoid cells in most organ-specific autoimmune diseases.

## HLA CLASS I AND II Ir-GENES AND DISEASE SUSCEPTIBILITY

As stated in the introduction Ir-genes code for differences in immune reactivity between individuals[1]. An important discovery has been the demonstration that MHC class I and II molecules are Ir-gene products[9]. Although the evidence for this mainly stems from studies in experimental animals, there is no reason to assume that this would not also be the case for the HLA class I and II molecules in man and in fact some evidence for this has been presented[2]. In other words the polymorphism discussed in the previous section is also functionally important.

The mechanism of HLA class I and II Ir-gene controlled differences in immune reactivity is unknown but animal studies suggest there are two obvious mechanisms which are certainly not mutually exclusive. The first mechanism follows directly from the role of these molecules as discussed in the previous section: the products of class I and II alleles may differ in their ability to present certain antigens to certain T-cell subsets. This difference may either be due to quantitative differences in expression of the products of these alleles or to qualitative differences resulting in more or less effective association of the antigen with the product of these alleles[10,11]. The second mechanism is that at least class II Ir-gene products may generate the T-cell repertoire of an individual in the thymus and their polymorphism will generate repertoires that differ between individuals. This mechanism may work basically in the same way as the first one, the (auto)-antigen-presenting cells in this case being accessory cells in the thymus[12,13].

There is evidence that the extreme polymorphism and perhaps also some of the striking linkage disequilibria of the HLA system are at least partly due to selection[14]. If it were the case that this selection occurred through HLA class I and II Ir-genes then infectious diseases are the most obvious candidates as the responsible selective force. Whatever the mechanism of HLA class I and II Ir-genes, it is easy to envisage that a high degree of polymorphism is advantageous not only for the individual but also and perhaps even more so, for the species attacked by many different and changing pathogens. There is some evidence to support this hypothesis[15,16]. However, we should realize that we can only study this for infectious diseases known today, which only became important some five millenia ago[17]. The evolution of the HLA system and other MHCs certainly took several thousand times this period. Therefore, it might well be that both the specialized function in the immune response and the subsequent possible selection by infectious diseases are only the last few steps in the long evolutionary journey of an already extremely polymorphic cell-communication system.

Most readers will be familiar with the fact that susceptibility to a large number of diseases is associated with alleles of the HLA system. A recent updating is to be found in Ref. 18. Most of these diseases have an immunopathological pathogenesis. It is striking that most associations are primarily with HLA class II markers and this is notably the case for the associations with autoimmune diseases. This may well reflect the fact that especially the HLA class II molecules have a central role in the regulation of the immune response as discussed in the previous section and thus HLA class II Ir-genes may play a more prominent role than class I Ir-genes in the development of immune regulation disorders like autoimmune diseases.

If we assume that these associations are due to HLA class I and II Ir-genes (which I do in this chapter), then the fact that HLA and disease associations do exist is in itself not surprising. However, why are there so many? I have little doubt that the function of the HLA system is not to confer susceptibility to (immunopathological) diseases, though I do believe that the HLA system has a function in protecting us from infectious diseases. Therefore, it might well be that selection by infectious diseases has left us with a set of class I and II Ir-genes which are useless in the absence of the selecting pathogens and even harmful in the presence of less virulent pathogens by conferring immunopathology and autoimmune disease. Such Ir-genes will not disappear soon because the disadvantage they confer usually results in morbidity after the reproductive age rather than in decreased Darwinian fitness, as is the case for most HLA-associated diseases.

## HLA AND ARTHRITIS

Table 3.2 lists the established associations between HLA antigens and arthritis as observed among Caucasians. Only significant associations confirmed in a number of other studies have been included. One should realize that the three HLA types listed (HLA-B27, DR5 and DR4) are only three out of at least 80 different HLA types (19 HLA-A, 39 HLA-B, 8 HLA-C and 19 HLA-DR) tested for associations. This makes the fact that HLA-B27 occurs so often the more remarkable. The strength of some of the B27-associations is quite strong, in fact the association between HLA-B27 and ankylosing spondylitis is one of the strongest associations between HLA and disease known thus far. If one compares Table 3.2 with any recent list of diseases associated with HLA antigens the preponderance of this particular class I antigen in arthritis is even more striking, because most other diseases are associated with class II rather than with class I antigens. So it seems appropriate to discuss the associations between HLA-B27 and the group of so-called sero-negative forms of arthritis separately from the associations of the HLA class II antigens HLA-DR4 and DR5 with, respectively, rheumatoid arthritis (RA) and juvenile rheumatoid arthritis. Because RA is both the most important and the most extensively studied association of the latter two, I will only discuss the association between HLA-DR4 and RA.

**Table 3.2**  Associations between HLA antigens and arthritis[a]

| HLA antigen | Type of arthritis | % Positive Patients | % Positive Controls | Relative risk[b] |
|---|---|---|---|---|
| HLA-B27 | ankylosing spondylitis | 89 | 9 | 69.1 |
| HLA-B27 | Reiter's disease | 80 | 9 | 37.1 |
| HLA-B27 | post-salmonella infection | 85 | 10 | 35.5 |
| HLA-B27 | post-yersinia infection | 77 | 11 | 21.4 |
| HLA-B27 | psoriatic | 27 | 8 | 3.8 |
| HLA-B27 | juvenile rheumatoid arthritis | 25 | 9 | 3.3 |
| HLA-DR5 | juvenile rheumatoid arthritis | 34 | 15 | 3.3 |
| HLA-DR4 | rheumatoid arthritis | 58 | 25 | 3.9 |

[a]Data selected from Ref. 18
[b]Relative risk is a measure of the strength of the association: it denotes how many times more often a particular type of arthritis is observed among individuals with a given HLA type (e.g. HLA-B27) as compared to individuals lacking that HLA type

## HLA-B27 and arthritis

Before concentrating on arthritis it seems worthwhile to ask the question: is HLA-B27 only associated with arthritis? If we check the list of B27-associated diseases[18], only iridocyclitis appears as a well established extra-articular condition. However this condition is clearly related to the accompanying (susceptibility to) arthritis (ankylosing spondylitis, Reiter's syndrome). Therefore, I prefer to ignore the unconfirmed reports of an association with asbestosis and meningococcal meningitis and to give a positive answer to this question: yes, HLA-B27 does seem to be associated specifically with susceptibility to arthritis. This specificity should probably be taken into account in any proposed mechanism for the association between B27 and each of the conditions listed in Table 3.2.

The strong association between B27 and arthritis following salmonella and yersinia infection seems potentially an ideal model for looking for an HLA class I Ir-gene, because it is one of the few HLA-associated conditions in which the inciting agent is known. One argument against an Ir-gene as the mechanism for HLA-B27-associated post-infectious arthritis might be the lack of antigen specificity. As discussed above, I assume that such an Ir-gene is antigen-specific and thus not any post-infectious arthritis should be associated with HLA-B27. This is apparently not the case, rheumatic fever probably being the best known example of a post-infectious arthritis not associated with B27. Other examples of post-infectious arthritis not associated with B27 are those following rubella vaccination[18] and parvovirus infections[19,20]. However, when we confine ourselves to enteric or urogenital infections, there is less evidence for specificity of the inciting pathogen. Apart from salmonella and yersinia, shigella, *Campylobacter jejuni* and the gonococcus have also been reported to trigger B27-associated post-infectious arthritis[18]. Of course there are many more enteric and urogenital pathogens than these five and negative studies tend to remain unpublished, but the possibility exists that the route of infection rather than the pathogen is specific for the B27-associated post-infectious arthropathies. Another argument against the Ir-gene hypothesis might be that a class I Ir-gene would not be likely to operate in a bacterial infection, because bacterial antigens are usually presented by class II molecules[21]. However, it has been reported that bacteria, including yersinia and salmonella, can bind to HLA class I molecules[22,23]. So it is easily conceivable that processed bacterial antigens might recycle together with class I antigens to the cell membrane and might be recognized by class I restricted cytotoxic T-cells and their precursors[21].

The vast majority of studies on HLA-B27 and arthritis have dealt with ankylosing spondylitis (AS). One of the reasons for this preference has certainly been the fact that this was one of the first associations discovered between HLA and disease and certainly the strongest[24,25]. The fact that this association was observed in all populations tested strongly suggests that the HLA-B27 molecule itself is the product of a susceptibility gene for AS[18]. It may not be a necessary factor for developing the disease because AS can exist in the absence of HLA-B27. However this is apparently a rare event[26]. Therefore I will from now on confine the discussion to HLA-B27-positive

AS. Family studies have demonstrated that the susceptibility to AS is inherited in a dominant fashion[27,28] which is compatible with the assumption that HLA-B27 itself is the susceptibility gene. Not everyone possessing B27 develops AS: for instance among the B27-positive population in the Netherlands the risk of developing AS seems to be less than 2%, which increases to more than 20% for B27-positive relatives of (B27-positive) AS patients[29]. These data clearly indicate that factors other than HLA-B27 are involved in the pathogenesis of AS. Apart from the clear preference for males, thus far no conclusive evidence for other genetic factors has been provided, so it seems attractive to postulate an environmental factor. Such a factor might be more abundant in families of (B27-positive) AS patients.

Thus the discovery of the association between HLA-B27 and AS, as well as other types of arthritis, and the genetic studies which followed this discovery have elucidated genetic factors of importance for the pathogenesis of these conditions. They have demonstrated a common genetic factor (HLA-B27) and suggested a common environmental factor (shared at least by salmonella and yersinia) as discussed above. Although the association is often quite strong, thus far the clinical implications have been limited. Probably the most important clinical application is that a negative HLA-B27 test in a first degree relative of a B27-positive patient virtually excludes the possibility that this relative will develop AS.

Ceppellini, one of the brains behind the HLA system, once made the historical statement that, 'there is little doubt that the motivation of Nature in selecting for a genetic polymorphism of this complexity was not an *a priori* hostility against transplantation surgeons'.

Sometimes I wonder whether hostility against immunogeneticists was the motive for nature being so reluctant to reveal the secret of the B27–AS association. As discussed before, I have little doubt that the susceptibility gene for AS is (at least in the majority of cases) HLA-B27 itself. The HLA-B27 gene is well characterized, its gene products are among the best characterized HLA molecules, and the association is one of the strongest HLA and disease associations known. There are however two problems: in the first place it is virtually impossible to study the substrate of the disease (spondylitis) and in the second place the hypothetical environmental factor triggering the disease has remained elusive. Therefore I think that we should put more effort into studying the mechanism of a B27-associated post-infectious arthritis in order to develop a testable model for the B27-AS association. A sophisticated way to do this would be by using HLA-transgeneic mice (P. Ivanyi and H. Ploegh, personal communication).

Two theories have been published as the explanation of (part of) the B27-AS association. The first is based on cross-reactivity observed between HLA-B27 and certain enteric bacteria[30,31], which has now also been demonstrated with the use of monoclonal antibodies[32]. It is assumed that this mimicry would result in an initially low responsiveness and thus a defective elimination of bacteria carrying the B27-cross-reactive determinant, which might then at a later stage lead to immunopathology. However, the basis for this assumption is rather weak[31,33,34]. The second theory is based on the observation that not just HLA-B27, but only HLA-B27-positive lymphocytes of AS patients

(B27⁺AS⁺) cross-react with an antigen present on klebsiella[35] and other enteric bacteria[36]. Whereas several other groups have not been able to obtain similar results, Geczy and his collaborators went on to show that culture filtrates of the B27⁺AS⁺ cross-reactive bacterial strains can modify B27⁺AS⁻ lymphocytes *in vitro* to become transiently susceptible to lysis by the antiserum reactive with B27⁺AS⁺ cells[37] as well as by B27-restricted cytotoxic lymphocytes of B27⁺AS⁻ individuals[38]. They isolated from these culture filtrates a factor carrying the cross-reactive determinant which appeared to be responsible for this *in vitro* modification[39] and suggested that this factor might be a plasmid[40]. They speculate that this plasmid might bind preferentially to the HLA-B27 molecule, in other words that HLA-B27 is the (only) receptor for this plasmid[40]. Because in this theory no mimicry or low responsiveness is involved, it is easy to envisage a role for antibodies and/or cytotoxic T lymphocytes recognizing B27 and a plasmid antigen in the effector phase of an immunopathological process resulting in ankylosing spondylitis[38,40]. If these observations could be confirmed, they would offer the basis for a most interesting Ir-gene mechanism: preferential binding to a polymorphic HLA class I molecule resulting not only in infection by but also presentation of an environmental agent as a triggering event for arthritis. If this were true, simple strategies to prevent ankylosing spondylitis might be devised, such as vaccination of individuals at risk (e.g. B27-positive family members of AS patients). Of course similar procedures might be envisaged for the post-infectious and reactive arthropathies.

## HLA-DR4 and rheumatoid arthritis

The association between rheumatoid arthritis (RA) and HLA-DR4 is – although certainly less strong than the B27 AS association – well established[18,41]. With few exceptions, it was also observed in all populations studied[18], suggesting that, as in the case of B27 and the sero-negative arthropathies, the DR4 determinant or a closely related epitope is causally related to disease susceptibility. This fits with the fact that, although certain DR4-containing haplotypes appear to be more strongly associated with RA than other ones[42,43], thus far no clearly better marker than DR4 or Dw4 (a T-cell epitope closely related to DR4) has been identified. Neither class I[18,44] nor MHC-coded complement polymorphisms[44] seem to be good candidates. Other class II markers, notably DQ, also seem no better than DR/Dw[45,46] and the same applies to class II restriction fragment length polymorphisms[47]. So it looks as if the best genetic marker(s) for susceptibility to RA may be found on HLA-DR molecules. One should probably consider such an HLA-associated susceptibility factor for RA as a relative rather than an absolute trait, in other words DR4 is associated with a relatively higher susceptibility than other DR types but is not the only DR phenotype associated with susceptibility. For instance DR1 also seems to confer susceptibility but to a lesser degree than DR4[48], whereas DR2 and perhaps also DR3 are associated with relative resistance[49,50]. Such a scale of relative degrees of susceptibility conferred by different HLA alleles has not only been observed for RA but for many HLA and disease associations, the B27—AS association probably being an exception to the rule.

Until recently, family studies had failed to clearly demonstrate increased haplotype sharing between affected siblings[44]. However, when one takes into account DR4- and RA-status of the parents a straightforward co-segregation analysis of both affected and unaffected siblings of a limited number of multi-case families could easily demonstrate that susceptibility to RA is controlled by an HLA-linked gene[51]. This has also been confirmed in larger material[48]. From our own[51] and other studies[44,52], it is clear that the mode of inheritance is not simply Mendelian, which is in agreement, for example, with the above-mentioned relative degree of susceptibility conferred by several HLA alleles or haplotypes. The situation may be even more complicated as the interested reader may learn from Ref. 51.

The HLA and RA studies have clearly demonstrated genetic heterogeneity in RA, DR4 being preferentially associated with extra-articular manifestations or so-called systemic RA[53]. Several reports have indicated that HLA-DR4 is not just associated with susceptibility to RA[54], but rather with severe RA as seen in the clinic (for references see Ref. 55). As shown in Table 3.3, RA with severe extra-articular symptoms (notably Felty's syndrome or vasculitis) particularly appeared to show a strong association with DR4, the relative risk (RR) for this subgroup being 23.8 as compared to the RR of 4.3 for RA without these severe extra-articular symptoms, which constituted a significant difference in DR4 frequency for these two groups[55]. This genetic heterogeneity has two important implications relevant for the present discussion. In the first place one could say that thus far the clinicians have done a better job than the immunogeneticists in defining the genetic susceptiblity to RA. Or, to put it in a practical perspective, immunogenetic studies for a better genetic marker than DR4 should take into account the clinical heterogeneity of RA and candidates for being better markers than DR4 should have an RR of considerably more than 25 for systemic RA (see Table 3.3). In the second place, any proposed mechanism for the association between RA and DR4 should take into account this preferential association with severe extra-articular manifestations.

Before concluding this chapter with a discussion on the mechanism of the association between DR4 and (systemic) RA, I will comment briefly on the implications of the HLA studies for patient management. Because — as discussed before — even the strong association between B27 and AS has limited diagnostic value, it is clear that the relatively weak association between

**Table 3.3** Genetic heterogeneity of rheumatoid arthritis

| Rheumatoid arthritis | Severe extra-articular manifestations[a] | DR4 positive (%) | Relative risk[b] |
|:---:|:---:|:---:|:---:|
| + | + | 92 | 23.8 |
| + | − | 63 | 4.3 |
| − | − | 28 | |

[a]Felty's syndrome and/or vasculitis
[b]Relative risk: see footnote to Table 3.2

DR4 and RA has no diagnostic application. The same applies to the preferential association of DR4 with systemic RA, because the DR4 frequency among the patients without these symptoms is still more than 50%. An interesting and potentially practically relevant observation was the strong association between HLA-DR3, particularly, and nephrotoxicity (proteinuria) due to therapy with gold salts among RA patients[56]. However this strong association could not be confirmed in other studies. Thus, generally speaking, the practical value of HLA-typing in the management of RA patients (or patients suspected of RA) is negligible. So in order for patients really to benefit from immunogenetic research we will have to unravel the mechanism of the association between DR4 and RA.

I will close this section with a discussion of the search for an Ir-gene which may explain the association between HLA-DR4 and RA since such an approach may offer leads to identifying (a) possible triggering antigen(s) of this terrible disease.

When we look at the scheme of the immunogenetic approach to arthritis outlined in Table 3.1, the starting situation for DR4 and RA is not very promising. Whereas for the B27–AS association we are rather sure that if an Ir-gene is involved it has to be B27 and thus we also know the potential Ir-gene product, this is less clear for DR4. As with the B27–AS association we also do not know the relevant immune response for the DR4–RA association and there is even less evidence pointing to a particular inciting or target antigen for RA. For the sake of the argument I will assume that a DR gene and product are, respectively, the Ir-gene and its product to be defined more accurately. So let us look for a relevant immune response. As discussed in several chapters elsewhere in this book (e.g. Chapters 4, 5 and 8) the immunohistology of RA strongly suggests that a delayed type hypersensitivity (DTH) reaction is the basis for this arthritis. Therefore it seems appropriate not to concentrate on antibodies and rheumatoid factor but rather on an abnormal T-cell response as the responsible mechanism for the DR4–RA association.

At this stage of the discussion it seems appropriate to ask whether the joint is indeed the most relevant location for the study of the mechanism of the DR4–RA association and if so what kind of an Ir-gene should we look for? As suggested by Panayi[57], RA may display an immunopathological spectrum similar to leprosy. At one end of this spectrum there would be joint destruction due to DTH (comparable to tuberculoid leprosy) and at the other end immune complex disease with extra-articular complications (comparable to lepromatous leprosy). The observation that total lymphoid irradiation (TLI) may relieve severe joint symptoms in RA without affecting autoantibody levels in serum[58] is interesting in this context. It may also be relevant that in some patients an increase of autoantibodies and an exacerbation of extra-articular symptoms has been observed after TLI (Ref. 58 and S. Strober, personal communication). Because DR4 is preferentially associated with these extra-articular complications, we have speculated that this immunological analogy may be extended to an immunogenetic one[55,59]. In leprosy the cell mediated immunity to the causative agent (*Mycobacterium leprae*) and thus the type of the disease may be controlled by HLA class II Ir-genes[60]. It is important to note here that we think that two types of Ir-genes are involved in leprosy: a classical Ir-gene coding for high responsiveness predisposing for tuberculoid leprosy and an immune suppression (Is-) gene coding for non-responsiveness due to suppressor T-cells predisposing to lepromatous leprosy[60,61]. Because the DR4-associated RA with extra-articular manifestations would be analogous to lepromatous leprosy, one might thus have to look for DR4-associated Is-gene rather than a classical Ir-gene.

What are the relevant triggering antigens to study for DR4-associated Ir- or Is-gene control? The only auto-antigen that has been studied for Ir-gene control is collagen, as far as I know. There is an interesting but unconfirmed report of a DR4-associated T-cell responsiveness to denatured collagen which is ascribed to the lack of suppressor T-cells[62]. Studies on a relationship between DR4 and anti-collagen antibodies have shown no association or equivocal results[63]. What about possible triggering environmental agents which might be under Ir-gene control? Many microbial agents, notably viruses and bacteria, have been suspected of triggering RA, but thus far no convincing evidence pointing towards a particular subject has been presented. I would like to repeat a suggestion made some years ago by Van Rood[59], namely that one may use the DR4-association as a lead for screening environmental agents suspected of triggering RA – and I provide one example resulting from this approach.

*Mycobacterium tuberculosis* has been shown by Irun Cohen and his associates to carry antigens cross-reactive with cartilage which cause adjuvant arthritis, an animal model with similarities to RA[64]. The same group has recently shown a preferential reactivity of synovial fluid T-lymphocytes from RA patients against these mycobacterial antigens[65], suggesting that these antigens might be relevant to the pathogenesis of RA. In support of this hypothesis is the evidence for a DR4-associated Ir-gene for *M. tuberculosis* published by our group in collaboration with John Stanford[66]. The fact that there does not seem to be a simple epidemiological correlation between tuberculosis and RA is certainly not evidence against this hypothesis. To study the possible effects of an *M. tuberculosis*-specific Ir-gene one might have to take into consideration the type of disease following infection as was demonstrated for leprosy[60]. For instance, the significantly decreased frequency of HLA-DR4 among patients with bone and joint tuberculosis as recently observed in India (J. Singh and J. C. Verma, personal communication) might offer a clue. However, it should be noted that the DR4-associated Ir-gene for *M. tuberculosis* postulated by us[66] would be difficult to fit into the previously mentioned extension of Panayi's hypothesis in which we suggested an Is- rather an an Ir-gene[59]. Studies in progress in our and several other laboratories may solve this issue.

## PROSPECTS

Why have I made such a point of the immunogenetic approach to arthritis? Certainly not because of the results shown in the two examples given, because these were not impressive. I do however believe that this approach may yield impressive results in future and the examples were discussed to show possible openings. Figure 3.2 shows schematically how the immunogenetic approach discussed by me may result in new strategies for therapy and prevention of immunopathological diseases in general and in arthritis in particular. I assume that the proposed Ir- and/or Is-gene products will function, in general, at the level of antigen presentation to T-cells. The first strategy, which has been rather extensively discussed in this chapter, is that the immunogenetic approach may identify an environmental triggering antigen for which we could device a vaccine. The second strategy, which has only been alluded to, is to define the Ir-gene product and specifically down-regulate it, thus preventing antigen presentation. This could either be performed by, for example, monoclonal antibodies directed against Ir-gene products[67] or by manipulating the expression regulation of these molecules[5]. Of course it might also be conceivable that the lack of an antigen-specific Is-gene product could be responsible for the disease susceptibility (e.g. Ref. 62). In that case one could perhaps upregulate that Is-gene product. The third approach is directed at the T-cell receptor for antigen + MHC. Assuming that there is a common feature (allotype or idiotype) to the receptors used by T-cells to recognize antigen + MHC in a given T-cell-mediated disease, one could use this

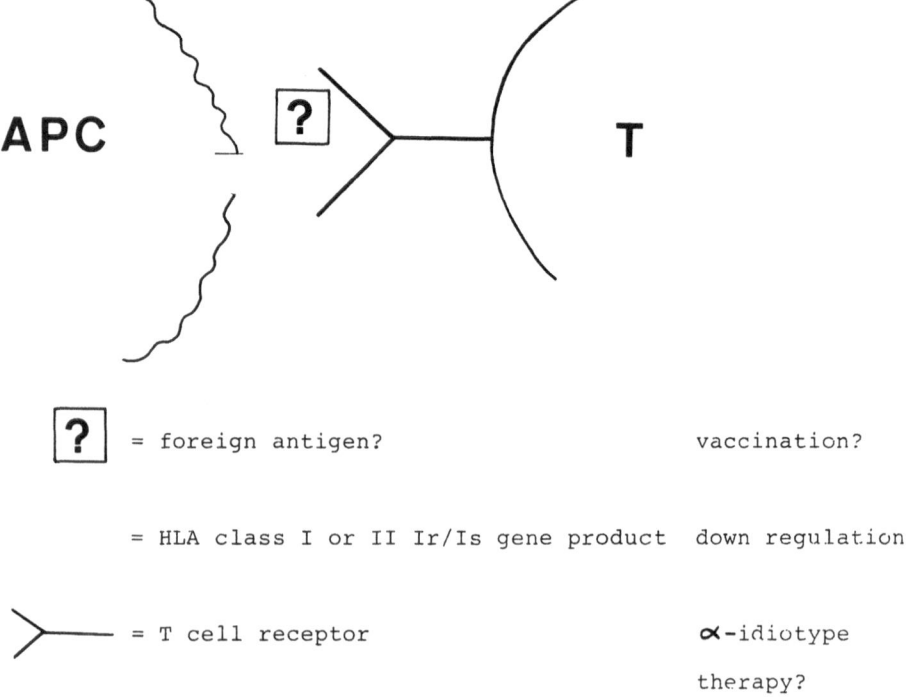

**Figure 3.2**  HLA class I and class II Ir- and Is-genes: new strategies for immunotherapy and prevention?

common antigen of the T-cell receptor to target intervention strategies. This last approach would be applicable even without knowing the triggering antigen.

## Acknowledgements

Tiny van Westerop helped in preparing this manuscript. The studies reviewed in this chapter have been in part supported by MEDIGON (The Dutch Foundation for Medical and Health Research).

## References

1. Benaccerraf, B. and McDevitt, H.O. (1972). The histocompatibility linked immune response genes. *Science*, **175**, 263–79
2. De Vries, R.R.P. and Van Rood, J.J. (1985). Introduction to Immunobiology of HLA class I and II molecules. *Progr. Allergy*, **36**, 1–9
3. De Vries, R.R.P. and Van Rood, J.J. (1987). Immunogenetics and common disease. In King, R.A., Rotter, J.I. and Motulski, A.G. (eds.), *The Genetics of Common Disease*. (In press)
4. Hood, L., Kronenberg, M. and Hunkapiller, T. (1985). T-cell antigen receptors and the immunoglobulin supergene family. *Cell*, **40**, 225–9
5. Botazzo, G.F., Pujoll-Borrell, R. and Hanfussa, T. (1983). Role of aberrant HLA-DR expression in induction of endocrine auto-immunity. *Lancet*, **2**, 1115–19
6. Unanue, E.R., Beller, D.I., Lu, C.Y. and Allen, P.M. (1984). Antigen presentation: comments on its regulation and mechanism. *J. Immunol.*, **132**, 1–5
7. Matis, L.A., Glimcher, L.H., Paul, W.E. and Schwartz, R.H. (1983). Magnitude of response of histocompatibility-restricted T-cell clones is a function of the product of the concentrations of antigen and Ia molecules. *Proc. Natl. Acad. Sci. USA*, **80**, 6019–23
8. The HLA Nomenclature Committee (1984). Nomenclature for factors of the HLA System 1984. In Albert, E. (ed.) *Histocompatibility Testing 1984*. pp. 4–8. (Berlin: Springer Verlag)
9. Benacerraf, B. (1981). Role of MHC products in immune regulation. *Science*, **212**, 1229–38
10. Matis, A., Jones, P.P. and Murphy, D.B. (1982). Immune response gene function correlates with the expression of an Ia antigen II. *J. Exp. Med.*, **155**, 508–23
11. Babbit, B.P., Allen, P.M., Matsueda, G., Haber, E., Unanue, E.R. (1985). Binding of immunogenic peptides to Ia histocompatibility molecules. *Nature*, **317**, 359–61
12. Longo, D.L. and Schwartz, R.H. (1980). T-cell specificity for H-2 and Ir-gene phenotype correlates with the phenotype of thymic antigen-presenting cells. *Nature*, **287**, 44–6
13. Kast, W.M., De Waal, L.P. and Melief, C.J.M. (1984). Thymus dictates major histocompatibility complex (MHC) specificity and immune response gene phenotype of class II MHC-restricted T-cells but not of class I MHC-restricted T-cells. *J. Exp. Med.*, **160** 1752–66
14. Bodmer, W.F. (1972). Evolutionary significance of the HLA system. *Nature*, **237**, 139–45
15. Piazza, A., Belvedere, M.C., Bernoco, D., Conighi, C., Contu, L., Curtoni, E.S., Mattiuz, P.L., Mayr, W., Richiardi, P., Scudeller, G. and Ceppellini, R. (1972). HLA-variation in four Sardinian villages under differential selective pressure by malaria. In Dausset, J. and Colombani, J. (eds.). *Histocompatibility Testing 1972*. pp. 73–84. (Copenhagen: Munksgaard)
16. De Vries, R.R.P., Meera Khan, P., Bernini, L.F., Van Loghem, E. and Van Rood, J.J. (1979). Genetic control of survival in epdiemics. *J. Immunogenet.*, **6**, 271–87
17. Haldane, J.B.S. (1949). Disease and evolution. *Ric. Sci.*, **19**, 68–76
18. Tiwari, L. and Terasaki, P.J. (1985). *HLA and Disease Associations*. (New York: Springer Verlag)
19. Klouda, P.T., Corbin, S.A., Bradley, B.A., Cohen, B.J. and Woolf, A.D. (1986). HLA and acute arthritis following human parvovirus infection. *Tissue Antigens*, **28**, 318–19
20. Dijkmans, B.A.C. and De Vries, R.R.P. (1986) *J. Rheum.*, **13**, 1192–3
21. Germain, R.N. (1986). The ins and outs of antigen presentation and processing. *Nature*, **322**, 687–9

22. Klaresborg, L., Bauck, G., Forsgen, A. and Peterson, P.A. (1978). Binding of HLA antigen-containing liposomes to bacteria. *Proc. Natl. Acad. Sci. USA*, **75**, 6197–201
23. Maeda, K., Kono, D., Kobayaski, S., Brenner, M.B. and Yu, D.T.Y. (1984). A study of the specificity of the direct binding between bacteria and HLA antigens. *Clin. Exp. Immunol.*, **57**, 694–702
24. Schlosstein, L., Terasaki, P.I., Bluestone, R. and Pearson, C.M. (1973). High association of HLA antigen w27 with ankylosing spondylitis. *N. Engl. J. Med.*, **288**, 704–6
25. Brewerton, D.A., Caffrey, M., Hart, F.D., James, D.C.O., Nicholls, A. and Sturrock, R.D. (1973). Ankylosing spondylitis and HLA-A27. *Lancet*, **i**, 904–7
26. Edmonds, J., Bashir, H., Thomson, G. and Carbonara, A.O. (1984). HLA-B27 negative ankylosing spondylitis. In Albert, E.D., Mayr, W.R. and Baur, M.P. (eds.). *Histocompatibility Testing 1984*. pp. 388–94. (Berlin: Springer Verlag)
27. Kidd, K.K., Bernozo, D., Carbonara, A.O., Daneo, V., Steiger, K. and Ceppellini, R. (1977). Genetic analysis of HLA-associated diseases: the 'illness susceptible' gene frequency and sex ratio in ankylosing spondylitis. In Dausset, J. and Svejgaard, A. (eds.). *HLA and Disease*. pp. 72–80. (Copenhagen: Munksgaard)
28. Van der Linden, S.M., Valkenburg, H.A., De Jongh, B.M. and Cats, A. (1984). The risk of developing ankylosing spondylitis in HLA-B27 positive individuals. *Arthr. Rheum.*, **27**, 241–9
29. Thomson, G. (1983). Investigation of the mode of inheritance of the HLA associated diseases by the method of antigen genotype frequencies among diseased individuals. *Tissue Antigens*, **21**, 81–104
30. Ebringer, A. (1978). The link between genes and disease. *New Scientist*, **79**, 865–7
31. Ogasawara, M., Kono, D.H. and Yu, D.T. (1986). Mimicry of human histocompatibility HLA-B27 antigens by *Klebsiella pneumoniae*. *Infect. Immun.*, **51**, 901–8
32. Van Bohemen, Ch.G., Grumet, F.C. and Zanen H.C. (1984). Identification of HLA-B27 M1 and M2 cross-reactive antigens in klebsiella, shigella and yersinia. *Immunology*, **52**, 607–10
33. Warren, R.E. and Brewerton, D.A. (1980). Fecal carriage of klebsiella by patients with ankylosing spondylitis and rheumatoid arthritis. *Ann. Rheum. Dis.*, **39**, 37–44
34. Eastmond, C.J., Willshaw, H.E., Burgess, S.E.P., Shimibaum, R., Cooke, E.M. and Wright, V. (1980). Frequency of fecal *Klebsiella aerogenes* in patients with ankylosing spondylitis and controls with respect to individual features of the disease. *Ann. Rheum. Dis.*, **39**, 118–23
35. Seager, K., Bashir, H.V., Geczy, A.F., Edmonds, J.P. and de Vere Tyndall, A. (1979). Evidence for a B27-associated cell surface marker on lymphocytes of patients with ankylosing spondylitis. *Nature*, **277**, 68–70
36. Predergast, J.K., Sullivan, J.S. and Geczy, A.F. (1983). Possible role of enteric organisms in the pathogenesis of ankylosing spondylitis and other seronegative arthropathies. *Infect. Immun.*, **41**, 935–41
37. Geczy, A.F., Alexander, K., Bashir, H.V. and Edmonds, J. (1980). A factor (s) in klebsiella culture filtrates specifically modifies an HLA-B27-associated cell-surface component. *Nature*, **283**, 782–4
38. Geczy, A.F. (1986). Cytotoxic T-lymphocytes against disease-associated determinant(s) in ankylosing spondylitis. *J. Exp. Med.*, **164**, 932–7
39. Druery, C., Bashir, H., Geczy, A.F., Alexander, K. and Edmonds, J. (1980). Search for klebsiella cell wall components cross-reactive with lymphocytes of B27⁺ AS⁺ individuals. *Hum. Immunol.*, **1**, 151–60
40. Upfold, L.I., Sullivan, J.S., Prendergast, J.K. and Geczy, A.F. (1985). HLA-B27: speculations on the nature of its involvement in ankylosing spondylitis. *Progr. Allergy*, **36** 177–89
41. Stastny, P. (1978). Association of the B-cell alloantigen DRw4 with rheumatoid arthritis. *N. Engl. J. Med.*, **298**, 869–74
42. Dawkins, R.L., Christiansen, F.T., Kay, P.H., Garlepp, M., McCluskey, J., Hollingworth, P.N. and Zilko, P.J. (1983). Disease associations with complotypes, supratypes and haplotypes. *Immunol. Rev.*, **70**, 5–22
43. Raum, D., Awdeh, Z., Glass, D., Kammer, G., Khan, M.A., Coblyn, J.S., Weinblatt, M., Holdsworth, D., Strong, L., Rossen, R.D., Brewer, E., Yunis, E. and Alper, C.A. (1984). Extended haplotypes of chromosome 6 in adult rheumatoid arthritis. *Arthr. Rheum.*, **27**, 516–21

44. Christiansen, F.T., Kelly, H. and Dawkins, R.L. (1984). Rheumatoid arthritis. In Albert, E.D., Mayer, W.R. and Baur, M.P. (eds.). *Histocompatibility Testing 1984*. pp. 378–83. (Berlin: Springer Verlag)
45. Duquesnoy, R.J., Marrari, M., Hackbarth, S. and Zeevi, A. (1984). Serological and cellular definition of a new HLA-DR associated determinant, MC1, and its association with rheumatoid arthritis. *Hum. Immunol.*, **10**, 165–76
46. Schreuder, G.M.Th., Tilanus, M.G.J., Bontrop, R.E., Bruining, G.J., Giphart, M.J., Van Rood, J.J. and De Vries, R.R.P. (1986). HLA-DQ polymorphism associated with resistance to type I diabetes detected with monoclonal antibodies, isoelectric point differences, and restriction fragment length polymorphism. *J. Exp. Med.*, **164**, 938–43
47. Festenstein, H., Awad, J., Hitman, G.A., Cutbush, S., Groves, A.V., Cassell, Ollier, W. and Cachs, J.A. (1986). New DNA polymorphisms associated with autoimmune diseases. *Nature*, **322**, 64–7
48. Ollier, W., Silman, A., Gosnell, N., Currey, H., Awad, J., Doyle, P., McCloskey, D., Alonso, A., Hossain, M.A. and Festenstein, H. (1986). HLA and rheumatoid arthritis: an analysis of multicase families. *Dis. Markers*, **4**, 85–98
49. Stastny, P. (1980). Joint Report on rheumatoid arthritis. In Terasaki, P.I. (ed.). *Histocompatibility Testing, 1980*. pp. 681–6. (Los Angeles: UCLA Tissue Typing Laboratory)
50. Jaraquemada, D., Ollier, W., Awad, J., Young, A., Silman, A., Roitt, I.M., Corbett, M., Hay, F., Cosh, J.A., Maini, R.N., Venables, P.J., Ansell, B., Holborow, J., Reeback, J., Currey H.L.F. and Festenstein, H. (1986). HLA and rheumatoid arthritis: a combined analysis of 440 British patients. *Ann. Rheum. Dis.*, **45**, 627–36
51. De Vries, R.R.P., Nijenhuis, L.E., Khan, M.A. and Mehra, N.K. (1985). Paradoxical inheritance of HLA-linked susceptibility to rheumatoid arthritis. *Tissue Antigens*, **26**, 286–92
52. Khan, M.A., Kushuer, I. and Weitkamp, L.R. (1983). Genetics of HLA-associated disease; rheumatoid arthritis. *Tissue Antigens*, **22**, 182–5
53. De Jongh, B.M., Westedt, M.L., De Vries, R.R.P., Valkenburg, H.A. and Cats, A. (1986). Genetic heterogeneity of rheumatoid arthritis. *Dis. Markers*, **4**, 29–33
54. De Jongh, B.M., Van Romunde, L.K.J., Valkenburg, H.A., De Lange, G.G. and Van Rood, J.J. (1984). Epidemiological study of HLA and GM in rheumatoid arthritis and related symptoms in an open Dutch population. *Ann. Rheum. Dis.*, **43**, 613–19
55. Westedt, M.L., Breedveld, F.C., Schreuder, G.M.Th., D'Amaro, J., Cats, A. and De Vries, R.R.P. (1986). Immunogenetic heterogeneity of rheumatoid arthritis. *Ann. Rheum. Dis.*, **45**, 534–8
56. Wooley, P.H., Griffin, J., Panayi, G.S., Batchelor, J.R., Welsh, K.I. and Gibson, T.J. (1980). HLA-DR antigens and toxic reaction to sodium aurothiomalate and D-penicillamine in patients with rheumatoid arthritis. *N. Engl. J. Med.*, **303**, 300–2
57. Panayi, G.S. (1982). Does rheumatoid arthritis have a clinicopathological spectrum similar to that of leprosy? *Ann. Rheum. Dis.*, **41**, 102–3
58. Tanay, A., Schiffman and Strober, S. (1986). Effect of total lymphoid irradiation on levels of serum autoantibodies in systemic lupes cythematosus and in rheumatoid arthritis. *Arthr. Rheum.*, **29**, 26–31
59. Van Rood, J.J. (1984). HLA as regulator. *Ann. Rheum. Dis.*, **43**, 665–72
60. De Vries, R.R.P., Van Eden, W. and Ottenhoff, T.H.M. (1985). HLA class II immune response genes and products in leprosy. *Progr. Allergy*, **36**, 95–113
61. Ottenhoff, T.H.M., Elferink, B.G., Klatser, P.R. and De Vries, R.R.P. (1986). Cloned suppressor T-cells from a lepromatous leprosy patient suppress *Mycobacterium leprae* reactive helper T-cells. *Nature*, **322**, 462–4
62. Solinger, A.M. and Stobo, J.D. (1982). Immune response gene control of collagen reactivity in man: collagen unresponsiveness in HLA-DR4 negative non responders is due to the presence of T-dependent suppressive influences. *J. Immunol.*, **129**, 1916–20
63. Rowley, M., Tait, B., Mackay, I.R., Cunningham, T. and Philips, B. (1986). Collagen antibodies in rheumatoid arthritis: significance of antibodies to denatured collagen and their association with HLA-DR4. *Arthr. Rhem.*, **29**, 174–84
64. Cohen, I.R., Holoshitz, J., Van Eden, W. and Frenkel, A. (1985). T-lymphocyte clones illuminate pathogenesis and affect therapy of experimental arthritis. *Arthr. Rheum.*, **28** 841–5
65. Holoshitz, J., Klajman, A., Drucher, I., Lapidst, Z., Yaretzky, A., Frenkel, A., Van Eden, W. and Cohen, I.R. (1986). T-lymphocytes of rheumatoid arthritis patients show augmented reactivity to a fraction of mycobacteria cross-reactive with cartilage. *Lancet*, **ii**, 305–9

66. Ottenhoff, T.H.M., Torres, P., De las Aguas, J.T., Fernandez, R., Van Eden, W., De Vries, R.R.P. and Stanford, J. (1986). Evidence for an HLA-DR4 associated immune response gene for *Mycobacterium tuberculosis? Lancet*, **ii**, 310–13

67. Steinman, L., Rosenbaum, J., Sriram, S. and McDevitt, H.O. (1981). *In vivo* effects of antibodies to immune response gene products: prevention of experimental allergic encephalo myelitis. *Proc. Natl. Acad. Sci. USA*, **78**, 7111–14

# 4
# Dendritic cells in inflammatory joint disease

S. C. KNIGHT

## INTRODUCTION

It is not known what initiates and perpetuates the immunological activity within the joints in inflammatory arthritis. Damage may result from the presence of cytokines such as interleukin-1 (IL-1)[1,2] or from the release of degradative enzymes from macrophages[1] but, whatever the final pathway for destruction of the joint, the underlying activation appears to be immunological. This chapter is not mainly concerned with the afferent or effector mechanisms causing damage but with the key question concerning possible mechanisms that start and promote the immunological activity.

Examination of other inflammatory reactions shows that antigen is presented to the lymphocytes by specialized, bone-marrow-derived dendritic cells (DC)[3-6]. Indeed, in the development of delayed hypersensitivity (DH) reactions which bear some resemblances to the lesions in inflamed joints, the DC may be the sole cell initiating the immunological activity during the early stages of sensitization[5]. Several properties of DC may contribute to their importance in initiating immune response. Antigens are acquired on the surface of these cells[5-7] which constituitively bear high levels of class II histocompatibility antigens[7]. *In vivo*, antigen may be preferentially located on the DC[5,6]. DC also form a physical focus where lymphocytes responsive to antigen accumulate[6-8] and this may be a prerequisite for starting an immune response. They have material on their cell membranes which has IL-1-like activity[9] and are potent activators of lymphocytes when present in extremely small numbers (i.e. less than 0.5% of the mononuclear cell population)[6,7]. The possibility that inflammation in the joints is initiated by antigen on DC has, therefore, been considered.

The circumstantial evidence that DC are involved in inflammatory arthritis in humans will be reviewed. In addition, the activity of DC with antigen in initiating various kinds of inflammatory reactions – including DH and autoimmunity – are considered to see what implications they may have for the understanding of the mechanisms producing inflammation within the joints. The cells under consideration, the DC, and some of the possible areas of confusion with other cell populations will firstly be defined before moving on to discuss the aberrant distribution of DC in patients with inflammatory arthritis.

## LIFE HISTORY OF DENDRITIC CELLS

The DC involved in the induction of immune responses to antigen are bone-marrow-derived cells[10-13] which are not dependent on the thymus for maturation since they occur in thymectomised pigs[14] and in athymic rats and mice[15,16]. Mature DC are present in small numbers in peripheral blood[17,18] and in most tissues of the body[19,20] where they may have a tissue-specific stage in their life history. This is exemplified by the Langerhans cells of the skin which belong to this class of antigen-presenting cells. These 'DC of the skin' have characteristic Birbeck granules[21] and, in the human, are labelled by the antibody OKT6[22]. The Langerhans cells of the skin are able to pick up foreign antigens and then travel as veiled cells in the afferent lymphatics to the lymph nodes[23]. There is strong evidence that these veiled cells entering via the lymph accumulate in the T-dependent areas of the lymph nodes[5,12,14,23,24] and become the interdigitating cells in the paracortex around which the T-lymphocytes aggregate during the onset of the immune response. They are almost certainly equivalent to the DC isolated from the tissues[7].

There has been debate about the relationship of these cells with classical phagocytic macrophages since the two cell types share some cell surface antigens[25]. However, there are also differences in the phenotypes of the two cell types and DC have little or no lysosomal enzyme activity[6,7]. DC also lack normal phagocytic function and have potency in presenting many antigens[6,7]. These factors, taken together with the differences in the development and distribution of macrophages and DC during ontogeny[26-28], make it likely that these two cell types are of different lineages.

There are two distinctions that need to be made to prevent confusion with other cell types described as 'dendritic'. Firstly, the follicular dendritic cells of the B-dependent areas of the lymph nodes are different from the DC being considered here. They arise within the lymph nodes and are derived from fibroblastic reticulum cells[26]. They acquire immune complexes and are believed to be involved in humoral immunity and the induction of B-cell memory[29]. The question as to whether they possess class II immune-associated (Ia) antigens is debated[29]. There are physical interactions within the lymph nodes between DC of the paracortex, lymphocytes and follicular reticulum cells at the edge of B-cell areas but the functional significance of these is unknown[26].

Within the synovial membranes the cell types likely to be confused with the immunological DC are again fibroblastic cells. These have been described as 'dendritic' or 'stellate'[30] and may contain large quantities of collagenase[31]. These cells become fibroblastic on culture[32]. In one study of cells isolated from the synovial membranes these fibroblast-related cells were the major 'dendritic' cells and transient expression of class II histocompatibility antigens on these cells was reported[33]. However, these non-phagocytic cells which lack constitutive class II antigens and are able to interconvert between a 'dendritic' shape and a morphology characteristic of fibroblasts have been distinguished both from the DC and from classical macrophages[34–36]. In histological studies Ia-negative fibroblasts are present not only in the synovial lining layer in rheumatoid arthritis (RA)[36] but have also been identified within the transitional zones of the synovium between the areas of T-lymphocyte infiltration and those rich in plasma cells[37]. From the descriptions of the fibroblast cells at the junction between T- and B-cell areas in the lymph nodes which give rise to follicular dendritic cells[26], it is tempting to speculate that a similar process is occurring in the joints, with 'tissue histiocytes' bearing many macrophage markers[37] being derived from fibroblast precursors. It is not clear whether cells equivalent to the follicular dendritic cells of lymph nodes which are able to acquire immune complexes on their surface are present. However, in addition to cells that have phagocytosed immune complexes, large mononuclear cells which probably bear immune complexes have been identified in synovial membranes from RA and juvenile chronic arthritis (JCA) patients but the cell type involved has not been identified[38,39]. The fibroblast-related cells will not be considered further in this article but it seems likely that, of the large mononuclear cells isolated from the synovial membranes of patients with arthritis, around one-third are likely to be these stellate fibroblastic cells, another third may be macrophages and the remainder are the DC of the type specialized to present antigen to T-cells[35].

## DENDRITIC CELLS IN SYNOVIAL MEMBRANES AND FLUIDS

In RA a striking feature of the cellular composition of synovial membranes is the increase in the numbers of large mononuclear cells which are highly positive for class II antigens, lack the markers and enzyme patterns of classical macrophages and have the phenotype and appearance of DC[35,37,40–44]. Positive identification of DC has been hindered by the lack of specific monoclonal antibody to human DC. Identification has, therefore, relied on the use of double-labelling techniques[35,45,46] and electron microscopy[37]. Thus, cells have been identified by a combination of cytochemical staining and staining with monoclonal antibodies[45,47–49]. Both macrophages and DC can express abundant class II antigens but only macrophages have high levels of lysosomal enzymes[50]. By contrast, DC have adenosine triphosphate on their membranes which is not present on macrophages[7]. The presence of DC has been confirmed in electron microscope studies identifying the characteristic morphology of these large cells with lobed nuclei, and having a pale cytoplasm with small vesicles and narrow tubules but with few lysosomes[37]. This latter study also confirmed the identity of the cell types by using stains for class II antigens and for monocytes and macrophages. A monoclonal antibody RFD1 which preferentially stains DC but is not usually present on monocytes and macrophages in histological sections has also aided the identification of DC[45].

71

The synovial lining cells consist mainly of classical macrophages which are class II positive and fibroblasts and these cell types also occur in the linings of non-inflamed joints[46]. The thickening which is found in this lining layer in inflammatory arthritis is probably secondary to the infiltration within the synovium[46]. The areas of heavy lymphocyte infiltration contain virtually no macrophages and the large cells in these areas consist of DC. In the transitional areas there are both macrophages and DC and the interstitial areas contain fibroblasts and cells with class II antigen and macrophage markers[37].

The DC in the areas of heavy lymphocyte infiltration have been found in contact with T-lymphocytes[46,51-54] and there are reports that cells with the so-called 'helper' phenotype predominate[40,43,53]. However, the predominance of T-helper cells in RA synovial tissues may not always occur since more variable distributions of T-cell types have been observed[46,51]. Different types of cells may, therefore, be present in different stages of the disease.

DC have also been isolated from the synovial fluid of patients with RA or JCA by virtue of their low density when separated on gradients of hypertonic metrizamide[55]. One-third to one-half of the cells isolated in this way are DC[55]. Electron microscopy of the cells from patients with JCA (Figure 4.1) show the characteristic DC morphology. The nucleus is irregular in shape and the pale cytoplasm has many polyribosomes. The cells have vesicles and show little evidence of lysosomal activity. The Golgi region is well developed and some of the cells also show well-developed endoplasmic reticulum. Many DC have microfilaments which presumably are related to the characteristic movement of these cells. They may be involved in the production of veils with their sweeping movements which can be seen in cultured cells[1214]. Figures 4.1 and 4.2 also show the presence of class II antigens on DC. In collaboration with Dr P. Fryer we have exposed the cells to monomorphic antibody to HLA-DR and then labelled them with 20 nm gold particles coated with protein A[53]. In electron microscopy pictures the gold shows the distribution of DR on the surface of the DC often covering the surface of the folds of the veils (Figure 4.1). The DC-enriched populations from synovial fluids also contain macrophages and occasional lymphocytes. Aggregates of cells occur in these samples and lymphocytes in contact with DC and with macrophages are found. The DR antigen is often preferentially located at the junctions between these cell types (Figure 4.2; S. C. Knight, P. Fryer, S. Griffiths and B. Harding, in preparation) suggesting that they are functional interactions and may be forming clusters of the type associated with lymphocyte activation[6-8].

Increase in DC in the synovial fluids is also a feature of inflammatory arthritides. DC were isolated from patients with RA, JCA and osteoarthritis (OA). In RA and JCA there were much higher numbers of DC than in OA[57]. Amongst the patients with OA there were many where no DC were isolated from the fluids and the numbers isolated from other patients was low. The numbers isolated from patients with RA and JCA were very variable and ranged from a proportion of the mononuclear cells similar to that seen in lymph nodes (0.1–0.5%) up to 10%. There was variability in the numbers of DC isolated on separate occasions from individual patients with JCA and up to 40-fold variations were seen in the number of DC isolated from the joint

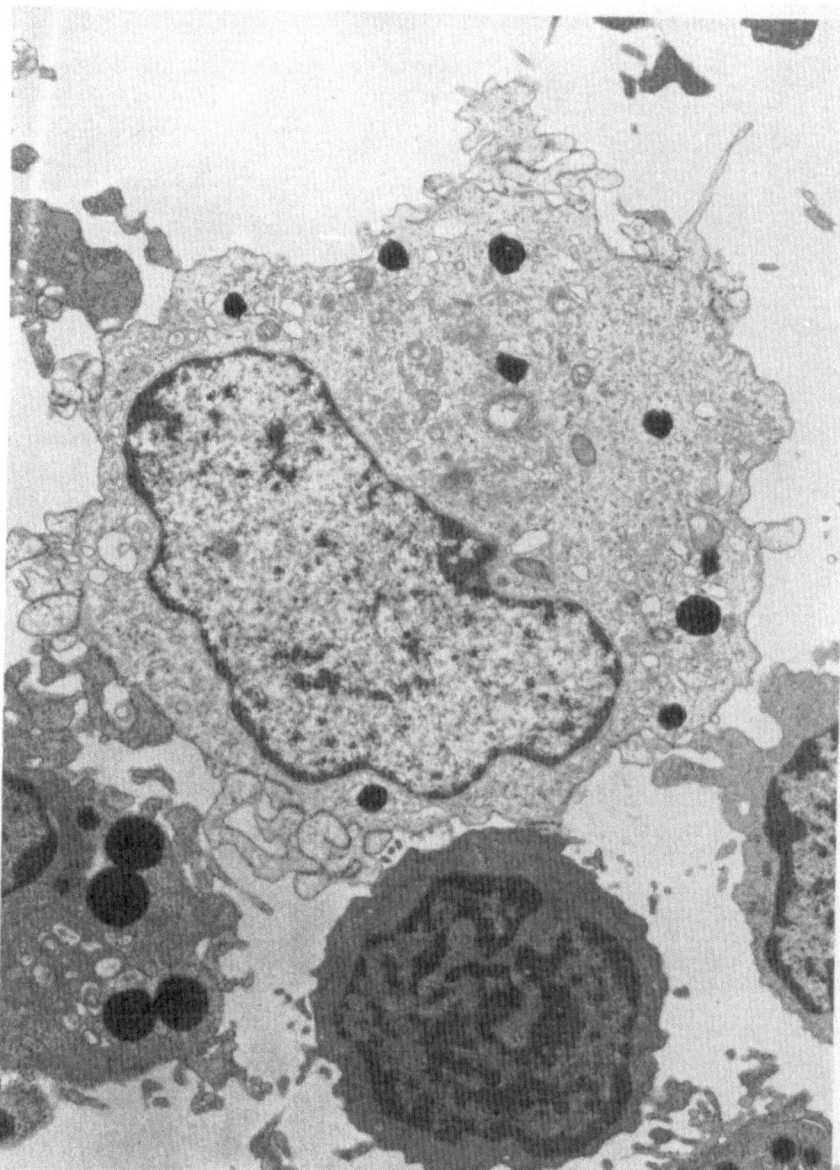

**Figure 4.1** shows a typical dendritic cell in contact with a lymphocyte and a macrophage. Gold labelling DR covers much of the cell surfaces including the edges of 'veils' (x 12 500) (Synovial fluid of a patient with juvenile chronic arthritis was kindly provided by Dr B. Ansell. Enriched populations of dendritic cells were prepared using hypertonic gradients of metrizamide[55,57]. Cells were incubated on ice in 0.1% azide with a monomorphic antibody to HLA-DR (Becton & Dickinson) for 30 min, exposed to colloidal gold particles (20 nm) coated with protein A, fixed in glutaraldehyde in cacodylate buffer and processed for electron microscopy[53])

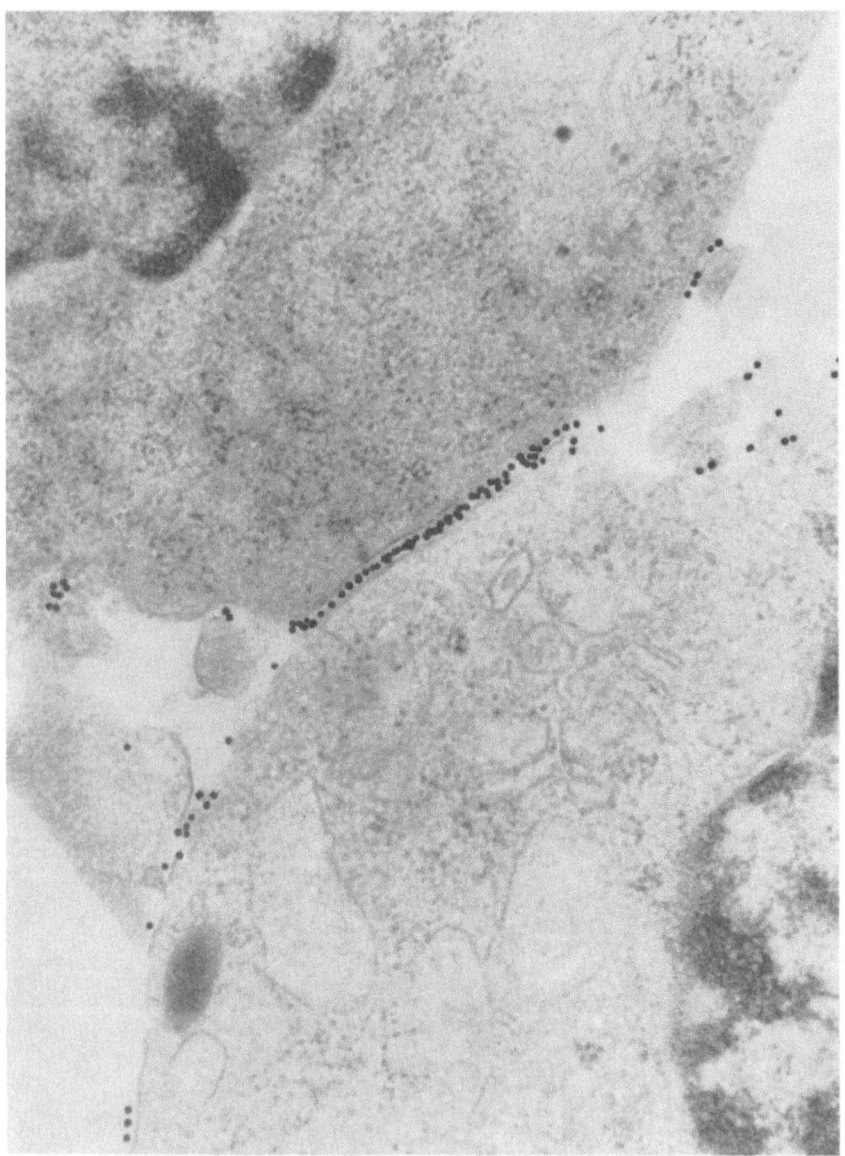

**Figure 4.2** is an area of contact between a dendritic cell and a macrophage showing an accumulation of DR antigen at the point of contact (× 62 500) (For method of preparation see legend to Figure 4.1)

fluids on different occasions several months apart. The underlying reasons for this variation are unknown but they did not relate to any obvious change in disease activity or to changes in treatment[5].

Another method more often used to isolate DC relies on the transient adherence of some DC. Many DC and macrophages adhere to plastic and after overnight incubation of these adherent cells the DC preferentially become non-adherent and can be purified by their low density on gradients of bovine serum albumin. Further purification can be achieved by cytolytic depletion of monocytes and lymphocytes using appropriate monoclonal antibodies and complement[58,59]. Using this technique the presence of DC in synovial fluids of RA patients (1–5%) was confirmed and their high frequency compared with that in peripheral blood was reported[60].

## FUNCTIONS OF DC FROM PATIENTS WITH INFLAMMATORY ARTHRITIS

The identity of the cells within RA joints which have the phenotype of DC was confirmed by functional studies. The DC, isolated from the synovial fluids of patients with RA, JCA or OA, assisted responses of lymphocytes to concanavalin A[55,57] with a similar potency to that shown by rabbit veiled cells in enhancing responses of syngeneic blood lymphocytes[24]. They also stimulated allogeneic lymphocytes to produce a potent mixed leukocyte reaction (MLR) which is known to depend mainly on stimulation by DC[61]. DC isolated from the synovial fluids of patients with RA also acted as accessory cells for the growth of periodate-modified T-lymphocytes[60], another response dependent on the action of DC[7]. When DC were isolated from the inflammatory tissue of the joint they were again efficient accessory cells for mitogen stimulation[62]. All these observations establish that cells with the phenotype of DC found in the synovial fluids or membranes of patients with inflammatory arthritis have the functions typical of DC.

In peripheral blood of patients with RA there is also a defect in the responsiveness to mitogens[63]. Since mitogen responses are dependent on the presence of DC[24] this lack of responsiveness might also result from a defect of DC function. However, there are high numbers of DC in the peripheral blood in patients with RA. In contrast, patients with JCA have hyper-responsive mononuclear cells in their peripheral blood[64,65] and in this disease there is a reduced number of DC in the peripheral blood (B. Harding, S. C. Knight and B. M. Ansell, unpublished). It appears from these studies that higher responsiveness is associated with lower numbers of DC and *vice versa*. There is a precedent for this in functional studies of DC when supraoptimal numbers of cells are used. Lymphocytes are stimulated by antigen on DC but as the numbers of DC used for stimulation are increased, responsiveness first increases, reaches a plateau and then decreases. Such a pattern of response is seen from *in vitro* studies[5,6] and *in vivo*[4]. The DC should, therefore, be considered not only as positive antigen-presenting cells switching on immune responses but also as regulatory cells.

75

DC are a major cell type causing the stimulation of syngeneic lymphocytes (SMLR)[66]. There is a defect in the SMLR in the peripheral blood of patients with RA[67] as well as in patients with other autoimmune and lymphoproliferative disorders[68]. However, DC from the synovial fluids of some patients with RA or JCA cause high levels of stimulation of syngeneic, peripheral blood lymphocytes[57]. Figure 4.3 shows the stimulation of autologous lymphocytes from peripheral blood by DC isolated from the joint fluids of two patients with JCA (B. Harding, S. C. Knight and B. M. Ansell, unpublished). The level of stimulation is compared with that caused by allogeneic DC from joint fluid. Low numbers of DC (2000) were used as a stimulus. The allogeneic stimulation was high using responder cells from both patients. However, DC from the joint of one patient showed syngeneic stimulation equivalent to the allogeneic effect while cells from the other caused little or no stimulation. The activated T-cells observed within joint fluids[69] and synovium[70] might be the result of syngeneic stimulation of lymphocytes by DC.

It may be useful at this juncture to discuss the nature of syngeneic stimulation in the SMLR. The characteristics for obtaining an SMLR are similar to those for producing stimulation by antigen, for example: DC are potent at producing stimulation; Ia is required; the responses are Ia-restricted; and the major responding cell is a T-cell[68,71]. The recognition of SMLR as a specific type of syngeneic stimulation relies on the finding that SMLRs occur in the absence of added antigen[71]. However, SMLR may be influenced very strongly not only by deliberate immunization but also by opportunistic exposure to antigen.

Figure 4.4 demonstrates the syngeneic stimulation observed using cells from deliberately immunized mice from the specific pathogen free unit at the Clinical Research Centre. It should be stressed that untreated animals had very small lymph nodes with lower numbers of DC than those usually reported for mice[72]. In these animals the number of DC isolated from the lymph nodes increased following sensitization by skin-painting with a contact sensitizer, picryl chloride (Figure 4.2)[5,72]. Normal DC caused no significant syngeneic stimulation of proliferation of lymphoid cells. However, DC from animals exposed to antigen carried surface antigen[5] and caused high syngeneic stimulation (Figure 4.4) which corresponded to the amount of antigen present on the surface of the DC[5,72]. The effect of expanding the number of responder lymphocytes is also shown in Figure 4.2 by the higher specific syngeneic stimulation when responder cells are from donors sensitized to the appropriate antigen (Figure 4.4)[72]. The highest SMLR thus occurs when there is antigen on the DC and an expanded population of specific responder lymphocytes.

In non-immunized mice there was usually no syngeneic stimulation by DC (Figure 4.4) but on several occasions for periods of 1–2 months the numbers of DC in lymph nodes increased and high syngeneic stimulation of lymphocytes was observed without any deliberate immunization. On two occasions this has coincided with infections by Sendai virus. A similar association of high SMLR with either deliberate immunization or with infection has been found in rabbits in studies of the syngeneic stimulation of peripheral blood lymphocytes by veiled cells (the dendritic cells in the afferent lymph)[6,24]. This is strong circumstantial evidence that high levels of autologous stimulation

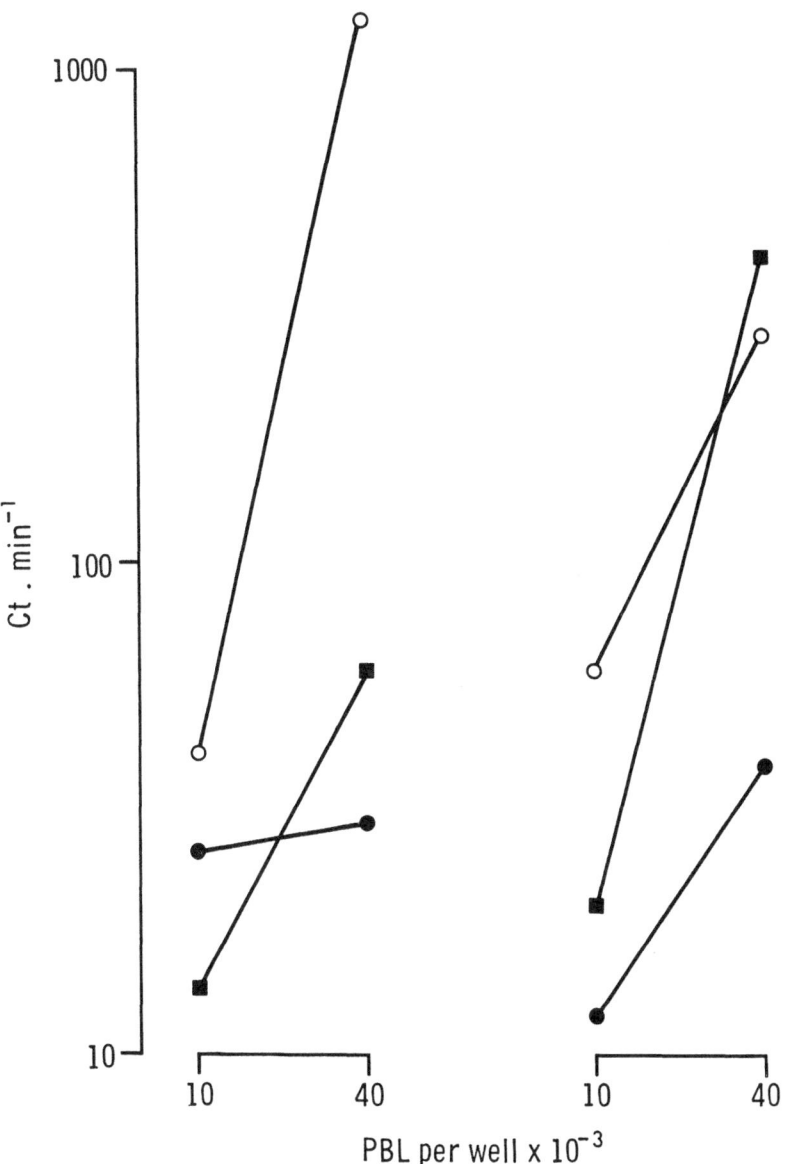

**Figure 4.3** Peripheral blood lymphocytes and dendritic cells from the joint fluids were prepared from two patients with juvenile chronic arthritis[55,56] (provided by Dr B. Ansell). Different numbers of lymphocytes were cultured with 2000 syngeneic (■) or allogeneic (○) dendritic cells in 20 $\mu$L hanging drop cultures and the uptake of [³H]thymidine assessed after 5 days in culture[57]. The DC caused marked stimulation of allogeneic lymphocytes. In one patient there was no syngeneic stimulation but syngeneic DC caused stimulation as marked as the allogeneic effect in the second patient

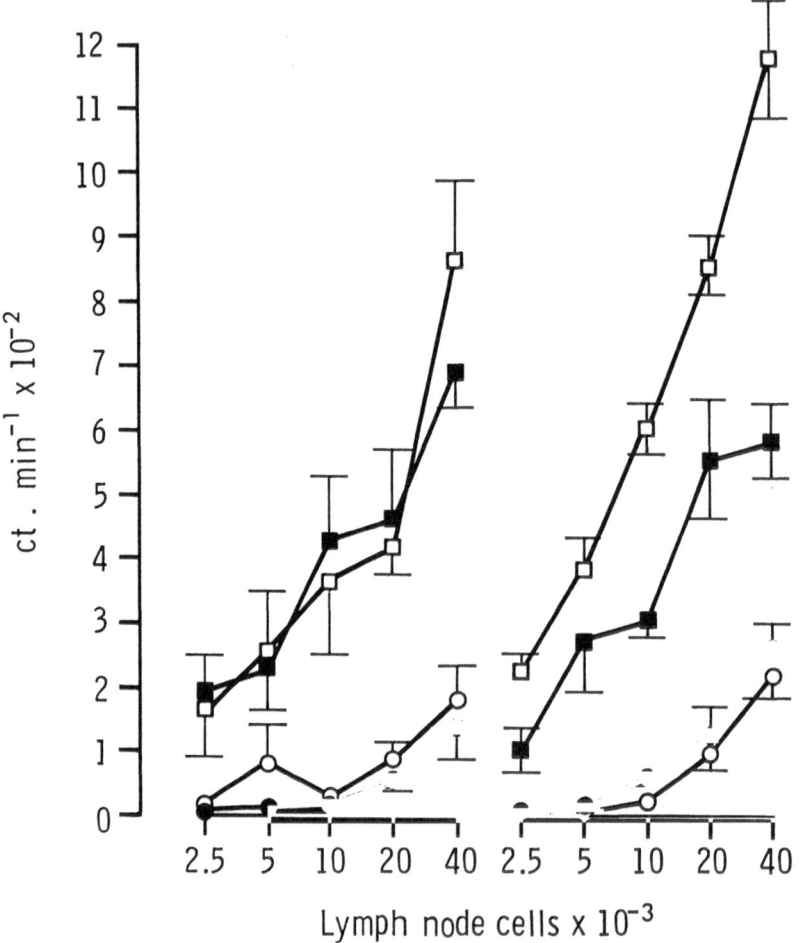

**Figure 4.4** Different numbers of lymph node cells from CBA mice (from the specific pathogen free unit at the Clinical Research Centre) were cultured in 20 μL hanging drops and the uptake of [³H]thymidine measured on day 3 of culture. Lymph node cells were from untreated mice (left) or mice sensitized 6 days earlier by skin painting with oxazalone (right). These cells were stimulated by the addition of irradiated (2500 rad) dendritic cells (DC). ● = no DC; ○ = 1000 normal DC; ■ = 1000 DC from animals skin-painted 1 day earlier with picryl chloride; □ = 1000 DC from animals skin-painted 1 day earlier with oxazalone. Details of the techniques are reported elsewhere[72]

of lymphocytes by DC is a demonstration of antigen presentation.

With this in mind we can return to the observations of SMLR with the cells from synovial fluids (Figure 4.3). If the presence of activated T-cells in the joints[69,70] does reflect the responsiveness of T-cells to autologous stimulation (as in Figure 4.3) then it may represent a response to antigen on DC. The distribution of lymphocytes responsive to antigen will also influence the level of syngeneic stimulation as demonstrated in Figure 4.4. There is evidence for compartmentalization of lymphocytes in reactive arthritis since lymphocytes from the joints, while not responding as well as peripheral lymphocytes to mitogenic stimulation[73,74], are more responsive to the putative causative agents[75].

Perhaps more surprising is the lack of syngeneic stimulation by DC in many patients (Figure 4.1) despite the increase in numbers of DC which suggests some involvement in antigen presentation. Here the narrow dosimetry requirements for antigen on DC or numbers of DC for optimal stimulation[6] and the inhibitory effects of 'over-stimulation' of immune responses by suppressor mechanisms including T-cells[76] or macrophages[77] may be relevant. Inhibitory effects of adding high numbers of adherent cells from synovial populations to T-cells have already been described[44] and the suggestion made that there is a population of adherent cells which is suppressive[78]. Further support for the presence of high levels of stimulatory activity compromised by a suppressor mechanism comes from the observations of the cytokines produced. Excessive amounts of interleukin-1 are produced by dendritic cells from synovial membranes and fluids of patients with RA[79,80]. Despite this, the levels of interleukin-2 are very low[81].

The fact that DC in the joints are producing interleukin-1 means that they are contributing a factor which is potentially damaging to the cartilage[82]. Products of DC may, therefore, be more directly involved in producing damage within inflamed joints in addition to their possible stimulatory effects on immunological activity.

The information described so far indicating that DC may be involved in initiating the damaging inflammatory activity in joints has all been circumstantial. However, the possibility has been studied directly in mice. *Chlamydia trachomatis* (chlamydiae) injected into the joints of mice initiated arthritis but when injected intravenously no arthritis was observed. When 100 000 DC exposed to a similar dose of antigen were injected intra-articularly the arthritis produced was more persistent than that resulting from antigen alone. Arthritis also developed in animals receiving intravenous injections of 100 000 DC exposed to chlamydiae (B. Thomas, S. C. Knight, M. Osborne, P. Bedford and D. Taylor-Robinson, in preparation). Chlamydial antigen on DC injected systemically can, therefore, produce arthritis in mice. In the light of these experiments, the circumstantial evidence for the involvement of DC in the development of human arthritis becomes more persuasive.

## DENDRITIC CELLS IN DELAYED HYPERSENSITIVITY AND AUTOIMMUNITY

There are similarities between the cellular components of delayed hypersensitivity (DH) reactions and inflammation in the joints[44,49,83,84] although the proportion of DC in DH reactions is considerably lower than that in RA[47]. DC are the prime cells in the initiation of DH to skin contact sensitizers. At early times following skin painting (1–48 h) there are increased numbers of DC in draining lymph nodes and antigen is preferentially located on these

DC[5,72]. The capacity of small numbers of these cells to stimulate lymphocytes is shown in Figure 4.4. Small numbers of DC from these lymph nodes (10–50 000) also initiate DH in syngeneic recipient mice. Involvement of the DC was confirmed in experiments where removal of DC using a specific anti-DC antibody abolished the capacity of lymph node cells to 'transfer' DH[5]. The DC from skin-painted mice initiate DH in recipient animals only up to 3 days after exposure to antigen. After this time DC have no effect and transfer of DH is then achieved with T-lymphocytes[90]. The DC are, therefore, essential to the development of DH but only during an early 3-day period following exposure to antigen before antigen-specific T-cells are stimulated.

DC also initiate autoimmune disease in animals. Rats given brain antigen in complete Freund's adjuvant developed symptoms of experimental allergic encephalomyelitis. DC from the spleens of these animals with disease (2–3 weeks after injection of antigen) initiated disease symptoms in syngeneic rats receiving intravenous injections of 80 000 DC[4]. Similar experiments in mice have initiated autoimmune thyroiditis by injection of 100 000 DC (depleted of residual T-cells) from animals with disease (induced using mouse thyroglobulin in adjuvant). Recipients produced anti-thyroglobulin antibodies and had focal thyroiditis (S. C. Knight, J. Farrant and J. Chan, in preparation). This suggests that autoantigen on DC was present in mice for long periods after injection of antigen in adjuvant. It also demonstrates that autoantigen on DC can initiate autoimmunity.

Taken together, these experiments show that antigen on DC can sensitize animals to give DH-type responses or present autoantigen to produce autoimmunity. In the development of DH the DC were central cells only for a limited period early in sensitization. In the autoimmune reactions to antigen in Freund's complete adjuvant, antigen was being continuously presented on DC. Experimental allergic arthritis can be produced by intra-articular injection with soluble antigen after prior immunization with the antigen in Freund's complete adjuvant[85]. The use of Freund's complete adjuvant results in the development of DH reactions[86] and this is important in the development of disease[87]. Elimination of antigen from joints is usually very rapid but is retarded when the joint is inflamed and is also delayed in animals specifically sensitized to the antigen in Freund's complete adjuvant. Antigen could thus be retained within joints for considerable periods of time[87,88]. The presence of persistent antigen in the form of immune complexes does not appear to be involved in the development of the disease[89]. However, both the development of DH reactions and of autoimmunity following exposure to autoantigen in adjuvant result from presentation of antigen on DC and it seems likely that continued presentation of antigen on DC could also be occurring in experimental allergic arthritis.

The evidence for involvement of DC in human arthritis remains circumstantial. These cells do play a central role in the development of other types of inflammatory reactions such as DH and autoimmunity and in post-chlamydial arthritis in mice. This provides support for the concept that DC presenting antigen are responsible for the initiation and maintenance of immunological activity in inflammatory arthritis in humans.

## Acknowledgements

I am grateful to my colleagues Drs P. Fryer, B. Harding, J. Farrant and S. Macatonia for agreeing to the discussion of our unpublished data. Studies with material from patients were approved by the Ethical Committee of Northwick Park Hospital.

## References

1. Henderson, B., Pettipher E.R. (1985). The synovial lining cell: Biology and pathobiology. *Semin. Arthr. Rheum.*, **14**, 1–32
2. Billingham, M.E.J. (1985). Interleukin 1: its relevance to rheumatoid arthritis. *Br. J. Rheumatol.*, **24**, 25–36
3. Lechler, R.I. and Batchelor, J.R. (1982). Restoration of immunogenicity to passenger-cell depleted kidney allografts by addition of donor strain dendritic cells. *J. Exp. Med.*, **155**, 31–41
4. Knight, S.C., Mertin, J., Stackpoole, A. and Clarke, J. (1983). Induction of immune response in vivo with small numbers of veiled cells. *Proc. Natl. Acad. Sci. USA*, **8**, 6032–5
5. Macatonia, S.E., Edwards, A. and Knight, S.C. (1986). Dendritic cells and contact sensitivity to fluorescein isothiocyanate. *Immunology*, **59**, 509–14
6. Knight, S.C. (1984). Veiled cells - 'dendritic' cells of the peripheral lymph. *Immunobiology*, **168**, 349–61
7. Steinman, R.M. and Nussenzweig, M.C. (1980). Dendritic cells: features and functions. *Immunol. Rev.*, **53**, 127–47
8. Inaba, K. and Steinman, R. (1986). Accessory cell–T lymphocyte interactions. Antigen-dependent and -independent clustering. *J. Exp. Med.*, **163**, 247–61
9. Nagelkerken, L.M. and Vriesman, J.C. van B. (1986). Membrane-associated IL-1 like activity on rat dendritic cells. *J. Immunol.*, **136**, 2164–70
10. Katz, S., Tamaki, K. and Sachs, D.H. (1979). Epidermal Langerhans cells are derived from cells originating in the bone marrow. *Nature*, **282**, 324–6
11. Pugh, C.W., Macpherson, G.G. and Steer, H.W. (1983). Characterisation of non-lymphoid cells derived from rat peripheral lymph. *J. Exp. Med.*, **157**, 1758–79
12. Drexhage, H.A., Lens, J.W., Cvetanov, J., Kamperdijk, E.W.A., Mullink, R. and Balfour, B.M. (1980). Veiled cells resembling Langerhans cells. In Van Furth, R. (ed.) *Mononuclear Phagocytes: Functional Aspects*. pp. 235–72. (The Hague: Martinus Nijhoff)
13. Bowers, W.E. and Berkowitz, M.R. (1986). Differentiation of dendritic cells in cultures of rat bone-marrow cells. *J. Exp. Med.*, **163**, 872–83
14. Drexhage, H.A., Mullink, H., De Groot, J., Clarke, J. and Balfour, B.M. (1979). A study of cells present in peripheral lymph of pigs with special reference to a type of cell resembling the Langerhans cell. *Cell. Tissue Res.*, **202**, 407–30
15. Fossum, S., Smith, M.E., Bell, E.B. and Ford, W.L. (1980). The architecture of rat lymph nodes. III. The lymph nodes and lymph borne cells of the congenitally athymic nude rat. *Scand. J. Immunol.*, **12**, 421–32
16. Knight, S.C., Bedford, P. and Hunt, R. (1985). The role of dendritic cells in the initiation of immune responses to contact sensitizers II. Studies in nude mice. *Cell. Immunol.*, **94**, 435–9
17. Knight, S.C., Farrant, J., Bryant, A., Edwards, A.J., Burman, S., Lever, A., Clarke, J. and Webster, A.D.B. (1986). Non-adherent, low-density cells from human peripheral blood contain dendritic cells and monocytes both with veiled morphology. *Immunology*, **57**, 595–603
18. Van Voorhis, W.C., Hair, L.S. and Steinman, R.M. (1982). Human dendritic cells: enrichment and characterization from peripheral blood. *J. Exp. Med.*, **155**, 1172–87
19. Hart, D.N.J. and Fabre, J.W. (1981). Demonstration and characterization of 1a-positive dendritic cells in the intestinal connective tissues of rat heart and other tissues but not brain. *J. Exp. Med.*, **154**, 347–61

20. Klinkert, W.E.F., LaBadie, J.H. and Bowers, W.E. (1982). Accessory and stimulating properties of dendritic cells and macrophages isolated from various rat tissues. *J. Exp. Med.*, **156**, 1–19

21. Thorbecke, G.J., Silberberg-Sinakin, I. and Flotte, J.J. (1980). Langerhans cells as macrophages in skin and lymphoid organs. *J. Invest. Dermatol.*, **75**, 32–43

22. Murphy, G.F., Bhan, A.K., Sato, S., Milm, M.C. and Harriet, T.J. (1981). A new immunological marker for human Langerhans cells. *N. Engl. J. Med.*, **304**, 791–2

23. Silberberg-Sinakin, I. and Thorbecke, G.J. (1980). Contact hypersensitivity and Langerhans cells. *J. Invest. Dermatol.*, **75**, 61–7

24. Knight, S.C., Balfour, B.M., O'Brien, J., Buttifant, L., Sumerska, T. and Clarke, J. (1982). Role of veiled cells in lymphocyte activation. *Eur. J. Immunol.*, **12**, 1057–60

25. Hogg, N., Takacs, L., Palmer, D.G., Selvendren, Y. and Allen, K. (1986). The P150-95 molecule is a marker of human mononuclear phagocytes: Comparison with the expression of class II molecules. *Eur. J. Immunol.*, **16**, 240–8

26. Villena, A., Zapata, A., Rivera-Pomar, J.M., Barrutia, M.G. and Fonfria, J. (1983). Structure of the non-lymphoid cells during post-natal development of the rat lymph nodes. *Tissue Res.*, **229**, 219–32

27. Wilders, M.M., Sminia, T., Plesch, B.E.C., Drexhage, H.A., Weiteureden, E.F. and Neuwissen, S.G.M. (1985). Large mononuclear 1a-positive veiled cells in Peyer's patches. *Immunology*, **48**, 461–7

28. Wilders, M.M., Sminia, T. and Janse, E.M. (1983). Ontogeny of non-lymphoid cells in the rat gut with special reference to large mononuclear 1a-positive dendritic cells. *Immunology*, **50**, 303–14

29. Klaus, G.G.B., Humphrey, J.H., Kunkl, A. and Dungworth, D.W. (1980). The follicular dendritic cells: its role in antigen-presentation in the generation of immunological memory. *Immunol. Rev.*, **53**, 3–28

30. Williamson, N., James, K. and Ling, N.R. (1966). Synovial cells: a study of the morphology and an examination of protein synthesis of synovial cells. *Ann. Rheum. Dis.*, **25**, 534–46

31. Woolley, D.E., Brinckerhoff, C.L. and Mainardi, C.O. (1979). Collagenase production by rheumatoid synovial cells: morphological and immunohistochemical studies of dendritic cells. *Ann. Rheum. Dis.*, **38**, 262–71

32. Baker, D.G., Dayer, J.M., Roelke, M. (1983). Rheumatoid synovial cell morphologic changes induced by a mononuclear cell factor in culture. *Arthr. Rheum.*, **26**, 8–14

33. Hendler, P.L., Lavoie, P.E., Werb, Z., Chan, J. and Seaman, W.E. (1985). Human synovial dendritic cells. Direct observation of transition to fibroblasts. *J. Rheumatol.*, **12**, 660–4

34. Winchester, R.J. and Burmester, G.R. (1981). Demonstration of 1a antigens on certain dendritic cells and on a novel elongate cell found in human synovial tissue. *Scand. J. Immunol.*, **14**, 439–43

35. Burmester, G.R., Dimitriu-Bona, A., Waters, S.I. *et al.* (1983). Identification of three major synovial lining cell populations by monoclonal antibodies directed to 1a antigens and antigens associated with monocytes/macrophages and fibroblasts. *Scand. J. Immunol.*, **17**, 69–82

36. Burmester, G.R., Locher, P., Koch, B. *et al.* (1983). The tissue architecture of synovial membranes in inflammatory and non-inflammatory joint disease. *Rheumatol. Int.*, **3**, 173–81

37. Iguchi, T., Kurosaka, M. and Ziff, M. (1986). Electron microscopic study of HLA-DR and monocyte/macrophage staining cells in the rheumatoid synovial membrane. *Arthr. Rheum.*, **29**, 600–13

38. Fish, A.J., Michael, A.F., Gewurz, H. and Good, R.A. (1966). Immunopathologic changes in rheumatoid arthritis synovium. *Arthr. Rheum.*, **9**, 267–80

39. Rodman, W.S., Williams, R.C., Bilka, P.J. and Muller-Eberhard, H.J. (1967). Immunofluorescent localisation of the third and fourth component of complement in synovial tissue from patients with rheumatoid arthritis. *J. Lab. Clin. Med.*, **69**, 141–50

40. Meijer, C.J.L.M., de Graaf-Reitsma, C.B., Lafeber, G.J.M. and Cats, A. (1982). *In situ* localisation of lymphocyte subsets in synovial membranes of patients with rheumatoid arthritis with monoclonal antibodies. *J. Rheumatol.*, **9**, 359–65

41. Janossy, G., Duke, O., Poulter, Panayi, G., Bofill, M. and Goldstein, G. (1981). Rheumatoid arthritis: A disease of T-lymphocyte/macrophage immunoregulation. *Lancet*, **ii**, 839–42

42. Klareskog, L., Forsum, V., Tjernlund, U.M., Kabelitz, D. and Wigren, A. (1981). Appearance of anti-HLA-DR-reacting cells in normal and rheumatoid synovial tissue. *Scand. J. Immunol.*, **14**, 183–92

43. Klareskog, L., Forsum, U., Wigren, A. and Wigzell, H. (1982). Relationships between HLA-DR-expressing cells and T lymphocytes of different subsets in rheumatoid synovial tissue. *Scand. J. Immunol.*, **15**, 501–7

44. Klareskog, L., Forsum, U. and Scheynius, A. (1982). Evidence in support of a self-perpetuating HLA-DR-dependent delayed-type cell reaction in rheumatoid arthritis. *Proc. Natl. Acad. Sci. USA*, **79**, 3632–6

45. Poulter, L.W., Duke, O., Hobbs, S., Janossy, G. and Panayi, G.S. (1982). Histochemical discrimination of HLA-DR positive cell populations in the normal and arthritic synovial linings. *Clin. Exp. Immunol.*, **48**, 381–8

46. Lindblad, S., Klareskog, L. and Hedfors, E. (1983). Phenotypic characterization of synovial tissue cells *in situ* in different types of synovitis. *Arthr. Rheum.*, **26**, 1321–32

47. Poulter, L.W. and Janossy, G. (1985). The involvement of dendritic cells in chronic inflammatory disease. *Scand. J. Immunol.*, **21**, 401–7

48. Forsum, U., Claesson, K., Hjelm, E., Karlsson-Parra, A., Klareskog, L., Scheynius, A. and Tjerniund, U. (1985). Class II transplantation antigens: Distribution in tissues and involvement in disease. *Scand. J. Immunol.*, **21**, 389–96

49. Poulter, L.W. (1983). Antigen-presenting cells *in situ*: their identification and involvement in immunopathology. *Clin. Exp. Immunol.*, **53**, 513–20

50. Turk, J.L., Rudner, E.J. and Heather, C.G. (1966). A histochemical analysis of mononuclear cell infiltrates of the skin. II. Delayed hypersensitivity in the human. *Int. Arch. Allergy*, **30**, 248–61

51. Førre, Ø., Thoen, J., Lea, T., Dobloug, J.H., Mellbye, O.J., Natuig, J.B., Pahle, J. and Solheim, B.G. (1982). In situ characterisation of mononuclear cells in rheumatoid tissues using monoclonal antibodies. *Scand. J. Immunol.*, **16**, 315–19

52. Førre, Ø., Thoen, J. and Dobloug, J.H. (1982). Detection of T-lymphocyte subpopulations in the peripheral blood and the synovium of patients with rheumatoid arthritis and juvenile arthritis using monoclonal antibodies. *Scand. J. Immunol.*, **15**, 221–6

53. Duke, O., Panayi, G.S., Janossy, G. (1982). An immunohistological analysis of lymphocyte subpopulations and their microenvironment in the synovial membranes of patients with rheumatoid arthritis by means of monoclonal antibodies. *Ann. Rheum. Dis.*, **42**, 357–61

54. Kurosaka, M. and Ziff, M. (1983). Immunoelectron microscopic study of the distribution of T cell subsets in rheumatoid synovium. *J. Exp. Med.*, **158**, 1191–210

55. Tyndall, A., Knight, S.C. and Edwards, A. (1983). Veiled (dendritic) cells in synovial fluid. *Lancet*, **i**, 472–3

56. van den Scheuren, B., Gasser, D., Marynen, P., van Leuven, F., David, G., Cassiman, J-J. and van den Berghe, H. (1985). Polymorphous endocytotic organelles in the receptor-mediated endocytosis of gold-labelled α2-macroglobulin complexes by human fibroblasts. *J. Cell. Sci.*, **75**, 411–21

57. Harding, B. and Knight, S. (1986). The distribution of dendritic cells in the synovial fluid of patients with arthritis. *Clin. Exp. Immunol.*, **63**, 594–600

58. van Voorhis, W.C., Hair, L.S., Steinman, R.M. and Kaplan, G. (1982). Human dendritic cells: enrichment and characterization from peripheral blood. *J. Exp. Med.*, **155**, 1172–87

59. van Voorhis, W.C., Steinman, R.M., Hair, L.S., Luban, J., Witmer, M.D., Koide, S. and Cohn, Z.A. (1983). Specific anti-mononuclear-phagocyte monoclonal antibodies: application to the purification of dendritic cells and the tissue localization of macrophages. *J. Exp. Med.*, **158**, 126–45

60. Zvaifler, N.J., Steinman, R.M., Kaplan, G., Lau, L.L. and Rivelis, M. (1985). Identification of immunostimulatory dendritic cells in the synovial effusions of patients with rheumatoid arthritis. *J. Clin. Invest.*, **76**, 789–800

61. Steinman, R.M., Gutchinov, B., Witmer, M.D. and Nussenzweig, M.C. (1983). Dendritic cells are the principal stimulators of primary mixed leukocyte reaction in mice. *J. Exp. Med.*, **151**, 613–27

62. Waalen, K., Førre, Ø., Pahle, J. and Natvig, J.B. (1986). Dendritic cells from human rheumatoid synovial inflammatory tissue and peripheral blood as accessory cells in mitogen stimulation of T lymphocytes. *Scand. J. Immunol.*, **23**, 373–81

83

63. Felder, M., Dore, C.J., Knight, S.C. and Ansell, B.M. (1985). In vitro stimulation of lymphocytes from patients with rheumatoid arthritis. Clin. Immunol. Immunopathol., 37, 253–61
64. Knight, S.C., Harding, B., Burman, S., O'Brien, J. and Farrant, J. (1979). Clinical applications of leucocyte culture: The importance of cell concentration. In Kaplan, J.C. (ed.) The Molecular Basis of Immune Cell Function. pp. 181–192. (Amsterdam: Elsevier/North Holland)
65. Tyndall, A., Knight, S.C., Burman, S., Denman, A.M. and Ansell, B.M. (1982). Lymphocyte responses in juvenile chronic arthritis and Behcet's disease – cell number requirements and effects of glucocorticosteroid therapy. Clin. Exp. Immunol., 50, 549–54
66. Nussenzweig, M.C. and Steinman, R.M. (1980). Contribution of dendritic cells to stimulation of the murine syngeneic mixed leukocyte reaction. J. Exp. Med., 151, 1196–212
67. Smith, J.B. and DeHoratius, R.J. (1982). Deficient autologous mixed lymphocyte culture reaction correlates with disease activity in systemic lupus erythematosus and rheumatoid arthritis. Clin. Exp. Immunol., 48, 155–62
68. Smith, J.B. and Talal, N. (1982). Significance of self-recognition and interleukin 2 for immunoregulation, autoimmunity and cancer. Scand. J. Immunol., 16, 269–78
69. Galili, U., Rosenthal, L. and Galili, N. (1979). Activated T cells in the synovial fluid of arthritic patients. Characterisation and comparison with in vitro activated human and murine T cells in co-operation with monocytes in cytotoxicity. J. Immunol., 122, 878–83
70. Burmester, G.R., Yu, D.T.Y. and Irani, A.M. (1981). Ia and T cells in synovial fluid and tissues of patients with rheumatoid arthritis. Arth. Rheum., 24, 1370–6
71. Hellman, D. and Stobo, J. (1982). The autologous mixed lymphocyte reaction: A precautionary note. Arthr. Rheum., 25, 121–5
72. Knight, S.C., Krejci, J., Malkovsky, M., Colizzi, V., Gautam, A. and Asherson, G.L. (1985). Role of dendritic cells in the initiation of immune responses to contact sensitizers. I. in vivo exposure to antigen. Cell Immunol., 94, 427–34
73. Petersen, J., Anderson, V. and Bendixen, G. (1982). Functional characteristics of synovial fluid and blood mononuclear cells in rheumatoid arthritis and traumatic synovitis. Scand. J. Rheumatol., 11, 75–80
74. Silver, R.M., Redelman, D., Zvaifler, N.J. (1983). Studies of rheumatoid synovial fluid lymphocytes. II. A comparison of their behaviour with blood mononuclear cells in the autologous mixed lymphocyte reaction and response to TCGF. Clin. Immunol. Immunopathol., 27, 15–27
75. Ford, D.K., Da Roza, D.M. and Schuizer, M. (1985). Lymphocytes from the site of disease but not blood lymphocytes indicate the cause of arthritis. Ann. Rheum. Dis., 44, 701–10
76. Knight, S.C. (1982). Control of lymphocyte stimulation in vitro: 'Help' and 'suppression' in the light of lymphoid population dynamics. J. Immunol. Methods, 50, R51–R63
77. Unanue, E., Beller, D.I., Lu, C.Y. and Allen, P.M. (1984). Antigen presentation: comments on its regulation and mechanism. J. Immunol., 132, 1–5
78. Klareskog, L., Holmdahl, R. and Rubin, K. (1985). Different populations of rheumatoid adherent cells mediate activation versus suppression of T lymphocyte proliferation. Arthr. Rheum., 28, 863–72
79. Waalen, K., Duff, G.W., Förre, Ø. (1986). Interleukin 1 activity produced by human rheumatoid and normal dendritic cells. Scand. J. Immunol., 23, 365–71
80. Nouri, A.M.E., Panayi, G.S., Waugh, P.W. and Waugh, A.P.W. (1985). Cytokines in rheumatoid arthritis: Production of IL-1. Br. J. Rheumatol., 24 suppl. 1, 191–6
81. Husby, G. and Williams, R.C. (1985). Immunohistochemical studies of interleukin-2 and γ-interferon in rheumatoid arthritis. Arthr. Rheum., 28, 174–81
82. Saklatvala, J., Sarsfield, S.J. (1985). Purification of pig IL-1 (catabolin) and its ability to cause cartilage proteoglycan resorption. Br. J. Rheumatol., 24 (Suppl. 1), 47–51
83. Poulter, L.W., Seymour, G.J. and Duke, O. (1983). Immunohistological analysis of delayed type hypersensitivity in man. Cell. Immunol., 74, 358–69
84. Scheynius, J., Klareskog, L. and Forsum, U. (1982). In situ identification of T lymphocyte subsets and HLA-DR expressing cells in the human skin tuberculin reaction. Clin. Exp. Immunol., 49, 325–30
85. Dumonde, D.C. and Glynn, L.E. (1962). The production of arthritis in rabbits by an immunological reaction to fibrin. Br. J. Exp. Pathol., 43, 373–83

86. Audibert, F., Chedid, L., Lefrancier, P. and Choay, J. (1976). Distinctive adjuvanticity of synthetic analogs of mycobacterial water-soluble components. *Cell. Immunol.*, **21**, 243–9
87. Glynn, L.E. (1968). The chronicity of inflammation and its significance in rheumatoid arthritis. *Ann. Rheum. Dis.*, **27**, 105–21
88. Consden, R., Doble, A., Glynn, L.E. and Nind, A.P. (1971). Production of a chronic arthritis with ovalbumin. Its retention in the rabbit knee joint. *Ann. Rheum. Dis.*, **30**, 307–15
89. Fox, A. and Glynn, L.E. (1977). Is persisting antigen responsible for the chronicity of experimental allergic arthritis? *Ann. Rheum. Dis.*, **36**, 34–8
90. Macatonia, S.E., Knight, S.C., Edwards, A.J., Griffiths, S. and Fryer, P. (1987). Delayed-type hypersensitivity to the contact sensitizer fluorescein isothiocyanate. *J. Exp. Med.* (in press)

# 5
# T-cell activation and function

A. M. SOLINGER

## INTRODUCTION

T lymphocytes play a major role in the immune response. They can recognize antigen with a significant degree of specificity, serve as effector cell and modify the immune response. Major recent advances regarding T-cell function and differentiation have led to the definition of unique sub-populations of T lymphocytes by characteristic cell surface glycoproteins (Table 5.1)[1-3]. Probably the most important breakthrough has resulted in major understanding of the structure and function of the T-cell receptor for antigen[4]. This chapter will deal exclusively with the activation and function of the human T lymphocyte.

## LYMPHOCYTE ONTOGENY AND FUNCTION

The stages of T-cell differentiation are associated with major changes in cell surface markers (Table 5.1). Most T-cell markers are missing from the earliest thymic lymphoid cells except for the sheep erythrocyte (E-rosette) receptor[3,5]. These cells do bear several antigens found on other bone-marrow derived cells[6]. With further maturation they lose the transferrin receptor (T9) but retain T10 and acquire a marker found on most thymocytes (T6). This molecule is associated with $\beta$2-microglobulin and is homologous with the murine TL. At approximately the same point in development, these cells first express the T4(CO4) and T8(CO8) glycoproteins. More than two-thirds of the thymic population co-express T4, T6, T8 and T10. With further differentiation, the thymocyte loses the T6 marker and develops several pan-T-cell antigens. Concomitant with this stage, these cells branch into two mutually exclusive populations bearing either T4 or T8. On release into the peripheral circulation, the T10 marker is lost[3,6].

Reinherz et al.[1,2,6] have suggested that normal T-cell differentiation involves several main stages, as defined by modulation of cell surface markers, but this

**Table 5.1** Definition of T-cell populations by surface antigens (adapted from Ref. 3)

| Surface antigens (cluster of differentiations) | Approximate MW of molecules (kDa) | | T-cell populations defined |
|---|---|---|---|
| | Non-reduced | Reduced | |
| T6, Leu 6 (CD1) | 49 (assoc. with β2-microgloblin) | 49 | 80% of thymocytes (Stage II)<br>0% of peripheral T-cells<br>homologous with the TL antigen in mice |
| T11$_{1,2,3}$, Leu 5 (CD2) | 50 | 50 | 95% of thymocytes<br>100% of E-rosette$^+$ lymphocytes (T-cells and null cells)<br>E-rosette receptor found on epitope T11 |
| T3, Leu 4 (CD3) | 25<br>20<br>20 | 25<br>20<br>20 | all mature T-cells<br>20–30% of thymocytes<br>T-cell receptor associated with Ti<br>$16 \times 10^4$ antibody molecules bound per cell |
| T4, Leu 3 (CD4) | 62 | 62 | 80–95% of thymocytes<br>40–60% of peripheral T-cells (inducer/helper T-cell) |
| T1, Leu 1 (CD5) | 67 | 67 | medullary thymocytes and some cortical thymocytes<br>100% peripheral T-cells<br>density on peripheral T-cells shows CD4 > CD8<br>$5 \times 10^4$ antibody molecules per cell |
| T8, T5, Leu 2 (CD8) | 76 | 33 + 30 (43 kDa in thymocytes) | 80% of thymocytes<br>35% of peripheral T-cells (cytotoxic/suppresser T-cell)<br>$14 \times 10^4$ antibody molecules per cell |
| T9, 5E9 | 180 | 90 | 100% of lymphoblasts and monocytes<br>transferrin receptor |
| T10 | 37 | 46, 12 } complex | early haematopoietic stem cells<br>activated T and B lymphocytes and circulating null cells (prothymocytes and thymocytes) |
| T12 | 120 | — | 10% of thymocytes (mature)<br>100% of peripheral T-cells<br>associated with onset of immunological competence |

**Table 5.1** (continued)

| Surface antigens (cluster of differentiations) | Approximate MW of molecules (kDa) | | T-cell populations defined |
|---|---|---|---|
| | Non-reduced | Reduced | |
| TQ1 | — | — | 50% of peripheral T cells, <7% of thymocytes<br>70–85% of CD4+ and 30–60% of CD8+ T-cells<br>CD4+TQ1−: helper for B-cells<br>CD4+TQ1+: suppressor/inducer (same as JRA+) |
| I2 | 28–34 | 28–34 | HLA-DR related Ia-like antigen on normal B-cells, monocytes and activated T-cells |
| Leu 10 | 27,32 | 27,32 | HLA-DC/DS but not DR, <2% of thymocytes<br>weakly found on most peripheral blood monocytes and activated T-cells |
| $\beta_2$-micro | 12 | 12 | associated with HLA-A,B,C molecules and CD1 as the invariant chain |
| Leu 8, 9.3 | | | 70% of peripheral blood lymphocytes<br>70–80% of E-rosette+ cells<br>10% of thymocytes<br>50% of B-cells<br>also binds with monocytes and granulocyte cells<br>75% of CD4+, 60% of CD8+ are Leu 8+<br>CD4+ Leu8− are T-helpers<br>CD4+ Leu8+ are T-suppressors |
| Leu 15 | | | 30% of peripheral lymphocytes<br>>90% of neutrophils, eosinophils and monocytes<br>CD8+ Leu 15+: suppress CD4+ antigen proliferation<br>CD8+ Leu 15−: cytotoxic effector cells specific for Class I-MHC responses |
| Ti | $\alpha$: 48–54<br>$\beta$: 40–44 | | antigen-specific (clonotypic) T-cell receptor<br>associated with T3 as a five chain complex |
| Tac | 55–60 | | interleukin-2 receptor<br>associated with T-cell activation |

88

theory does not take into account kinetic or precursor–product evidence. Although the common thymocyte has been found in the thymus, there is little information describing the presence of T6 positivity on peripheral blood. Only three investigators have described the simultaneous expression of T4 and T8 on circulating cells[7-9]. These cells were further predicted by several investigators who noted that the T4[1] population plus the number of T8[1] cells was significantly increased over the number of cells which were E-rosette[+] or T3[+7-12]. Others, however, have noted that the T4[+] population plus the T8[+] population were identical in frequency to those found in peripheral blood[13,14]. These same authors also showed an increased T4/T8 ratio in cord blood in contrast to the previously noted decreased T4/T8 ratio. These contradictory findings may be explained by the variation in marker expression which correlates with the gestational age of the newborn infant[9]. We have demonstrated the existence in cord blood of a sizeable population of cells which bear the common thymocyte marker T6 and co-express the T4 and T8 antigens. The frequency of these unique cells correlates negatively with gestational age. If the cord blood samples used in our previous studies had all come from 40-week gestation newborn infants, several of the findings found in our work would not have been discovered.

Studies by Scollay et al.[15], Herrod and Valenski[16] and Asma et al.[17], postulate that the final stages of T-cell maturation and differentiation may occur outside the thymus in peripheral organs such as peripheral blood and spleen. Scollay et al.[15] noted that the murine thymus migrant cells found in the periphery tended to resemble medullary thymocytes and were distinct from the majority of T-cells that surrounded them. They suggested that the migrants originated in the thymus medulla. They postulated that these cells leave the thymus with a medulla-like phenotype and acquire a normal peripheral T-cell phenotype only after their arrival in the periphery. They felt that although these cells left the thymus in an immunocompetent state and were phenotyp-ically mature by most criteria, there were a few final maturation steps that occurred after arrival in the periphery. Our data are consistent with these theories. Furthermore, the presence of Ia on the majority of the aforementioned immature uncommitted cells is consistent with previous reports which showed increased Ia positivity in an immature population of cord cells thought not to be due to activation artifacts[7,18-21]. Durandy et al.[12] did not find an increased expression of DR on cells from cord blood harvested from infants at 18 to 22-week gestation. However, he noted an increased frequency of T4[+] and T8[+] cells over E-rosette[+] cells. Therefore, it would appear that during the terminal stages of differentiation in the periphery, Ia may be a newly expressed antigen which correlates with a loss of autoreactive cells, in the development of a good mixed lymphocyte reaction. Our preliminary studies looking at the presence of Tac (IL-2-receptor expression associated with activated T-cells) indicate that there is a population of peripheral blood cells (10–15%) from 30 to 35-week gestation infants positive for this marker. Further studies to define the overlap between this population and the 'dual labelled' cells are in progress.

The functional status of the T4[+] T6[+] T8[+] uncommitted cell is unknown at this time. However, previous studies indicate the presence of a T4[+]

89

suppressor/suppressor-inducer cell in cord blood which correlates well with the presence of a good mixed lymphocyte reaction in neonatal cord blood but poor cell-mediated lympholysis[22,23]. Scudelletti et al.[21] have shown that a lower percentage of cord lymphocytes acquired Ia antigens following stimulation with phytohaemagglutinin (PHA) on comparison with normal adult lymphocytes. There do not appear to be any abnormalities in the sensitivity to PHA stimulation and/or kinetics of induction of Ia antigens. These cells also showed a low stimulatory activity in autologous mixed lymphocyte reactions. This did not reflect a non-specific abnormality in the stimulatory activity of the PHA-treated cells in cord blood since these cells did not differ from allogeneic T-cells from adults. They felt that this was not a reflection of a non-specific abnormality in the proliferative response to PHA-activated cells from adults. They also showed that the defect in the proliferative response is not restricted to the autologous mixed lymphocyte reaction from PHA-stimulated cells, since it was also found in autologous mixed lymphocyte reactions from non-T-cells as stimulators. However, cell surface marker studies correlated well with these functional studies. Only one study to date has shown normal cell-mediated immunity in neonates[22]. Dezutter-Dambuyant et al.[24] have shown by indirect immunofluorescence and ultrastructural immunogold labelling that the T6 antigen exists on the membrane surface. This cell is found in a higher proportion of subjects aged 1 to 13 years, compared to those aged 20 to 26 years ($1.8 \pm 1.2\%$ versus $0.6 \pm 0.6\%$). Although this frequency of T6$^+$ cells is not of the degree noted in our studies, it does further substantiate the presence of a cortical thymocyte-like cell present in the peripheral blood detected by surface marker studies.

The exact nature of these uncommitted T-cells is still unclear. They may represent the pool of immunocompetent (early, post-thymic or precursor) cells which differentiate in an extra-thymic site and eventually migrate to organs such as the spleen, bone marrow, or other sites of the lymphoreticular system. The presence of these unique cells in the peripheral blood may be the initial exposure of these immature cells to self-antigens outside the thymus.

The majority of the peripheral T-cells (50–70%) bear the T4 marker, while 25–45% have the T8 antigen[23,25–27]. These lymphocytes are predominantly the helper/inducer and suppressor populations, respectively. Both groups will express T11 (E-rosette), a receptor which permits easy isolation of all T-cell lineage cells in vitro.

The T4$^+$ cells function as helper/inducers for T–T, T–B, and T–macrophage interactions[2]. They are the only cells to respond directly to soluble antigen or to non-T-cells in the autologous mixed lymphocyte reaction. These lymphocytes are also of prime importance in supplying necessary signals for B-cell proliferation and differentiation into immunoglobulin secreting cells. Cytotoxic function can be elicited in T4$^+$ cells in response to major histocompatibility antigens in a mixed lymphocyte reaction if T8$^+$ are absent[3]. Antigen-responsive T4$^+$ cells produce several non-specific helper factors including interleukin-2 and $\gamma$-interferon. They are also central in the release of factors which affect hematopoietic development, as well as secreting osteoclast activating factor, inducing fibroblast proliferation and collagen synthesis, and influencing a number of inflammatory responses and autoimmune phenomena.

The T8$^+$ lymphocyte is also capable of responding to allogeneic determinants of the major histocompatibility complex and becoming the major source of cytotoxic T lymphocyte effectors. However, these cells need the interaction with T4$^+$ lymphocytes of their products for optimal development[3,27]. Except for interleukin-2 and $\gamma$-interferon, they do not secrete the factors common to the T4$^+$ cells noted above. In contrast with the T4$^+$ cell, the T8$^+$ subset has mature suppressor and cytotoxic function without significant evidence of inducer function. T8$^+$ cells function as suppressors of both mitogen-induced and antigen-specific antibody production but also require T4$^+$ inducers. These T8$^+$ lymphocytes can be induced with moderate levels of histamine.

Through the use of other newly recognized markers, further complexity of these major subsets has been appreciated. A segment of T4 cells reactive with sera from selected patients with juvenile chronic arthritis (JRA$^+$) or with anti-Ia reagents or sensitive to moderate doses of irradiation function as the suppressor inducer population[3]. The TQ1 antisera identifies most of the JRA$^+$ cells, but the TQ1$^-$ population serves as the predominant help for immunoglobulin production. These two markers have aided in showing the distinction between autoreactivity and antigen reactivity since marker positive T4 (suppressor inducer-containing) cells proliferate more readily in autologous mixed lymphocyte reactions than the reciprocal population. The commercially available Leu 8 antisera may recognize a similar population of T4$^+$ cells.

Heterogeneity also appears to exist in the T8$^+$ population of lymphocytes[3,28]. They include precursors to cytotoxic, pre-suppressor, and both specific and non-specific suppressor effector T-cells. Phenotypic markers have been somewhat successful in distinguishing these subsets. However, most of the work has been based on functional assays. The Ia status of these cells has been helpful. Activated Ia$^-$ cells are cytotoxic in a routine cell-mediated lympholysis assay, while activated Ia$^+$ cells are suppressive and collaborate with fresh T8$^+$ cells to induce further suppression. Evidence also exists that a T8$^+$ cell is responsible for contrasuppression, i.e. a cell which is capable of suppressing a suppressor population.

## THE T-CELL RECEPTOR

### Structure

Advances in molecular biology have permitted an understanding of the complexity of the antigen-specific T-cell receptor[29-51]. The T-cell receptor is shown in Figure 5.1. There appear to be three polypeptide chains constituting this structure. The molecules encoded by the $\alpha$, $\beta$ and $\gamma$ genes have significant homology with the immunoglobulin genes[29-33]. Many of the fine structural features of these polypeptide chains have been inferred from the translated sequences of cDNA clones. The $\alpha$, $\beta$ and $\gamma$ chains appear to be 30–37 kDa prior to their modification by glycosylation and cleavage of the leader

91

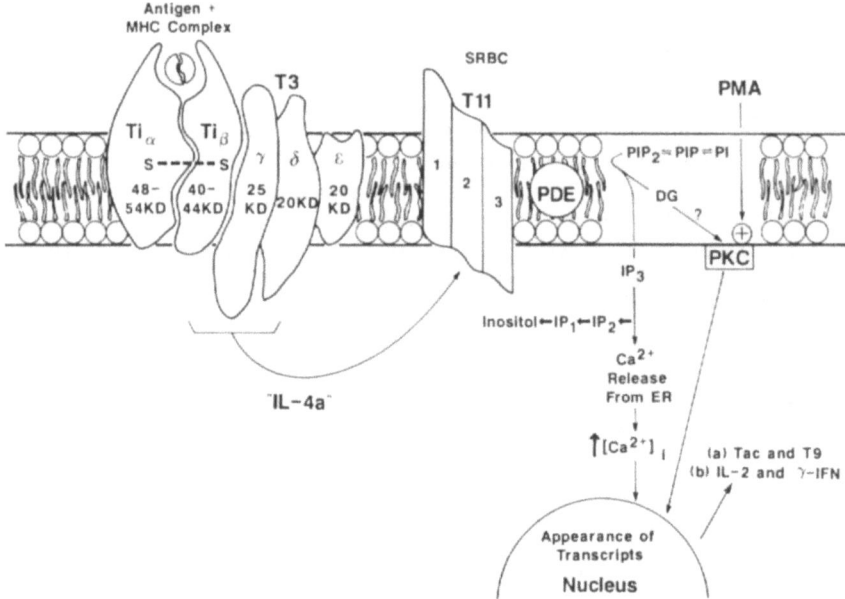

**Figure 5.1** The T-cell receptor. $Ca^{2+}$ = calcium ion; DG = diacylglycerol; ER = endo-plasmic reticulum; $\gamma$-IFN = $\gamma$-interferon; IL-2 = interleukin-2; IL-4a = proposed lymphokine which stimulates T11; $IP_1$ = inositol phosphate; $IP_2$ = inositol biphosphate; $IP_3$ = inositol triphosphate; $K^+$ = potassium ion; MHC = major histocompatibility complex; $Na^+$ = sodium ion; PDE = phosphodiesterase; PI = phosphatidylinositol; PIP = phosphatidylinositol phosphate; $PIP_2$ = phosphatidylinositol biphosphate; PKC = protein kinase C; PMA = phorbol myristate acetate; T3 = nonpolymorphic T-cell receptor associated with Ti; T9 = transferrin receptor; T11 = sheep red blood cell receptor; Tac = IL-2 receptor; Ti = clonotypic antigen receptor. (Adapted from Refs. 4 and 31)

sequence[31,47]. All three chains can be divided into seven regions[51]: a hydrophobic leader region (18–29 amino acids) characteristic of all cell surface and secreted proteins; a variable (V) region of 88–98 amino acids; an 87–113 amino acid sequence which resembles the immunoglobulin constant (C) region; a variable length connecting peptide; a segment localized to the transmembrane region (20–24 amino acids); and a 5–12 amino acid cytoplasmic region.

The combined V and J segments show significant structural homology with immunoglobulin V regions including a 110 amino acid segment, an important disulphide bridge and several other conserved amino acids vital to chain structure. The carboxyl terminus of both the $\alpha$ and $\beta$ chains are bridged by a disulphide bond making a stable heterodimer. The $\gamma$ chains also have a similarly placed cysteine which allows them to form homo- or heterodimers. All three chains have positively charged amino acids in the hydrophobic stretch of the transmembrane region. This is not unique but somewhat unusual. The additional positively charged amino acids of the $\alpha$ and $\beta$ chains may allow for ionic interactions with the negatively charged aspartic acid in the parallel region of the $\delta$ chain of the T3 complex or other membrane proteins. This accounts for part of the stability of this region.

The chromosomal locations of the $\alpha$, $\beta$ and $\gamma$ genes have been elucidated recently. The $\alpha$ locus is found in bands of q11–12 of chromosome 14 near, but not linked to the immunoglobulin heavy-chain genes[35–37,39,44,51]. In situ hybridization techniques have localized the $\beta$ genes to the q32–35 bands of the seventh chromosome with some hybridization to the p15–21 short arm bands of the same chromosome[34,40–42,45,51]. A good review of the fine details of the receptor structure and the molecular genetics involved in its construction on the T-cell surface has just been published by Kronenberg et al.[51].

An important aspect of the antigen-specific T-cell response involves the interaction of the $\alpha$, $\beta$ and $\gamma$ chains of the receptor with the non-polymorphic T3 (CD3) molecule[31,32]. It is comprised of a 20 kDa chain which carries the major antigenic determinant of this structural dimer. The other chain is a 25 000 molecular weight protein associate' non-covalently. Antibody to T3 can be strongly mitogenic and it blocks antigen-specific T-cell proliferative responses as well as cytotoxic effector functions[31]. These antisera lead to the loss of T3 from the cell surface along with the antigen-specific receptor molecule as a co-modulated unit. Resynthesis of the T3 receptor leads to recovery of the lost functions. Between 30 000 and 40 000 molecules of both the T3 and antigen receptor molecules are found on the surface of a human T lymphocyte and appear at the same time of T-cell ontogeny. Acuto et al.[4,30,32,52] made significant advances in the ontogeny of the antigen-specific T-cell receptor (Ti) by use of a thymus-derived tumour cell line. SDS-PAGE and peptide map analysis showed that a homologous T3-associated heterodimer was synthesized and expressed by the tumour line. This association is found only in late intrathymic and post-thymic states of ontogeny. The appearance of immunologic competence is acquired only among the population of cells which express T3. Further evidence for the importance of this complex is found through studies of DNA rearrangements preceding the expression of the Ti–T3 unit[51]. Ti $\beta$ gene rearrangement occurs in the common (cortical) and late (medullary) thymocyte stages but not in the early thymocytes. However, surface expression of the antigen-specific T-cell receptor $\alpha$ and $\beta$ chains does not occur until the late (medullary) thymocyte stage. Transcriptional studies also indicate that $\alpha$ mRNA does not appear during intrathymic ontogeny until after initiation of activation of the Ti $\beta$ genes. Although the T4 and T8 molecules play a significant role in antigen recognition, possibly as stabilizing elements to facilitate cell–cell interactions, the T3-antigen receptor complex most likely is the critical structure in antigen-specific T-cell activation.

## Major Histocompatibility Complex interaction

T-cells only recognize antigen when it is present on the surface of cells in the context of the appropriate allele of a polymorphic major histocompatibility complex (MHC) molecule[3,4]. Therefore, T-cells have specificity for both antigen and MHC molecules, and the antigen recognition is said to be MHC-restricted. A major debate has ensued during the last decade as to an explanation for this dual specificity – a single T-cell antigen receptor which recognizes a combined antigen/MHC determinant *versus* a model which needs separate binding sites for antigen and the MHC molecule. Evidence is accumulating against the second model[49].

A correlation exists between T-cell recognition of MHC class-I (HLA-A, B or C) molecules, expression of $\gamma$ gene RNA, and cytotoxic function. A similar correlation is found between T-cell recognition of antigen in the context of MHC class-II (HLA-DR, SB or DC) molecules and helper function and/or interleukin-2 (IL-2) on the other[3,53]. The structure of the T-cell antigen receptor is not felt to be responsible for this dichotomy[53-57]. Both classes of T-cells express $\alpha$ and $\beta$ constant (C) region RNA, indicating that unlike immunoglobulins there are no function-related T-cell-receptor constant-region isotypes. Furthermore, the same $\beta$ gene V region pool is utilized in both functional classes of T-cells. The exact role that the MHC molecule plays in antigen recognition, its recognition by T-cells, and its association with the Ti/T3 complex remains to be clarified.

### Antigen interaction

Hypervariable regions of the T-cell receptor $\alpha$ and $\beta$ chains are expected to represent those portions of the molecule involved in antigen and MHC contact[31,51]. These regions have more diversity than the parallel V regions of immunoglobulins. For this reason, it has been hypothesized that the T-cell receptor has a greater area interacting with nominal antigen. The $\alpha/\beta$ heterodimer interacts as in antibody to generate a single binding site[49,55].

It is possible to construct a model of antigen recognition by lymphocytes. The structure responsible for recognition of antigen in the context of MHC is a clonally categorical Ti molecule, which is associated with the T3 glycoproteins[31,32,52]. Depending upon the functional subset of the T lympho-cyte, either T4 or T8 serves as auxillary binding site for an invariant portion of class II or class I MHC gene products respectively. These glycoprotein markers are not felt to be critical for T-cell activation and thus are considered to serve as an anchored structure which facilitates the cell–cell contact necessary for efficient interaction. This is especially important for killer-target-cell functioning as well as the triggering of primary immune responses which are necessary prior to clonal expansion of high-affinity antigen-responsive cells. Experimental data indicates that effector cells do exist which exhibit high-affinity Ti/T3 receptors for specific antigen and do not require T4/T8 for interaction with their respective targets. Clones may also exist which recognize antigen in contradiction of the T4-class II and T8-class I correlation.

### T-CELL ACTIVATION

The process of T-cell activation is a complex story involving several levels of sophistication[58-69]. The major emphasis in the current literature centers on the interaction between the Ti molecule and the T3 receptor[31]. The antigen receptor appears to be a molecular complex between the $\alpha/\beta$ heterodimer of the Ti complex and the heterotrimer of the T3 peptides: T3-$\delta$ (25 kDa), T3-$\gamma$ (20 kDa glycoprotein), and T3-$\epsilon$ (20 kDa protein)[31]. The T3-$\gamma$ molecule is transmembrane and may serve as a critical part of the signal transmission. Several pieces of evidence support the close association between these five chains:

(1) Ti co-modulates with T3 on T-cell lines and clones[52,58,59];

(2) Diminished expression of T3 is associated with antigen-induced T-cell unresponsiveness of clones[70–73];

(3) The appearance of T3 and Ti are linked in ontogeny[2,3];

(4) T3 and Ti will, under some circumstances, co-isolate on immunopreci-pitation[31];

(5) Bifunctional reagents will cross-link T3 and Ti[31].

However, their structure and functional relationship has not been fully delineated. Cross-linking studies do indicate a spatial relationship between Ti-$\beta$ and T3-$\gamma$.

Activation of the T3/Ti complex by antigen, monoclonal antibodies directed against T3, or mitogens such as phytohemagglutinin (which binds to Ti molecules)[31] appears to be mediated through a common pathway. These early events activate a phosphodiesterase[31,64] that in turn catalyzes the hydrolysis of phosphatidylinositol biphosphate to inositol triphosphate and diacylglycerol. Cytoplasmic release of the inositol triphosphate mobilizes $Ca^{2+}$. The fungal metabolite cyclosporin A interferes with the signalling events of T-cell activation related to intracellular increase in $Ca^{2+}$ by binding to calmodulin and not at the level of IL-2 gene expression[74–76]. Inositol tri-phosphate is degraded to inositol biphosphate, inositol phosphate and ulti-mately inositol, which can be recycled to phosphatidylinositol. Diacylglycerol has been proposed as the physiological activator of protein kinase C, the site of phorbol myristate acetate non-specific activation of T-cells[31]. These pro-cesses induce the appearance of transcripts for IL-2 and $\gamma$-interferon[58,59,64,66–68]. These transcripts are first detectable 2 h after stimulation, reach a peak at 4–6 h, and decline so that they reach baseline at 24 h. The activation of protein kinase C also seems to play a role in the initial transcription of the IL-2 receptor (Tac). This induction is inhibited by cycloheximide, actinomycin D and desferoxamine but not by mitomycin C or X-irradiation[31,77]. This is consistent with the requirement for de novo RNA and protein synthesis but not DNA synthesis. The enzyme is translocated from the cytoplasm to the membrane. The Tac receptor reaches a maximum at 48–72 h. This is followed by a progressive decline in the number of receptors by 7–21 days to 20% of the peak expression. These observations support the view that IL-2 receptor expression in combination with IL-2 secretion controls the expansion and subsequent cessation of the normal cellular immune response[31,58].

An alternative pathway for the activation of T-cells has been described by Reinherz et al. and others[78–80]. This mode of stimulation is quite primitive and independent of both antigen and accessory cells. The theoretical existence of this pathway has been postulated due to the lack of the T3/Ti molecule on early thymocytes in the presence of expansion of these precursor cells to an activated state. This also helps explain the rapid expansion of antigen non-specific T-cells in the immediate vicinity of antigen-specific T-cell stimulation. This alternative pathway makes use of the 50 kDa T11 sheep erythrocyte (SRBC) binding molecule. T11 consists of at least three distinct epitopes[78]: $T11_1$, the SRBC binding site present on all T-cells and thymocytes; $T11_2$, an epitope unrelated to the SRBC binding site but found on the same cells; and $T11_3$, an epitope not found on resting T-cells but expressed rapidly with activation or exposure of T-cells to anti-$T11_2$. Monoclonal antibodies to $T11_2$ and $T11_3$ epitopes induce intense T-cell proliferation. The T11 structure probably plays a role in differentiation and/or activation of intrathymic cells before expression of the T3/Ti antigen receptor complex[78,81]. Triggering of the T11 molecule leads to IL-2 receptor induction suggesting that this may be the final common pathway for activation. A molecule called IL-4a by Reinherz et al.[81] has been proposed as the messenger which relays the antigen-MHC induced activation from the T3/Ti complex to the $T11_{2-3}$ molecule.

## Acknowledgements

I would like to thank Evelyn V. Hess, MD, for reviewing this manuscript and helping in the organization of this chapter. I would also like to thank my wife, Carol, for her excellent art work and Susan Hansen and Jan Shulman for their excellent secretarial help in the preparation of this manuscript.

## References

1. Reinherz, E.L., Kung, P.C., Goldstein, G., Levey, R.H. and Schlossmann, S.F. (1980). Discrete stages of human intrathymic differentiation: Analysis of normal thymocytes and leukemic lymphoblasts of T-cell lineage. Proc. Natl. Acad. Sci. USA, 77, 1588–92
2. Reinherz, E.L. and Schlossman, S.F. (1980). The differentiation and function of human T lymphocytes. Cell, 19, 821–7
3. Romain, P.L. and Schlossman, S.F. (1984). Human T lymphocyte subsets. Functional heterogeneity and surface recognition structures. J. Clin. Invest., 74, 1559–65
4. Acuto, O. and Reinherz, E.L. (1985). The human T-cell receptor. N. Engl. J. Med., 312, 1100–11
5. Janossy, G., Tidman, N., Papageorgiou, E.S., Kung, P.C. and Goldstein, G. (1981). Distribution of T lymphocyte subsets in the human bone marrow and thymus: An analysis with monoclonal antibodies. J. Immunol., 126, 1608–13
6. Schlossman, S.F., Meuer, S.C., Acuto, O., Morimoto, C. and Reinherz, E.L. (1983). Human T lymphocytes: Their differentiative history and functional program. In Progr. Immunol., V, 1069–78
7. Johnson, C. and Dwyer, J.M. (1983). Comparative analysis of the heterogeneity of mononuclear cells present in adult and cord blood by simultaneous examinations of multiple phenotypic characteristics. Cell. Immunol., 81, 88–98
8. Griffiths-Cheu, S., Patterson, J.A.K., Berger, C.L., Edelson, R.L. and Chu, A.C. (1984). Characterization of immune T cell subpopulations in neonatal blood. Blood, 64, 296–300
9. Solinger, A.M. (1985). Immature T lymphocytes in human neonatal blood. Cell. Immunol., 92, 115–22
10. Lucivero, G., Dell'Osso, A., Iannone, A., Selvaggi, L., Antonoci, S., Bettocchi, S. and Bonomo, L. (1983). Phenotypic immaturity of T and B lymphocytes in cord blood of full-term normal neonates. Biol. Neonate, 44, 303–8

11. Zola, H., Moore, H.A., Bradley, J., Need, J.A. and Beverley, P.C.L. (1983). Lymphocyte sub-populations in human cord blood: Analysis with monoclonal antibodies. *J. Reprod. Immunol.*, **5**, 311–17

12. Durandy, A., Oury, C., Griscelli, C., Dumez, Y., Oury, J.F. and Henrion, R. (1982). Prenatal testing for inherited immune deficiencies by fetal blood sampling. *Prenatol. Diagn.*, **2**, 109–13

13. Jacoby, D.R. and Oldstone, M.B.A. (1983). Delineation of suppressor and helper activity within the OKT4-defined T lymphocyte subset in human newborns. *J. Immunol.*, **131**, 1765–70

14. Waltzer, W.C., Baker, D.A., Pullis, C.K., Bachvaroff, R.J. and Rapaport, F.T. (1982). Alterations in lymphocyte subpopulations during human pregnancy. *Transplant*, **34**, 307–8

15. Scollay, R., Wilson, A. and Shortman, K. (1984). Thymus cell migration: Analysis of thymus emigrants with markers that distinguish medullary thymocytes from peripheral T cells. *J. Immunol.*, **132**, 1089–94

16. Herrod, H.G. and Valenski, W.R. (1982). Impaired T-lymphocyte colony formation by cord blood mononuclear cells. *J. Clin. Immunol.*, **2**, 319–26

17. Asma, G.E.M., Van Den Bergh, R.L. and Vossen, J.M. (1983). Uşe of monoclonal antibodies in a study of the development of T lymphocytes in the human fetus. *Clin. Exp. Immunol.*, **53**, 429–36

18. Miyawaki, T., Yachie, A., Nagaoki, T., Mukai, M., Yokoi, T., Uwadana, W. and Taniguchi, N. (1982). Expression ability of Ia antigens on T-cell subsets defined by monoclonal antibodies on pokeweed mitogen stimulation in early human life. *J. Immunol.*, **128**, 11–15

19. Koizumi, S., Yamagami, M., Miura, M., Horita, S., Sano, M., Ikuta, N. and Taniguchi, N. (1982). Expression of Ia-like antigens defined by monoclonal OKIa1 antibody on hemopoietic progenitor cells in cord blood: A comparison with human bone marrow. *Blood*, **60**, 1046–9

20. Zimmerman, R., Ozer, H., DeWolf, H.C., Evans, R.L., Yunis, E.J. and Schlossman, S.F. (1979). The detections of Ia-like and DRw antigens on activated T cells. *Transplant. Proc.*, **11**, 1770–3

21. Scudelletti, M., Torrielli, F., Pende, D., Piccardo, C., Indiveri, F. and Ferrone, S. (1984). Human T cells in cord blood: Abnormalities in Ia antigens induction by phytohemagglutinin and in autologous mixed lymphocyte reactions. *Cell. Immunol.*, **88**, 521–30

22. Hawes, C.S., Kemp, A.S. and Jones, W.R. (1980). *In vitro* parameters of cell-mediated immunity in the human neonate. *Clin. Immunol. Immunopathol.*, **17**, 530–6

23. Rayfield, L.S., Brent, L. and Rodeck, C.H. (1980). Development of cell-mediated lympholysis in human foetal blood lymphocytes. *Clin. Exp. Immunol.*, **42**, 561–70

24. Dezutter-Dambuyant, C., Schmitt, D., Faure, M., Cordier, G. and Thivolet, J. (1984). Detection of OKT-6-positive cells (without visible Birbeck granules) in normal peripheral blood. *Immunol. Lett.*, **8**, 121–6

25. Damle, N.K., Mohagheghpour, N., Kansas, G.S., Fishwild, D.M. and Engleman, E.G. (1985). Immunoregulatory T cell circuits in man: Identification of a distinct T cell subpopulation of the helper/inducer lineage that amplifies the development of alloantigen-specific suppressor T cells. *J. Immunol.*, **134**, 235–43

26. Kozbor, D., Finan, J., Nowell, P.C. and Croce, C.M. (1986). The gene encoding the T4 antigen maps to human chromosome 12. *J. Immunol.*, **136**, 1141–3

27. Damle, N.K., Fishwild, D.M. and Engleman, E.G. (1985). Antigen-specific suppressor T lymphocytes in man make use of the same set of surface molecules as do cytolytic T lymphocytes: Role of Leu-2/T8, Leu-4/T3, Leu-5/T11, LFA-1 molecules. *J. Immunol.*, **135**, 1724–30

28. Sansoni, P., Silverman, E.D., Khan, M.M., Melmon, K.L. and Engleman, E.G. (1985). Immunoregulatory T cells in man – histamine-induced suppressor T cells are derived from a Leu 2$^+$ (T8$^+$) subpopulation from that which gives rise to cytotoxic T cells. *J. Clin. Invest.*, **75**, 650–6

29. Marrack, P. and Kappler, J. (1986). The antigen-specific, major histocompatibility complex restricted receptor on T cells. *Adv. Immunol.*, **38**, 1–30

30. Meuer, S.C., Acuto, O., Hercend, T., Schlossman, S.F. and Reinherz, E.L. (1984). The human T-cell receptor. *Annu. Rev. Immunol.*, **2**, 23–50

31. Weiss, A., Imboden, J., Hardy, K., Manger, B., Terhorst, C. and Stobo, J. (1986). The role of the T3/antigen receptor complex in T-cell activation. *Annu. Rev. Immunol.*, **4**, 593–619

97

32. Acuto, O., Fabbi, M., Bensussan, A., Milanese, C., Campen, T.J., Royer, H.D. and Reinherz, E.L. (1985). The human T-cell receptor. *J. Clin. Immunol.*, **5**, 141–57
33. Williams, A.F. (1984). The T-lymphocyte antigen receptor – elusive no more. *Nature*, **308**, 108–9
34. Barker, P.E., Ruddle, F.H., Royer, H.D., Acuto, O. and Reinherz, E.L. (1984). Chromosomal location of human T-cell receptor gene Tiβ. *Science*, **226**, 348–9
35. Marx, J.L. (1985). The T-cell receptor – the genes and beyond. *Science*, **227**, 733–5
36. Kranz, D.M., Saito, H., Disteche, C.M., Swisshelm, K., Pravtcheva, D., Ruddle, F.J., Eisen, H.N. and Tonegawa, S. (1985). Chromosomal location of the murine T-cell receptor α-chain gene and the T-cell γ gene. *Science*, **227**, 941–5
37. Croce, C.M., Isobe, M., Palumbo, A., Puck, J., Ming, J., Tweardy, D., Erikson, J., Davis, M. and Rovera, G. (1985). Gene for α-chain of human T-cell receptor: Location on chromosome 14 region involved in T-cell neoplasm. *Science*, **227**, 1044–7
38. Howard, J.C. (1985). Immunological help at last. *Nature*, **314**, 494–5
39. Jones, C., Morse, H.G., Kao, F-T., Carbone, A. and Palmer, E. (1985). Human T-cell receptor α-chain genes: Location on chromosome 14. *Science*, **228**, 83–5
40. Isobe, M., Erickson, J., Emanuel, B.S., Nowell, P.C. and Croce, C.M. (1985). Location of gene for β subunit of human T-cell receptor at band 7q35, a region prone to rearrangement in T-cells. *Science*, **228**, 580–2
41. Morton, C.C., Duby, A.D., Eddy, R.L., Shows, T.B. and Seidman, J.G. (1985). Genes for β-chains of human T-cell antigen receptor map to regions of chromosomal rearrangement in T cells. *Science*, **228**, 582–5
42. Duby, A.D., Klein, K.A., Murre, C. and Seidman, J.G. (1985). A novel mechanism of somatic rearrangement predicted by a human T-cell antigen receptor β-chain complementary DNA. *Science*, **228**, 1204–6
43. Ritz, J., Campen, T.J., Schmidt, R.E., Royer, H.D., Hercend, T., Hussey, R.E. and Reinherz, E.L. (1985). Analysis of T-cell receptor gene rearrangement and expression in human natural killer clones. *Science*, **228**, 1540–3
44. Erikson, J., Williams, D.L., Finan, J., Nowell, P.C. and Croce, C.M. (1985). Locus of the α-chain of the T-cell receptor is split by chromosome translocation in T-cell leukemias. *Science*, **229**, 784–6
45. Berliner, N., Duby, A.D., Morton, C.C., Leder, P. and Seidman, J.G. (1985). Detection of a frequent restriction fragment length polymorphism in the human T cell antigen receptor β-chain locus. *J. Clin. Invest.*, **76**, 1283–5
46. Waldmann, T.A., Davis, M.M., Bongiovanni, B.S. and Korsmeyer, S.J. (1985). Rearrangements of genes for the antigen receptor on T cells as markers of lineage and clonality in human lymphoid neoplasms. *N. Engl. J. Med.*, **313**, 776–83
47. Robertson, M. (1985). The present state of recognition. *Nature*, **317**, 768–71
48. Quertermous, T., Murre, C., Dialynas, D., Duby, A.D., Strominger, J.L., Waldmann, T.A. and Seidman, J.G. (1986). Human T-cell chain genes: Organization, diversity and rearrangement. *Science*, **231**, 252–5
49. Ashwell, J.D., Fox, B.S. and Schwartz, R.H. (1986). Functional analyses of the interaction of the antigen-specific T cell receptor with its ligands. *J. Immunol.*, **136**, 757–68
50. Boylston, A.W. (1986). Monoclonal antibodies to the T cell antigen receptor. *Immunol. Today*, **7**, 40–1
51. Kronenberg, M., Siu, G., Hood, L.E. and Shastri, N. (1986). The molecular genetics of the T-cell antigen receptor and T-cell antigen recognition. *Annu. Rev. Immunol.*, **4**, 529–91
52. Royer, H.D., Campen, T.J., Ramarli, D., Chang, H-C., Acuto, O. and Reinherz, E.L. (1985). The human T lymphocyte receptor complex for antigen and MHC. *Behring Inst. Mitt.*, **77**, 1–21
53. Durandy, A., Fischer, A., Charron, D. and Griscelli, C. (1986). Specific binding of antigen onto human T lymphocytes. *J. Clin. Invest.*, **77**, 1557–64
54. Brown, M.A., Glimcher, L.A., Nielsen, E.A., Paul, W.E. and Germain, R.N. (1986). T-cell recognition of Ia molecules selectively altered by a single amino acid substitution. *Science*, **231**, 255–8
55. Heber-Katz, E., Hansburg, D. and Schwartz, R.H. (1983). The Ia molecule of the antigen-presenting cell plays a critical role in immune response gene regulation of T-cell activation. *J. Mol. Cell. Immunol.*, **1**, 3–14

56. Linch, D.C., Nadler, L.M., Luther, E.A. and Lipton, J.M. (1984). Discordant expression of human Ia-like antigens on hematopoietic progenitor cells. *J. Immunol.*, **132**, 2324–9
57. Gay, D., Coeshott, C., Golde, W., Kappler, J. and Marrack, P. (1986). The major histocompatibility complex-restricted antigen receptor on T cells IX. Role of accessory molecules in recognition of antigen plus isolated Ia. *J. Immunol.*, **136**, 2026–32
58. Waldmann, T.A. (1986). The structure, function, and expression of interleukin-2 receptors on normal and malignant lymphocytes. *Science*, **232**, 727–32
59. Manger, B., Weiss, A., Weyand, C., Goronzy, J. and Stobo, J.D. (1985). T cell activation: Differences in the signals required for IL-2 production by nonactivated and activated T cells. *J. Immunol.*, **135**, 3669–73
60. Manger, B., Weiss A., Hardy, K.J. and Stobo, J.D. (1986). A transferrin receptor antibody represents one signal for the induction of IL-2 production by a human T cell line. *J. Immunol.*, **136**, 532–8
61. Miller, R.A., Rozans, M.K., Ythier, A.A. and Strom, T.B. (1986). Stages of T cell activation: Continued antigen dependence of IL-2 producing cells after IL-2 receptor expression. *J. Immunol.*, **136**, 977–83
62. Martin, P.J., Ledbetter, J.A., Morishita, Y., June, C.H., Beatty, P.G. and Hansen, J.A. (1986). A 44 kilodalton cell surface homodimer regulates interleukin-2 production by activated human T lymphocytes. *J. Immunol.*, **136**. 3282–7
63. Uchiyama, T., Hori, T., Tsudo, M., Wano, Y., Umadome, H., Tamori, S., Yodoi, J., Maeda, M., Sawami, H. and Uchino, H. (1985). Interleukin-2 receptor (Tac-antigen) expressed on adult T cell leukemia cells. *J. Clin. Invest.*, **76**, 446–53
64. Farrar, W.L. and Ruscetti, F.W. (1986). Association of protein kinase C activation with IL2 receptor expression. *J. Immunol.*, **136**, 1266–73
65. Taylor, D.S., Kern, J.A. and Nowell, P.C. (1986). IL-2 alone is mitogenic only for Tac-positive lymphocytes in human peripheral blood. *J. Immunol.*, **136**, 1620–4
66. Gaulton, G.N. and Eardley, D.D. (1986). Interleukin-2-dependent phosphorylation of interleukin-2 receptors and other T cell membrane proteins. *J. Immunol.*, **136**, 2470–7
67. Nakagawa, T., Nakagawa, N., Volkman, D.J. and Fauci, A.S. (1986). Sequential synergistic effect of interleukin-2 and interferon-γ on the differentiation of a Tac-antigen-positive B cell line. *J. Immunol.*, **136**, 164–8
68. Tadmori, W., Kant, J.A. and Kamoun, M. (1986). Down regulation of IL-2 mRNA by antibody to the 50-kd protein associated with E receptors on human T lymphocyte. *J. Immunol.*, **136**, 1155–60
69. Hercend, T., Ritz, J., Schlossman, S.F. and Reinherz, E.L. (1981). Comparative expression of T9, T10 and Ia antigens on activated human T cell subsets. *Hum. Immunol.*, **3**, 247–59
70. June, C.H., Ledbetter, J.A., Rabinovitch, P.S., Martin, P.J., Beatty, P.G. and Hansen, J.A. (1986). Distinct patterns of transmembrane calcium flux and intracellular calcium mobilization after differentiation antigen cluster 2 (E-rosette receptor) or 3 (T3) stimulation of human lymphocytes. *J. Clin. Invest.*, **77**, 1224–32
71. Weber, W.E.J., Buurman, W.A., Vandermeeren, M.M.P.P. and Raus, J.C.M. (1985). Activation through CD3 molecule leads to clonal expansion of all human peripheral blood T lymphocytes: Functional analysis of clonally expanded cells. *J. Immunol.*, **135**, 2337–42
72. Fox, D.A., Schlossman, S.F. and Reinherz, E.L. (1986). Regulation of the alternative pathway of T cell activation by anti-T3 monoclonal antibody. *J. Immunol.*, **136**, 1945–50
73. Ceuppens, J.L., Meurs, L., Baroja, M.L. and Van Waurwe, J.P. (1986). Effect of T3 modulation on pokeweed mitogen-induced T cell activation: Evidence for an alternative pathway of T cell activation. *J. Immunol.*, **136**, 3346–50
74. Colombani, P.M., Robb, A. and Hess, A.D. (1985). Cyclosporin A binding to calmodulin: A possible site of action on T lymphocytes. *Science*, **228**, 337–9
75. Szamel, M., Berger, P. and Resch, K. (1986). Inhibition of T lymphocyte activation by cyclosporin A: Interference with the early activation of plasma membrane phospholipid metabolism. *J. Immunol.*, **136**, 264–9
76. Manger, B., Hardy, K.J., Weiss, A. and Stobo, J.D. (1986). Differential effect of cyclosporin A on activation signaling in human T cell lives. *J. Clin. Invest.*, **77**, 1501–6
77. Carotenuto, P., Pontesilli, O., Cambier, J.C. and Hayward, A.R. (1986). Desferoxamine blocks IL-2 receptor expression on human T lymphocytes. *J. Immunol.*, **136**, 2342–7
78. Fox, D.A., Hussey, R.E., Fitzgerald, K.A., Bensussan, A., Daley, J.F., Schlossman, S.F. and Reinherz, E.L. (1985). Activation of human thymocytes via the 50 kd T11 sheep erythrocyte

99

binding protein induces the expression of interleukin 2 on both T3$^+$ and T3$^-$ populations. *J. Immunol.*, **134**, 330–5

79. Schmidt, R.E., Hercend, T., Fox, D.A., Bensassan, A., Bartley, G., Daley, J.F., Schlossman, S.F., Reinherz, E.L. and Ritz, J. (1985). The role of interleukin-2 and T11 E-rosette antigen in activation and proliferation of human NK clones. *J. Immunol.*, **135**, 672–8

80. Hünig, T.R. (1986). The ligand of the erythrocyte receptor of T lymphocytes: Expression on white blood cells and possible involvement in T cell activation. *J. Immunol.*, **136**, 2103–8

81. Milanese, C., Richardson, N.E. and Reinherz, E.L. (1986). Identification of a T helper cell-derived lymphokine that activates resting T lymphocytes. *Science*, **231**, 1118–22

# 6
# Soluble mediators of immunity: interleukins

F. S. DI GIOVINE, J. A. SYMONS, J. MANSON and G. W. DUFF

## INTRODUCTION

Interleukins were defined originally as inducible peptide cytokines that mediated interactions between leukocytes[1]. This definition was soon revised when it became clear that interleukin-1 (IL-1), in particular, was active on many non-leukocytic cell types and was not made exclusively by leukocytes[2].

The huge impetus that molecular cloning gave to the field of cytokine research made it possible to define the biological properties of individual recombinant-produced proteins. One consequence of this has been the erosion of the conventional distinction between inflammatory and antigen-specific immune responses. Underlying the immune response is a selective growth and differentiation of one or a small number of lymphocyte clones. The binding of antigen to the lymphocyte antigen receptor (T- or B-cells) selects that cell for clonal expansion and makes it responsive to a range of peptide growth factors. These cytokine growth factors are produced by antigen-presenting cells (including endothelial cells) and by lymphocytes themselves. In many cases they have powerful pro-inflammatory effects in addition to their activities on lymphocytes.

Cytokine actions are mediated by high affinity receptors on target cells and the number of receptor sites seems to be regulated. Receptor expression for some growth or differentiation factors may be cell-cycle linked and therefore dependent on the cells' previous history including previous exposure to other cytokine growth factors. It may well be that the sequence and timing of cytokine action are as important as cytokine concentration in determining the functional outcome.

Cytokines such as interferons and tumour necrosis factors would certainly qualify as interleukins if discovered and characterized today but it is unlikely that their names will now be changed. To qualify for the designation

101

'interleukin' a cytokine should satisfy the following recommended criteria:

(1)  Inducible production by leukocytes (but not necessarily exclusively);

(2)  It should function during inflammatory responses;

(3)  Availability of amino acid sequence.

So far there are five well-characterized interleukins and several molecules have been proposed as further interleukins. There has undoubtedly been confusion over nomenclature and the identities of various soluble factors that were initially defined by biological activity. The availability of sequence data and the production of large quantities of recombinant proteins for biological testing have now largely resolved these problems. What emerges is a system of transiently-expressed genes encoding proteins with powerful biological effects on multiple tissue targets. Interleukins may operate either as autocrine, paracrine or endocrine soluble mediators or may be active during cell contact when present as membrane components of the producing cell.

The main biological function of interleukins would seem to be as mediators of host defence but clearly they themselves have a major pathogenic potential if their production (or target cell responsiveness) becomes deregulated. There is increasing evidence for cytokine abnormalities in several autoimmune diseases and, in particular, in rheumatic diseases. Whether these abnormalities contribute to or are consequent on the disease process is still unknown. However, the injection of IL-1 intra-articularly in animals[3] leads within hours to cartilage proteoglycan breakdown and recruitment of inflammatory cells into the joint space suggesting that IL-1 may be an important mediator of arthritis. In this chapter each of the established interleukins will be briefly discussed. Inevitably there is more information available on the earlier interleukins than on those characterized more recently.

## INTERLEUKIN-1

Interleukin-1 (IL-1) is a primary mediator of the host response to infection and injury. Originally IL-1 was thought to be a product of activated macrophages but it is now known that several different cell types can produce it (Table 6.1). It was first described as a T-lymphocyte activating factor (LAF) because of its ability to potentiate thymocyte proliferation[4] based on the induction of T-cell growth factors and/or their receptors − e.g. interleukin 2 (IL-2), interleukin 4 (IL-4)[5]. The LAF activity of IL-1 on murine thymocytes is used in the conventional bioassay for measuring IL-1 *in vitro*. The cloning of IL-1[6] and subsequent availability of recombinant protein has now made it possible to assign confidently an extensive range of biological properties to IL-1[7] including: stimulation of B-lymphocyte maturation and proliferation; induction of fever; stimulation of acute phase protein synthesis by hepatocytes; stimulation of collagenase and $PGE_2$ release by synovial cells; and induction of cartilage and bone resorption (Table 6.2).

102

**Table 6.1**   Cells reported to produce IL-1

| | |
|---|---|
| Blood monocytes | |
| Tissue macrophages | alveolar macrophages |
| | Kupffer cells |
| | synovial cells |
| Lymphocytes | murine and human helper T-cell clones |
| | human B-cell lines (EBV-transformed) |
| | NK/LGL cells |
| Vascular cells | smooth muscle cells |
| | endothelial cells |
| Brain cells | astrocytes |
| | microglia |
| | glioma cell lines |
| Skin cells | keratinocytes |
| | Langerhans cells |
| Miscellaneous | synovial dendritic cells |
| | kidney mesangial cells |

## IL-1 molecules

IL-1 proteins are produced by at least two genes. IL-1 cDNA has been cloned and sequenced from three species, rabbit[8], mouse[9] and human[6]. Human IL-1$\beta$ cDNA codes for an acidic propeptide of 269 amino acids (MW 30.75 kDa) that is processed to a mature neutral peptide of 153 amino acids (MW 17.3 kDa). IL-1$\alpha$ cDNA codes for a protein of 271 amino acids (MW 30.6 kDa) which is then processed to a mature acidic peptide (pI 5) of 159 amino acids (MW 17.5 kDa). Both IL-1$\alpha$ and IL-1$\beta$ cDNAs have been shown to produce biologically active IL-1 in xenopus oocytes, *Escherichia coli* and simian COS cell systems[10].

The sequence homology between human IL-1$\alpha$ and IL-1$\beta$ is 26% for amino acids and 45% for nucleotides. Of the identical positions, 53% are in the C-terminal region of the biologically active 17 kDa molecules and the sequence between residues 164 and 266 shows greatest conservation suggesting that this region may mediate biological activity. The N-terminal sequences of mature (17 kDa) IL-1 peptides show little homology suggesting either that this region is not involved in biological function or that IL-1$\alpha$ and IL-1$\beta$ have different biological functions in this region. The N-terminal region of the propeptide which is cleaved to produce the bioactive 17 kDa peptide has no known biological function but shows 47% homology between human IL-1$\alpha$ and IL-1$\beta$. Human and murine IL-1$\alpha$ share 72% peptide homology in this region and IL-1$\beta$ shows more homology with both human and murine $\alpha$ than in the biologically active part of the molecule, implying that the conserved sequences of the cleaved portion may also serve some biological function.

The genomic sequences of human IL-1$\alpha$[11], human IL-1$\beta$[12] and murine IL-1$\alpha$[13] have now been characterized. The human IL-1$\alpha$ gene is 12 kb containing seven exons and six introns. The first exon encodes a 5′-untranslated mRNA region. Most of the IL-1 propeptide cleaved fragment is coded in exons 2, 3 and 4 and the mature form is coded in exons 5, 6 and 7. Exon 7 also encodes 3′-untranslated regions that may influence transcript stability. The genomic

**Table 6.2** Some reported biological activities of interleukin-1 *in vitro*

| | |
|---|---|
| *Immune system* | |
| T-cells: | IL-2 induction |
| | IL-2 receptor expression |
| | IL-4 release |
| | BSF-2 release |
| B-cells: | BCGF activity (proliferation) |
| | BCDF activity (antibody production) |
| | chemotaxis |
| Monocytes | $PGE_2$ synthesis |
| | IL-1 induction |
| | cytotoxicity |
| | chemotaxis |
| NK cells: | synergism with IL-2 in NK activity |
| Basophils: | degranulation |
| Neutrophils: | chemotaxis |
| | adhesion to endothelial cells |
| | increased thromboxane synthesis |
| | augments reactive oxygen production |
| *Central nervous system* | |
| | Astrocyte proliferation |
| | Production of $PGE_2$ in rabbit hypothalamic and other cells |
| *Liver* | |
| | Decreased hepatocyte albumin synthesis |
| | Increased synthesis of some acute phase glycoproteins |
| *Musculo-skeletal tissues* | |
| Bone: | resorption |
| | osteoclast activation |
| | osteoblast mitogenesis |
| Cartilage: | resorption |
| | decreased proteoglycan and collagen synthesis |
| | increased proteoglycan release |
| Fibroblasts: | proliferation |
| | $PGE_2$ production |
| | collagenase induction |
| | phospholipase activation (chondrocytes) |
| Synoviocytes: | $PGE_2$ production |
| | collagenase induction |
| *Vascular Tissues* | |
| Endothelial cells: | proliferation |
| | $PGI_2$ production |
| | procoagulant activity |
| | increased adhesiveness |
| Vascular smooth muscle cells: | IL-1 production in response to IL-1 |
| *Cytotoxic/cytostatic effects* | Thyroid cells |
| | Human pancreatic islet $\beta$-cells |
| | Some transformed cell lines |

sequence of IL-1$\beta$ has been reported by two groups[12,14]. This gene also contains seven exons and has a primary transcript of 7–7.5 kb. The two reported IL-1$\beta$ sequences have identical coding regions but show some differences in 3'- and 5'-untranslated regions and also in the introns, raising the possibility of polymorphism. The genomic organization of the human IL-1$\alpha$ and $\beta$ genes, with respect to number and size of exons and conservation of amino acids at the exon junctions, suggest that they may have diverged from a common ancestor. The extensive sequence homology found in the introns suggests they may have regulatory function in IL-1 gene expression. Southern analysis of human–mouse somatic cell hybrids and *in situ* hybridization to human metaphase chromosomes has assigned the human IL-1$\beta$ gene to the long arm of chromosome 2 at position 2q13–2q21. The chromosomal localisation of IL-1$\alpha$ has not yet been reported.

## Biological properties of IL-1

The many biological activities of IL-1 are concerned either with local inflammatory responses at the site of a lesion or generalized (systemic) reactions to injury or infection (Table 6.2 and Table 6.3). Recombinant IL-1 has been shown to regulate a number of genes at the transcription level. Addition of recombinant IL-1$\alpha$ or purified IL-1$\beta$ to human hepatoma cells induces increased levels of mRNA for factor B and other acute phase reactants, supporting a role for IL-1 in induction of acute phase protein synthesis[15]. Both recombinant IL-1s have also been shown to increase chondrocyte levels of mRNA for collagenase[16] and decrease mRNA levels for albumin in hepatocytes[15]. In endothelial cells and smooth muscle cells recombinant IL-1 itself has been shown to induce IL-1 gene expression[17] suggesting a mechanism by which IL-1 production by smooth muscle may amplify and sustain local inflammatory responses. Recombinant IL-1 also activates endothelial cells to produce procoagulant activity[18], $PGI_2$ and $PGE_2$ and increases cellular adhesiveness.

The role of IL-1 in T-cell activation has also been confirmed using recombinant proteins. Addition of IL-1$\alpha$ or $\beta$ to T-cell clones produces an increase in RNA synthesis, leading to an increase in expression of IL-2 and

**Table 6.3**  Biological activities of IL-1 *in vivo*

Hypotension
Fever
Slow wave sleep
Anorexia and weight loss
Neutrophilia
Acute phase proteins production: SAA, SAP,
 fibrinogen, CRP, $\alpha$1-AT
Plasma metal level: hypozincaemia, hypoferraemia
Increased hormone levels: cortisone, ACTH
Increased survival in immune-suppressed mice
Bone-marrow cell radioprotection
Articular proteoglycan degradation

IL-2 receptor followed by an increase in DNA synthesis[19]. Rabbits and mice injected intravenously with recombinant IL-1 develop typical monophasic fevers[7], confirming the role of IL-1 as an endogenous pyrogen. These and other properties of either purified native IL-1 or recombinant IL-1 are given in Tables 6.2 and 6.3. Many of the biological properties of IL-1 have also been shown with tumour necrosis factor (TNF), a distinct macrophage-derived product. TNF is not only capable of stimulating the same cellular and biochemical events as IL-1 but can also induce the production of IL-1 itself. One important difference between IL-1 and TNF is that TNF does not act as a classical inter-species lymphocyte activating factor[20].

## Activation of IL-1 production

In monocytes stimulated with lipopolysaccharides (LPS), mRNAs appear that hybridize to IL-1$\beta$ cDNA and IL-1$\alpha$ cDNA[21]. These mRNAs were at very low levels or absent from unstimulated monocytes indicating that gene expression required an extrinsic activation signal. The IL-1$\beta$ mRNA is present at ten times the level of IL-1$\alpha$ in LPS-stimulated human monocytes and this correlates with the levels of biologically active IL-1$\alpha$ and IL-1$\beta$. IL-1 production may therefore be predominantly controlled at transcription level but the release of biologically active protein may also be under post-transcriptional control which determines peptide processing, intracellular translocation and extracellular release. Microbial products such as bacterial cell wall lipopolysaccharides are very potent stimulators of IL-1 production at pg mL$^{-1}$ concentrations. IL-1 production can be induced or augmented by IL-1 itself[17], TNF[22] and other cytokines such as $\gamma$-interferon and colony stimulating factors, suggesting potential mechanisms for sustained inflammatory responses. Monosodium urate is a potent IL-1 inducer[20] supporting the hypothesis that IL-1 may play an important role in urate crystal arthropathy. Many other substances, e.g. immune complexes, have been reported to stimulate the production of IL-1 but whether these stimuli act directly or indirectly through an intermediate such as TNF has not been established.

## Release of IL-1

Unlike other secreted proteins, IL-1$\alpha$ and $\beta$ have no hydrophobic signal sequence either at the N-terminal or internally. The mechanism of IL-1 release from cells is not well understood. It has been suggested that IL-1 is only released from damaged cells[23] or intracellular processing enables its release from cells by a mechanism different from that of other secreted proteins.

## IL-1 receptors

The wide range of biological activities of IL-1 involves a number of different target cell types. All of these cells have been shown to have specific cell surface receptors for IL-1[24]. A single class of IL-1 receptor has been found, the number per cell varying from less than 10 in some T-cell lines to over 500 in highly responsive cells such as monocytes and 5000 in some fibroblast cell lines. Competitive binding studies indicate that IL-1$\alpha$ and $\beta$ share the same receptor[25]. Both the IL-1$\alpha$ propeptide (MW 30 kDA) and the mature peptide (17 kDA) are reported to bind the murine T-cell IL-1 receptor whereas only mature IL-1$\beta$ has been found to bind to the receptor[26].

The receptor has been characterized as a 79–82 kDA molecular weight protein[24,27]. Elucidation of receptor structure and regulation of its expression awaits the cloning of the cDNA.

## INTERLEUKIN-2

Interleukin-2 (IL-2) is a genetically unrestricted, peptide growth factor produced by T-cells following activation with either mitogen or antigen. The definitive biological assay for IL-2 measures its ability to maintain the growth of IL-2-dependent cytotoxic T-cell lines[28]. However, as will be discussed, a broad spectrum of biological activities have now been ascribed to IL-2 in addition to its role as a T-cell growth factor (TCGF).

IL-2 is released from T-cells in response to two signals provided by antigen-presenting cells (APC): antigen (in association with major histocompatibility complex products) and IL-1. T-cell mitogens such as concanavalin A (con A) substitute for antigen in the process of T-cell activation. All subclasses of T-cells have been shown to release IL-2 under appropriate conditions, but T helper cells appear to be the major *in vivo* source[29]. Upon secretion, IL-2 causes proliferation of any IL-2 receptor-bearing T-cell, regardless of its subclass or antigenic specificity. Specificity is maintained at the level of IL-2 receptor expression since only T-cells stimulated through antigen receptor seem to synthesize IL-2 receptors (IL-2R). It also appears that IL-2R expression is dependent on APC and the presence of IL-1[19].

## IL-2 molecules

As with many other lymphokines, IL-2 exhibits considerable size and charge heterogeneity[30]. Human IL-2 is secreted as a single polypeptide (MW 15–17 kDA) with a range of pIs from 6.5 to 8.2. Initially these differences were interpreted as multimolecular forms of IL-2, but it is now clear that the heterogeneity is due to a variable carbohydrate component, particularly sialic acid, which appears to have no effect on the bioactivity of the molecule. There appears to be a single gene for IL-2 present in the human genome on chromosome 4. This is 8 kb long with four exons and three introns. The first exon encodes the 20 amino acid hydrophobic leader sequence and an untranslated region. The three remaining exons contain the sequences for the mature peptide. The amino acid sequence of human IL-2 predicted from cDNA gives a protein of MW 15.4 kDa[31,32].

107

## IL-2 receptors

As with other polypeptide hormones and growth factors, IL-2 exerts its action through a specific cell surface receptor. Resting T-cells do not express high affinity IL-2R but membrane receptors appear rapidly on T-cells after activation through the antigen receptor. Analysis of the IL-2R was facilitated by a monoclonal anti-IL-2R antibody (anti-Tac)[33] which competes with IL-2 for receptor protein binding sites. Initial receptor binding studies with radiolabelled anti-Tac and IL-2 suggested that activated T-cells express 5 to 20-fold more binding sites for anti-Tac than for IL-2. However, this situation was resolved[34] by the finding that there were two affinity classes of IL-2 receptors. It was found that approximately 10% of the IL-2 receptors bound IL-2 with high affinity ($K_d = 10^{-11}$ mol L$^{-1}$), whereas the remaining receptors had an apparent 1000-fold lower affinity ($K_d = 10^{-8}$ mol L$^{-1}$). Since anti-Tac reacts with both IL-2 binding sites this accounts for the discrepancy between high affinity IL-2 receptors and Tac epitopes. Although IL-2 binding causes a 10-fold up-regulation of the Tac protein, binding of IL-2 to its high affinity receptors actually reduces receptor expression by 20–30%[35]. Recently it has been discovered that the high affinity receptor comprises two non-covalently linked proteins ($\alpha$ and $\beta$ chains)[36].

Resting T-cells, B-cells and macrophages do not display IL-2 receptors. Most T-cells, however, can be induced to express IL-2 receptors by interaction with antigen, mitogen or monoclonal antibodies directed at the T-cell antigen receptor. However, IL-2R expression is not limited to activated T-cells but has been noted on other activated mononuclear cell populations. Normal peripheral blood B-cells stimulated with a range of agents can be induced to express IL-2 receptors. Tac protein has also been detected on monocytes and tissue macrophages such as Kupffer cells in the liver and Langerhans cells in the skin. Interestingly, IL-2R have also been described on oligodendrocytes[37], the myelinating cells of the central nervous system.

## Biological activities of IL-2

As previously mentioned, the major action of IL-2 is to stimulate mitogenesis of activated T-cells. This action may be mediated by translocation of C kinase to the plasma membrane with subsequent phosphorylation of membrane proteins correlated with[38] inhibition of adenylcyclase and increased cell proliferation. By stimulating adenylcyclase, prostaglandins (E series) have the opposite (i.e. inhibitory) effect on T-cell activation. Though IL-2 is a key T-cell growth factor it is not restricted to this role. IL-2 induces other T-cell lymphokines such as $\gamma$-interferon ($\gamma$-IFN)[39]. $\gamma$-IFN has a range of immune functions that include stimulation of natural killer (NK) cell activity, generation of cytotoxic T-lymphocytes, macrophage activation and increased expression of major histocompatibility antigens. The use of anti-Tac strongly inhibits the production of $\gamma$-IFN[40] indicating that this property of IL-2 is also mediated by the IL-2 receptor. IL-2 may play a direct role in stimulating non-T-cell immunity. Studies have shown that IL-2 causes an increase in natural killer (NK) cell activity beyond that attributable to induction of $\gamma$-IFN[41]. IL-2 appears to promote function and possibly also the proliferation of these cells. IL-2 also expands lymphokine activated killer (LAK) cell populations, a property that has been exploited in the treatment of human cancer (see below). IL-2 stimulates B-cell growth indirectly by inducing B-cell growth factors such as IL-4 from T-cells and also directly via IL-2 receptors on B-cells[42]. A variety of activated and transformed B-cells have been found to display IL-2 receptors that are found to be of similar size and affinity to the receptors present on T-cells. A recent report[43] suggests that IL-2 augments the cytotoxicity of human monocytes. This is compatible with the observation that monocytes express IL-2 receptors on their surface[44] and together with the report of IL-2 receptors on oligodendrocytes[37] shows that IL-2 is not exclusively a lymphocytotropic hormone.

IL-2 can be regarded as one of the most important humoral factors in the regulation of cellular immunity and many human disease states are characterized by deficient production and/or responsiveness to IL-2. Decreased production of IL-2 has been described in patients with metastatic cancer[45] and Hodgkin's disease[46]. In chronic inflammatory conditions a deficient production of IL-2 or defective response is seen in chronic active hepatitis[47], systemic lupus erythematosus, rheumatoid arthritis, Sjogren's syndrome[48] and multiple sclerosis[49]. These *in vitro* defects can often be reversed by the addition of exogenous IL-2 or by the removal of suppressor cells[50].

The use of IL-2 as a therapeutic agent in the treatment of cancer has been reviewed by Rosenberg and Lotze[51]. IL-2 can be used therapeutically in a number of regimens. Initially, after IL-2 injection, all lymphoid cells decrease in the peripheral blood but, with continuous administration of IL-2, recovery and then expansion of lymphoid populations occur with total numbers of lymphocytes sometimes increasing 16-fold. A problem with this form of therapy is the toxicity which is usually reversible with the discontinuation of treatment. It is reported that this therapy caused significant tumour shrinkage in a number of melanoma patients. Another form of therapy for cancer uses LAK cells and IL-2. LAK cells are generated *in vitro* by 3 to 5 days incubation of the patient's blood cells with IL-2. The cells are then injected back into the patient along with recombinant IL-2. The use of LAK cells plus IL-2 appears to hold significant promise for the treatment of some forms of human malignancy.

## INTERLEUKIN-3 AND OTHER HAEMATOPOIETIC GROWTH FACTORS

Haematopoietic growth factors or colony stimulating factors (CSFs) are a family of glycoprotein growth factors that control proliferation and differentiation of haemopoietic stem cells and influence functional activities of mature cells[52]. All four CSFs stimulate the formation of haematopoietic colonies in agar cultures. Colony formation is initiated from an undifferentiated blast cell which proliferates and produces differentiated progeny whose phenotype depends on the type of CSF present. The CSFs were originally named after their effects on haematopoietic progenitor cells *in vitro*. Multi-CSF or interleukin-3 (IL-3) is produced by activated T-cells and stimulates proliferation of pluripotent stem cells. GM-CSF (CSF-2), derived from macrophages, T-cells, endothelial cells and fibroblasts, acts on stem cells to produce either granulocytes or monocytes. G-CSF causes granulocyte proliferation and M-CSF (CSF-1) is a growth factor for monocyte precursors[52,53].

## IL-3 molecules

In each case, cDNA encoding biologically active CSF protein has been expressed in *E. coli*. Although the various CSFs interact with, and cause proliferation and differentiation of the same responder cell populations, they possess no obvious structural homology. The gene for human IL-3 has only recently been cloned[54]. Both the IL-3 and GM-CSF genes have been assigned to chromosome 11 within 230 kb of each other[55] and it is possible that the tight linkage facilitates coordinate regulation in activated T-cells. The complete nucleotide sequence of IL-3 contains a single long open reading frame of 456 nucleotides encoding a polypeptide of 152 amino acids. The first nineteen residues form a characteristic signal peptide leaving a mature peptide of 133 amino acids with a predicted MW of 14.6 kDa. Biochemical sizing gives rise to different MW estimates probably due to variable glycosylation. The human IL-3 sequence retains approximately 30% peptide homology with murine IL-3 and the structures of the genes are obviously related, with five exons and two introns of similar size[54]. The following discussion mainly refers to murine IL-3.

## Biological activities of IL-3

Initial observations indicated that T-cells of helper phenotype were the predominant source of IL-3[56]. Confirmation of this has been obtained with cloned T-cell lines from mixed lymphocyte reactions[57] and the lymphoma cell line EL-4. Additionally, IL-3 is produced by the WEHI-3B, myelo-monocytic leukaemia cell line, and rat C6 glioma cells[58]. The latter raises the possibility that production of IL-3 by astrocytes contributes to the development and maintenance of lymphopoietic cells within inflammatory brain lesions.

Experiments with homogenous populations of target cells and with single cells have defined IL-3-responsive target cells. Pure IL-3 directly stimulated the growth of cloned mast cell lines[59] and single isolated haemopoietic stem cells respond to IL-3 by generating macrophages, neutrophils, mast cells and megakaryocytes as well as erythroid colonies. However, the action of IL-3 is not restricted to immature haemopoietic cells. Purified IL-3 stimulates the division of differentiated mast cells and antagonizes the action of γ-interferon in the regulation of major histocompatibility complex (MHC) expression[60]. IL-3 also stimulates peritoneal macrophage division and phagocytosis. At present the bioactivity that distinguishes IL-3 from the other CSFs is the stimulation of colony formation in isolated mast cells and megakaryocytes.

110

## IL-3 effects on mature immune cells

IL-3 has been reported to promote the growth of helper T-cell clones[61] but the findings that thymocytes and T-cells do not possess detectable receptors for IL-3[62], and that thymocytes showed no responses to the molecule argues against a direct action of IL-3 on T-cells. However, the action of IL-3 on mature macrophages, as discussed previously, allows IL-3 to influence immune responses by altering accessory cell function. Evidence for a direct action of IL-3 on B-cells is also lacking though IL-3-dependent pre-B-cells have been isolated from foetal liver[63]. The observations that IL-3 has no effect on the growth and differentiation of mature antigen-stimulated B-cells[64] and that splenic cells do not absorb IL-3 suggests that they do not express IL-3 receptors.

The interaction of IL-3 with its target occurs via a 75 kDa cell surface receptor. The characteristics of CSF receptors have been recently reviewed[62] and it appears that most IL-3 dependent lines possess approximately 1000 IL-3 receptors per cell with a binding affinity between $5 \times 10^{-11}$ and $5 \times 10^{-12}$ mol L$^{-1}$. Consumption of IL-3 at $37°C$ can be blocked by metabolic inhibitors consistent with internalization of receptors. The role of IL-3 in normal human physiology is not yet defined. *In vivo* experiments showed IL-3 effects compatible with its known *in vitro* properties[65]. The effects of IL-3 are usually localized and only intense immunological stimulation such as occurs in graft-*versus*-host disease produces IL-3 in the serum[66]. IL-3 appears to link the immune system with the haemopoietic system to stimulate an adequate production of cells for normal immune function. There is no evidence yet that IL-3 produced by T-cells plays any role in the steady-state production of any haemopoietic cells. Biologically active CSFs are not normally detectable in stromal culture supernatants, but it was recently reported[67] that GM-CSF bound to glycosaminoglycans of the extracellular matrix which might explain its absence in these supernatants.

Aberrant expression of the IL-3 gene may play a role in oncogenesis. Evidence for this has come from three sources. Initially it was noted that the release of IL-3 by the leukaemic cell line WEHI-3B differed from that by T-cells in that it was constitutive rather than inducible and was not accompanied by the secretion of IL-2, GM-GSF or γ-IFN. Secondly, IL-3-dependent mast cell lines grown in the absence of IL-3 occasionally gave rise to colonies that produced and used IL-3 in an autocrine fashion[68] via the cell surface receptor. Further, unlike the parental line, these variants caused a disseminated mast cell leukaemia when injected into syngeneic animals. Finally, viral-induced monocytic leukaemic cells both produce and require IL-3 for growth[53] suggesting that aberrant expression of the IL-3 gene may be involved in leukaemogenesis.

The CSFs may have considerable therapeutic potential and are well-tolerated. GM-CSF induces leukocytosis in monkeys and could perhaps be used both before and after cytoreductive drug therapy to maintain host defence. GM-CSF has also been shown to have macrophage activating functions, promoting tumoricidal activity of macrophages. In addition, the CSFs show some clinical promise in the management of certain parasitic and bacterial infections. Treatment of mice with GM-CSF leads to diminished parasitaemia associated with *Trypanosoma cruzi* infection and also protects mice from an otherwise lethal infection with *Salmonella typhimurium*[69].

## B-CELL GROWTH FACTORS

Both proliferation and differentiation of B-cells are at least partially driven by lymphokine growth factors from activated T-cells[70]. After activation of the resting B-cell by crosslinking of surface IgM (experimentally induced by anti-IgM antibody), B-cells enter the G1 phase of the cell cycle but then need progression factors from other cells to enter the S phase and T-cell products are required to pass through the G2 phase to mitosis[71].

T-cell-derived IL-4 or B-cell stimulating factor-1 (BSF-1) was the first B-cell growth factor (BCGF-1) to be described. The second (BCGF-2) is now called IL-5 or T-cell replacing factor (TRF). A third growth factor, BSF-2 (B-cell stimulating factor-2) has recently been characterized. Molecular cloning of BSF-2 has shown identity with $\beta$2-interferon and this may be given the name interleukin-6.

## INTERLEUKIN-4

IL-4 has had a variety of previous names based on functional characterizations: BSF-1 (B-cell stimulating factor-1); BCDF-$\gamma$ (B-cell differentiation factor-$\gamma$); BCGF-1 (B-cell growth factor-1) and $IgG_1$ induction factor.

It was described originally as a T-cell-derived glycoprotein that augmented proliferation of anti-IgM-activated B-cells[72,73] which are now known to require IL-4 to enter the S phase of the cell cycle[74]. IL-4 alone does activate B-cells[75] but it is more potent as a co-stimulus with antigen or anti-IgM[76].

### IL-4 molecules

Murine[77,78] and human[79] IL-4 cDNA have been cloned and expressed. At the time of writing, chromosome location and genomic sequences have not been published. The IL-4 cDNA consists of a single open reading frame for 153 residues. The N-terminal of the predicted polypeptide is hydrophobic, as expected for a secreted protein. Analysis of hydrophobicity and consensus sequences for processing of signal peptides suggest that the cleavage site of the propeptide is at position 24. The mature polypeptide would then be 129 residues long (predicted MW would be approx. 15 kDa). The molecule has two potential glycosylation sites. Purified native IL-4 was found to be a glycosylated protein with pIs of 6.4, 6.7 and 7.4 on isoelectric focussing which, on SDS-PAGE, showed a major band at 19 kDa with a second at 14 kDa[80]. Comparison of human and mouse IL-4 cDNA revealed that the regions encoding amino acids 1–90 and 129–149 share 50% peptide homology and 70% nucleotide homology. The region 91–128 shows no homology. The 24 N-terminal residues of both purified and recombinant IL-4 were identical[81].

## Biological activities of IL-4

Purified murine IL-4[81] demonstrates species-dependent[82], high-affinity surface binding to many target cells (B-cells, T-cells, mast cells, macrophages, undifferentiated haematopoietic cells).

The number of receptors on resting B- and T-cells was calculated to be about 300 per cell[81], increasing by five- to seven-fold on cell activation. This observation is of particular interest as resting B- and T-cells apparently express *no* high affinity IL-2 receptor[83]. The binding of iodinated murine IL-4 to its receptor is not inhibited by IL-2 or γ-IFN but γ-IFN blocks the action of BSF-1 on resting B-cells[84]. The effects of IL-4 acting alone on resting B-cells include induction of surface class II molecules[85-87] and an increase in cell diameter[88].

IL-4 alone also induces proliferation of some cloned B-cell tumour lines. All of these actions are consistently enhanced in the presence of a polyclonal activator (anti-IgM, Protein A, LPS) or in the case of antigen-primed B-cells, by antigen itself[88].

IL-4 also promotes $IgG_1$[89] and IgE[90] production in B-cells stimulated with LPS and induces low affinity Fc receptors on 40–70% of tonsil B-cells and also on Burkitt's lymphoma lines. This last action occurs at concentrations 10 to 50 times lower than that required to stimulate cellular proliferation[91] and is also enhanced by polyclonal B cell activators and inhibited by γ-IFN.

Cells other than B-cells are targets for IL-4. It has been described as a mast cell growth factor[92] distinct from IL-3 (MCGF-2) and is a T-cell growth factor distinct from IL-2 (TCGF-2)[92-95]. IL-4 induces proliferation of phytohaemagglutinin-activated T-cells and both $T4^+$ and $T8^+$ T-cell clones[94]. This action is not blocked by anti IL-2 or anti-TAC antibody. The effect of IL-4 appears to be weaker and shorter lasting than IL-2 but, unlike IL-2, IL-4 does not select for $T8^+$ cells and $T4^+/T8^+$ ratios remain unchanged after IL-4 stimulation. At suboptimal concentrations IL-4 synergizes with IL-2. IL-4 also induces proliferation of $T3^-$ NK clones but does not induce LAK-cell generation alone or in synergy with IL-2[93].

It has recently been shown that in some murine helper T clones[95] IL-4 can act as an autocrine signal, independently of IL-2 production. Another interesting activity of IL-4 is its reported action on growth and differentiation of precursor cells: recombinant IL-4 promotes differentiation of normal mouse thymic T-cell precursors[96], and apparently acts on haemopoietic cells to produce granulocytes, megakaryocytes and erythroid colonies in soft agar seeded with anti-Thy-1-treated mouse bone marrow[81]. *In vivo*, induction of a T dependent polyclonal $IgG_1$ response in mice[97] was associated with splenic T-cell IL-4 release from day 3 to a peak at day 9. Further, anti-BSF-1 antibody injected into mice, inhibited IgE production during *Nippostrongylus brasiliensis* infection[76].

## INTERLEUKIN-5

As early as 1972, it was noted that B-cell differentiation and proliferation can occur in the absence of T-cells, provided that supernatants of activated T-cells were present[98]. The activity present in these supernatants was called T-cell replacing factor (TRF). TRF action on B-cells is not MHC-restricted[99], but

TRF production (from helper T-cells) occurred only in the presence of H2 compatible antigen-presenting cells. The polypeptide responsible for this activity has been purified and cloned and has been given the name interleukin-5 (IL-5).

## IL-5 molecules

Both human[100] and murine[101] IL-5 cDNAs have been cloned. The murine cDNA was cloned from a library of a T-cell line producing TRF activity and encodes a polypeptide of 133 amino acids, with three possible N-glycosylation sites. There is a 21 residue hydrophobic signal peptide. The secreted polypeptide has a MW of 12.3 kDa. Using this mouse IL-5 cDNA as a probe, cDNA was cloned from a human T-cell leukaemia line. The cloned human DNA encoded human IL-5 propeptide of 134 amino acids (predicted MW 12.84 kDa) containing 22 N-terminal hydrophobic amino acids and two possible N-glycosylation sites with two C-terminal cysteine residues. Nucleotide and amino acid sequences of human and murine IL-5 cDNA are respectively 77% and 70% homologous. The homology is greater in the C-terminal half (80% homology) than in the N-terminal half (66%).

Biochemical characterization of the natural protein was facilitated by the establishment of a T-cell hybrid clone (B.151)[102]: TRF bioactivity was produced by this line[102] and purified to homogeneity[103]. It was characterized as a molecule of 50–60 kDa[102] on gel chromatography and 18 kDa in denaturing conditions (SDS-PAGE). The molecule was highly hydrophobic, glycosylated and trypsin-sensitive.

## Biological activities of IL-5

IL-5 is the molecule responsible for TRF activity[100] – a B-cell growth factor (BCGF-2) distinct from IL-4. It also co-purifies (and may be identical) with Eosinophil Differentiation Factor (EDF)[104,105]. IL-5 can therefore be tested in bioassays for either TRF or BCGF-2. TRF activity is measured in antibody-production experiments where T-cells are limiting. This usually involves either induction of anti-DNP IgG plaque-forming cells (in B-cells from DNP/KLH treated mice) or induction of IgM-PFC in BCL$_1$ (murine B-cell chronic leukaemia line). BCGF-2 activity is usually assayed as induction of proliferation of the BCL$_1$ cell line, or proliferation of purified normal B-cells in the presence of dextran sulphate.

Both TRF and BCGF-2 activity are expressed by the recombinant IL-5 product, matching data obtained with purified natural TRF[102]: TRF and BCGF-2 were not separable by various purification procedures and removal of TRF by absorption on BCL$_1$ cells was accompanied by BCGF-2 removal. A monoclonal antibody blocking TRF activity always blocked BCGF-2 activity[102]. Most reports indicate that the mitogenic effect of IL-5 on B-cells is dependent on co-stimulation of B-cells through their surface IgM (see Table 6.4)[106].

114

Table 6.4   Effects of interleukins on antigen-specific B-cells (based on Refs. 64, 88)

| | Interleukin alone | | Interleukin + antigen | |
|---|---|---|---|---|
| | Proliferation | Antibody formation | Proliferation | Antibody formation |
| IL-1 | − | ± | + + | + + |
| IL-2 | − | ± | + + | + + |
| IL-3 | − | − | ± | ± |
| IL-4 | + + | ± | + + + | ± |
| IL-5 | − | ± | + + + | + + + |
| Medium | − | − | ± | ± |

## Candidates for future interleukins?

In the most recent literature, several leukocyte peptides with actions on the immune system have been described. These include a T-cell factor that induces IL-1[107], a B-cell product that inhibits lymphocyte Fc receptor expression[108] and the proposed IL-6, a factor identified variously as BSF-2 (B-cell stimulating factor-2), IFN-$\beta$2 (interferon-$\beta$2) or HPGF (hybridoma-plasmacytoma growth factor)[109] or HSF (hepatocyte simulating factor). Human BSF-2 has now been cloned[110]. This factor is constitutively produced by HTLV-1 infected human T-cell lines, cardiac myxoma cells and a bladder carcinoma line (T24). BSF-2 induces Ig production in Epstein-Barr virus-transformed B-cell lines[111].

## CONCLUSIONS

The number of well-characterized cytokines is growing. To be designated an 'interleukin', cytokines of known peptide sequence should be produced by leukocytes and have a role in inflammation. Interleukin-1 has many pro-inflammatory and catabolic activities as well as providing a powerful co-stimulus for lymphocyte production of lymphokine growth factors and their receptors (e.g. IL-2,3,4 and 5). IL-1 therefore acts as a common mediator of inflammation and specific immunity. The availability of nucleotide probes, recombinant interleukins, receptor proteins and monoclonal antibodies should ensure rapid progress in defining the interactions among cytokines that are important in normal homeostasis and the pathogenesis of inflammatory and immune diseases.

## References

1. Aarden, L.A., Brunner, T.K., Cerottini, J.C. et al. (1979). Revised nomenclature for antigen-non-specific T cell proliferation and helper factors (letter). J. Immunol., 123, 2928−9
2. Oppenheim, J.J. and Gery, I. (1982). Interleukin 1 is more than an interleukin. Immunol. Today., 3, 113−19
3. Pettipher, E.R., Higgs, G.A. and Henderson, B. (1986). Interleukin 1 induces leukocyte infiltration and cartilage proteoglycan degradation in the synovial joint. Proc. Natl. Acad. Sci. USA, 83, 8749−53
4. Gery, I., Gershon, R.K. and Waksman, B.H. (1972). Potentiation of the T-lymphocyte response to mitogens. I. The responding cell. J. Exp. Med., 136, 128−42

5. Durum, S.K., Schmidt, J.A. and Oppenheim, J.J. (1985). Interleukin 1: an immunological perspective. In Paul, W.E., Fathman, C.G. and Metzger, H. (eds.) *Annual Review of Immunology*. pp. 263–87. (California: Annual Reviews Inc)
6. Dinarello, C.A. (1986). Interleukin-1: Amino acid sequences, multiple biological activities and comparison with tumour necrosis factor (cachectin). In Cruse, J.M., Lewis, R.E. and Jackson, M. (eds.) *The Year in Immunology*. Vol. 2, pp. 68–89. (Basel: Karger)
7. Dinarello, C.A., Cannon, J.G., Mier, J.W., Bernheim, H.A., LoPreste, G., Lynn, D.L., Love, R.N., Webb, A.C., Auron, P.E., Reuben, R.C., Rich, A., Wolff, S.M. and Putney, S.D. (1986). Multiple biological activities of human recombinant interleukin 1. *J. Clin. Invest.*, **77**, 1734–9
8. Furutani, Y., Notake, M., Yamayoshi, M., Yamagishi, J., Nomura, H., Ohue, M., Fukui, T., Yamada, M. and Nakamura, S. (1985). Cloning and characterizaton of the cDNAs for human and rabbit interleukin-1 precursor. *Nucl. Acids Res.*, **13**, 5869–82
9. Lomedico, P., Gubler, U., Hellman, C.P., Dukovitch, M., Giri, J.G., Pan, Y.E., Collier, K., Semionow, R., Chua, A.O. and Mizel, S.B. (1984). Cloning and expression of murine interleukin 1 cDNA in *Escherichia coli. Nature*, **312**, 458–62
10. Rosenwasser, L.J., Webb, A.C., Clark, B.D., Ihrie, S., Dinarello, C.A., Gehrk, L., Wolff, S.M., Rich, A. and Auron, P.E. (1986). Expression of biologically active human interleukin 1 subpeptides by transfected simian COS cells. *Proc. Natl. Acad. Sci. USA*, **83**, 5243–46
11. Furutani, Y., Notake, M., Fukui, T., Ohue, M., Nomura, H., Yamada, M. and Nakamura, S. (1986). Complete nucleotide sequence of the gene for human interleukin-1α. *Nucl. Acids Res.*, **14**, 3167–79
12. Clark, B.D., Collins, K.L., Gandy, M.S., Webb, A.C. and Auron, P.E. (1986). Genomic sequence for human pro-interleukin-1β – possible evolution from a reverse transcribed pro-interleukin-1α gene. *Nucl. Acids Res.*, **14**, 7897–914
13. Telford, J.L., Macchia, G., Massone, A., Carinci, V., Palla, E. and Melli, E. (1986). The murine interleukin-1β gene: structure and evolution. *Nucl. Acids. Res.*, **14**, 9955–63
14. Bensi, G., Raugei, G., Palla, E., Carinci, V., Buonamassa, D. and Melli, M. (1987). Human interleukin-1β gene. *Gene*, **52**, 95–101
15. Perlmutter, D.H., Goldberger, G., Dinarello, C.A., Mizel, S.B. and Colton, H.R. (1986). Regulation of class III major histocompatibility complex gene products by interleukin 1. *Science*, **232**, 850–2
16. Krane, S.M. (1987). Modulation of matrix synthesis and degradation in joint inflammation. Presented at the *Strangeways Research Laboratory 75th Anniversary Symposium*, April 6–8, Cambridge
17. Warner, S.J., Auger, K.R. and Libby, P. (1987). Human interleukin 1 induces interleukin 1 gene expression in human vascular smooth muscle cells. *J. Exp. Med.*, **165**, 1316–31
18. Bevilacquea, M.P., Pober, J.S., Majeau, G.R., Contran, R.S. and Gimbrone, M.A. (1984). Interleukin 1 (IL1) induced biosynthesis and cell surface expression of procoagulation activity in human vascular endothelial cells. *J. Exp. Med.*, **160**, 618–23
19. Lowenthal, J.W., Cerottini, J.C. and MacDonald, H.R. (1986). Interleukin 1 dependent induction of both interleukin 2 secretion and interleukin 2 receptor expression by thymoma cells. *J. Immunol.*, **137**, 1226–31
20. Di Giovine, F., Malawista, S.E., Nuki, G. and Duff, G.W. (1987). Interleukin 1 (IL-1) as a mediator of crystal arthritis. Stimulation of T cell and synovial fibroblast mitogenesis by urate crystal-induced IL-1. *J. Immunol.*, **138**, 3213–8
21. March, C.J., Mosley, B., Larsen, A., Cerretti, D.P., Braedt, G., Price, V., Gillis, S., Henney, C., Kronheim, S.R., Grabstein, K., Conlon, P.J., Hopp, T.P. and Cosman, D. (1985). Cloning, sequence and expression of two distinct human interleukin 1 complementary DNAs. *Nature*, **315**, 641–7
22. Dinarello, C.A., Cannon J.G., Wolff, S.M., Bernheim, H.A., Beutler, B., Cerami, A., Figari, I.S., Palladino, M.A. and O'Connor, J.V. (1986). Tumor necrosis factor (cachectin) is an endogenous pyrogen and induces production of interleukin 1. *J. Exp. Med.*, **163**, 1433–50
23. Gery, I., Davies, P., Derr, J., Kreh, N. and Barranger, J.A. (1981). Relationship between production and release of lymphocyte-activating factor (interleukin 1) by murine macrophages. I. Effects of various agents. *Cell Immunol.*, **64**, 293–303
24. Dower, S.K., Kronheim, S.R., March, C.J., Conlon, P.J., Hopp, T.D., Gillis, S. and Vral, D. (1985). Detection and characterisation of high affinity plasma membrane receptors for human interleukin 1. *J. Exp. Med.*, **162**, 501–15

25. Bird, T.A. and Saklatvala, J. (1986). Identification of a common class of high affinity receptors for both types of porcine interleukin-1 on connective tissue cells. *Nature*, **324**, 263–6

26. Mosley, B., Urdal, D.L., Prickett, K.S., Larsen, A., Cosman, D., Conlon, P.J., Gillis, S. and Dower, S.K. (1987). The interleukin 1 receptor binds the human interleukin-1α precursor but not the interleukin-1β precursor. *J. Biol. Chem.*, **262**, 2941–4

27. Lowenthal, J.W. and MacDonald, H.R. (1986). Binding and internalization of interleukin 1 by T cells. Direct evidence for high- and low-affinity classes of interleukin 1 receptor. *J. Exp. Med.*, **164**, 1060–74

28. Gillis, S., Ferm, M.M., Ou, W. and Smith, K.A. (1978). T cell growth factor: Parameters of production and a quantitative microassay for activity. *J. Immunol.*, **120**, 2027–32

29. Pfizenmaier, K., Scheurich, P., Daukener, W., Kronke, M., Rollinghoff, M. and Wagner, H. (1984). Quantitative representation of all T cells committed to develop into cytotoxic effector cells and/or interleukin 2 activity-producing helper cells within murine T lymphocyte subsets. *Eur. J. Immunol.*, **14**, 33–9

30. Robb, R.J. and Smith, K.A. (1981). Heterogeneity of human T-cell growth factor(s) due to variable glycosilation. *Mol. Immunol.*, **18**, 1087–94

31. Taniguchi, T., Matsui, H., Fujita, T., Takaoka, C., Kashima, N., Yoshimoto, R. and Hamuro, J. (1983). Structure and expression of a cloned cDNA for human interleukin-2. *Nature*, **302**, 305–10

32. Mita, S., Maeda, S. and Shimada, K. (1986). Characterization of human genomic DNA sequences homologous to the interleukin 2 cDNA. *Biochem. Biophys. Res. Commun.*, **138**, 966–73

33. Uchiyama, T., Broder, S. and Waldmann, T.A. (1981). A monoclonal antibody (anti-Tac) reactive with activated and functionally mature human T cells. 1. Production of anti-Tac monoclonal antibody and distribution of Tac ( + ) cells. *J. Immunol.*, **126**, 1393–7

34. Robb, R.J., Greene W.C. and Rusk, C.M. (1984). Low and high affinity cellular receptors for interleukin 2. Implications for the level of Tac antigen. *J. Exp. Med.*, **160**, 1126–46

35. Smith, K.A. and Cantrell, D.A. (1985). Interleukin 2 regulates its own receptors. *Proc. Natl. Acad. Sci. USA*, **82**, 864–8

36. Smith, K.A. (1987). The two-chain structure of high-affinity IL-2 receptors. *Immunol. Today*, **8**, 11–13

37. Benveniste, E.N. and Merrill, J.E. (1986). Stimulation of oligodendroglial proliferation and maturation by interleukin-2. *Nature*, **321**, 610–13

38. Farrar, W.L. and Taguchi, M. (1985). Stimulation of protein kinase C membrane association: evidence for IL-2 receptor phosphorylation. *Lymphokine Res.*, **4**, 87–93

39. Farrar, W.L., Johnson, M.M. and Farrar, J.J. (1981). Regulation of the production of immune interferon and cytotoxic T lymphocytes by interleukin-2. *J. Immunol.*, **126**, 1120–5

40. Vilcek, J., Henriksen-DeStefano, D., Siegel, D., Klion, A., Robb, R.J. and Le, J. (1985). Regulation of IFN-γ induction in human peripheral blood cells by exogenous and endogenously produced interleukin 2. *J. Immunol.*, **135**, 1851–6

41. Henney, C.S., Kuribayashi, K., Kern, D.E. and Gillis, S. (1981). Interleukin 2 augments natural killer cell activity. *Nature*, **291**, 335–7

42. Mingari, M.C., Gerosa, F., Carra, G., Accolla, R.S., Moretta, A., Zubler, R.H., Waldmann, T.A. and Moretta, L. (1984). Human interleukin-2 promotes proliferation of activated B cells via surface receptors similar to those of activated T cells. *Nature*, **312**, 641–3

43. Malkovsky, M., Loveland, B., North, M., Asherson, G.L., Garo, L., Ward, P. and Fiers, W. (1987). Recombinant interleukin-2 directly augments the cytotoxicity of human monocytes. *Nature*, **325**, 262–5

44. Herrmann, F., Cannistra, S.A., Levine, H. and Griffin, J.D. (1985). Expression of interleukin 2 receptors and binding of interleukin 2 by γ-interferon-induced human leukemic and normal monocytic cells. *J. Exp. Med.*, **162**, 1111–16

45. Nakayama, E., Asano, S., Takuwa, N., Yokota, J. and Miwa, S. (1983). Decreased TCGF activity in the culture medium of PHA stimulated peripheral mononuclear cells from patients with metastatic cancer. *Clin. Exp. Immunol.*, **51**, 511–16

46. Zamkoff, K.W., Reeves, W.G., Paolozzi, F.P., Poiesz, B.J., Comis, R.L. and Tomar, R.H. (1985). Impaired interleukin regulation of the phytohemagglutinin response in Hodgkin's disease. *Clin. Immunol. Immunopathol.*, **35**, 111–24

117

47. Yoshioka, K., Kakumu, S., Murakami, H. and Fukui, K. (1984). Interleukin 2 activity in chronic active liver diseases: response by T cells and in the autologous mixed lymphocyte reaction. *Clin. Exp. Immunol.*, **54**, 668–76
48. Miyasaka, N., Nakamura, T., Russell, I.J. and Talal, N. (1984). Interleukin 2 deficiencies in rheumatoid arthritis and systemic lupus erythematosus. *Clin. Immunol. Immunopathol.*, **31**, 109–17
49. Merrill, J.E., Mohlstrom, C., Uittenbogaart, C., Kermani-Arab, V., Ellison, G.W. and Myers, L.W. (1984). Response to and production of interleukin 2 by peripheral blood and cerebrospinal fluid lymphocytes of patients with multiple sclerosis. *J. Immunol.*, **133**, 1931–7
50. Linker-Israeli, M., Bakke, A.C., Quismorio, F.P. and Horwitz, D.A. (1985). Correction of interleukin-2 production in patients with systemic lupus erythematosus by removal of spontaneously activated suppressor cells. *J. Clin. Invest.*, **75**, 762–8
51. Rosenberg, S.A. and Lotze, M.T. (1986). Cancer immunotherapy using interleukin-2 and interleukin-2-activated lymphocytes. In Paul, W.E., Fathman, C.G. and Metzger, H. (eds.) *Annual Review of Immunology.* pp. 681–709. (California: Annual Reviews Inc.)
52. Metcalf, D. (1985). The granulocyte–macrophage colony-stimulating factors. *Science*, **229**, 16–22
53. Schrader, J.W. (1986). The panspecific hemopoietin of activated T lymphocytes (interleukin 3). In Paul, W.E., Fathman, C.G. and Metzger, H. (eds.) *Annual Review of Immunology.* pp. 205–230. (California: Annual Reviews Inc.)
54. Yang, Y.C., Ciarletta, A.B., Temple, P.A., Chung, M.P., Kovacic, S., Witek-Giannotti, J.S., Leary, A.C., Kriz, R., Donahue, R.E., Wong, G.G. and Clark, S.C. (1986). Human IL-3 (multi-CSF): Identification by expression cloning of a novel hematopoietic growth factor related to murine IL-3. *Cell*, **47**, 3–10
55. Barlow, D.P., Bucan, M., Lehrach, H., Hogan, B.L.M. and Gough, N.M. (1987). Close genetic and physical linkage between murine haemopoietic growth factor genes GM-CSF and multi-CSF (IL-3). *EMBO J*, **6**, 617–23
56. Ihle, J.N., Lee, J.C. and Rebar, L. (1981). T cell recognition of Moloney leukemia virus proteins. III T cell proliferative responses against gp 70 are associated with the production of a lymphokine inducing 20 alpha hydroxysteroid dehydrogenase in splenic lymphocytes. *J. Immunol.*, **127**, 2565–70
57. Glasebrook, A.L. and Fitch, F.W. (1980). Alloreactive T cell lines. I. Interactions between cloned amplifier and cytotoxic T cell lines. *J. Exp. Med.*, **151**, 876–95
58. Frei, K., Bodmer, S., Schwerdel, C. and Fontana, A. (1985). Astrocytes of the brain synthesize interleukin-3-like factors. *J. Immunol.*, **135**, 4044–7
59. Clark-Lewis, I., Kent, S.B.H. and Schrader, J.W. (1984). Purification to apparent homogeneity of a factor stimulating the growth of multiple lineages of haemopoietic cells. *J. Biol. Chem.*, **259**, 7488–94
60. Wong, G.H.W., Clark-Lewis, I., Hamilton, J.A. and Schrader, J.W. (1984). P-cell stimulating factor and glucocorticoids oppose the action of interferon-γ in inducing Ia antigens on T-dependent mast cells (P cells). *J. Immunol.*, **133**, 2043–50
61. Hapel, A.J., Lee, J.C., Farrar, W.L. and Ihle, J.N. (1981). Establishment of continuous cultures of Thy-1.2$^+$ Lyt-1$^+$,2$^-$ T cells with purified interleukin-3. *Cell*, **25**, 179–86
62. Nicola, N.A. (1987). Why do haemopoietic growth factor receptors interact with each other? *Immunol. Today*, **8**, 134–40
63. Palacios, R., Henson, G., Steinmetz, M. and McKearn, J.P. (1984). Interleukin-3 supports growth of mouse pre-B-cell clones *in vitro. Nature*, **309**, 126–31
64. Pike, B.L. and Nossal, G.J.V. (1985). A high efficiency cloning system for single hapten-specific B lymphocytes that is suitable for assay of putative growth and differentiation factors. *Proc. Natl. Acad. Sci. USA*, **82**, 3395–9
65. Crapper, R.M., Clark-Lewis, I. and Schrader, J.W. (1984). The *in vivo* functions and properties of persisting cell stimulating factor. *Immunology*, **53**, 33–42
66. Crapper, R.M. and Schrader, J.W. (1986). Evidence for the *in vivo* production and release into the serum of a T cell lymphokine, persisting-cell stimulating factor (PSF) during graft-vs-host reactions. *Immunology*, **57**, 553–8
67. Gordon, M.Y., Riley, G.P., Watt, S.M. and Greaves, M.F. (1987). Compartmentalization of a haematopoietic growth factor (GM-CSF) by glycosaminoglycans in the bone marrow microenvironment. *Nature*, **326**, 403–5

68. Schrader, J.W and Crapper, R.M. (1983). Autogenous production of a hemopoietic growth factor 'P cell stimulating factor' as a mechanism for transformation of bone-marrow derived cells. *Proc. Natl. Acad. Sci. USA*, **80**, 6892–6
69. Henney, C. (1986). Therapeutic potential for colony stimulating factors. Presented at the conference on *Cytokines and Other Mediators in Inflammatory Diseases*, December 1–2, London
70. Kishimoto, T. (1985). Factors affecting B-cell growth and differentiation. In Paul, W.E., Fathman, C.G. and Metzger, H. (eds.), *Annual Review of Immunology*, pp. 133–57. (California: Annual Reviews Inc.)
71. Melchers, F. and Andersson, J. (1986). Factors controlling the B-cell cycle. In Paul, W.E., Fathman, C.G. and Metzger, H. (eds.), *Annual Review of Immunology*, pp. 13–36. (California: Annual Reviews Inc.)
72. Howard, M., Farrar, J., Hilfiker, M., Johnson, B., Takatsu, K., Hamaoka, T. and Paul, W.E. (1982). Identification of a T-cell-derived B cell growth factor distinct from interleukin 2. *J. Exp. Med.*, **155**, 914–23
73. Ohara, J., Lahet, S., Inman, J. and Paul, W.E. (1985). Partial purification of murine B cell stimulatory factor (BSF)-1. *J. Immunol.*, **135**, 2518–23
74. Muraguchi, A., Kasahara, T., Oppenheim, J.J. and Fauci, A.S. (1982). B cell growth factor and T cell growth factor produced by mitogen stimulated normal human peripheral blood T lymphocytes are distinct molecules. *J. Immunol.*, **129**, 2486–9
75. Rabin, E.M., Ohara, J. and Paul, W.E. (1985). B cell stimulatory factor 1 activates resting B cells. *Proc. Natl. Acad. Sci. USA*, **82**, 2935–9
76. Oliver, K., Noelle, R.J., Uhr, J.W., Krammer, P.H. and Vitetta, E.S. (1985). B cell growth factor (B cell growth factor 1 or B cell-stimulating factor provisional 1) is a differentiating factor for resting B cells and may not induce cell growth. *Proc. Natl. Acad. Sci. USA*, **80**, 2465–7
77. Noma, Y., Sideras, P., Naito, T., Bergstedt-Lindqvist, S., Azuma, C., Severinson, E., Tanabe, T., Kinashi, T., Matsuda, F., Yaoita, Y. and Honjo, T. (1986). Cloning of cDNA encoding the murine IgG1 induction factor by a novel strategy using SP6 promoter. *Nature*, **319**, 640–6
78. Lee, F., Yokota, T., Otsuka, T., Meyerson, P., Villaret, D., Coltman, R., Mosmann, T., Rennick, D., Roehm, N. and Smith, C. (1986). Isolation and characterization of a mouse interleukin cDNA clone that expresses B cell stimulatory factor 1 activities and T cell and mast cell stimulating activities. *Proc. Natl. Acad. Sci. USA*, **83**, 2061–5
79. Yokota, T., Otsuka, T., Mosmann, T., Banchereau, J., DeFrance, T., Blanchard, D., Vries, J.E., Lee, F. and Arai, K.I. (1986). Isolation and characterization of human interleukin cDNA clone, homologous to mouse B-cell stimulatory factor 1, that express B cell and T cell stimulating activities. *Proc. Natl. Acad. Sci. USA*, **83**, 5894–8
80. Farrar, J.J., Howard, M., Fuller-Farrar, J. and Paul, W.E. (1983). Biochemical and physicochemical characterisation of mouse B cell growth factor: a lymphokine distinct from interleukin 2. *J. Immunol.*, **131**, 1838–42
81. Ohara, J. and Paul, W.E. (1987). Receptors for B-cell stimulating factor-1 expressed on cells of haematopoietic lineage. *Nature*, **325**, 537–40
82. Mosmann, T.R., Yokota, T., Kastelein, R., Zurawski, S.M., Arai, N. and Takebe, Y. (1987). Species-specificity of T cell stimulating activities of IL 2 and BSF-1 (IL-4): comparison of normal and recombinant, mouse and human IL 2 and BSF-1 (IL-4). *J. Immunol.*, **138**, 1813–16
83. Vitetta, E.S., Brooks, K., Chen, Y.W., Isakson, P., Jones, S., Layton, J., Mishra, G.C., Pure, E., Weiss, E., Word, C., Yuan, D., Tucker, P., Uhr, J.W. and Krammer, P.H. (1984). T cell derived lymphokines that induce IgM and IgG secretion in activated murine B cells. *Immunol. Rev.*, **78**, 137–57
84. Rabin, E.M., Mond, J.J., Ohara, J. and Paul, W.E. (1986). Interferon gamma inhibits the action of B cell stimulatory factor (BSF)-1 on resting B cells. *J. Immunol.*, **137**, 1573–6
85. Noelle, R., Krammer, P.H., Ohara, J., Uhr, J.W. and Vitetta, E.S. (1984). Increased expression of Ia antigens on resting B cells: an additional role for B cell growth factor. *Proc. Natl. Acad. Sci. USA*, **81**, 6149–53
86. Roehm, N.W., Leibson, H.J., Zlotnik, A., Kappler, J., Marrack, P. and Cambier, J.C. (1984). Interleukin induced increase in Ia expression by normal mouse B cells. *J. Exp. Med.*, **160**, 679–94

87. Yokota, T., Otsuka, T., Takebe, Y., Mosmann, T., Banchereau, J., DeVries, J., Arai, N., Miyaijima, A., Lee, F. and Arai, K. (1987). Isolation and characterisation of mouse and human IL-4 genes that express B cell, T cell and mast cell stimulating activities. *Lymphokine Res.*, **6**, 1817A

88. Alderson, M.R., Pike, B.L. and Nossal, G.J.V. (1987). Effects of antigens and lymphokines on early activation of single hapten-specific B lymphocytes. *J. Immunol.*, **138**, 1056–63

89. Vitetta, E.S., Ohara, J., Myers, C.D., Layton, J.E., Krammer, P.H. and Paul, W.E. (1985). Serological, biochemical and functional identity of B cell-stimulatory factor 1 and B cell differentiation factor for $IgG_1$. *J. Exp. Med.*, **162**, 1726–31

90. Coffman, R.L. and Carty, J. (1986). A T cell activity that enhances polyclonal IgE production and its inhibition by interferon-$\gamma$. *J. Immunol.*, **136**, 949–54

91. Banchereau, J., DeFrance, T., Rousset, F., Aubry, J.P., Vaubervliet, B., Bonnefoy, J.Y., Arai, N., Takebe, Y., Yokota, T., Lee, F., Arai, K. and de Vries, J.E. (1987). The pleiotropic effects of recombinant human IL-4 on B lymphocytes. *Lymphokine Res.*, **6**, 1816A

92. Mosmann, T.R., Bond, M.W., Coffman, R.H., Ohara, J. and Paul, W.E. (1986). T cell and mast cell lines respond to B cell stimulatory factor 1. *Proc. Natl. Acad. Sci. USA*, **83**, 5654–8

93. Hu-Li, J., Shevach, E.M., Mizuguchi, J., Ohara, J., Mosmann, T. and Paul, W.E. (1987). B cell stimulatory factor 1 (interleukin 4) is a potent costimulant for normal resting T lymphocytes. *J. Exp. Med.*, **165**, 157–72

94. Spits, H., Yssel, H., Aray, K., Takebe, Y., Yokota, T., Lee, F., Arai, N., Banchereau, J. and de Vries, J.E. (1987). The effects of recombinant human IL-4 on T cells. *Lymphokine Res.*, **6**, 1815A

95. Lichtman, A.H., Kurt-Jones, E.A. and Abbas, A.K. (1987). B cell stimulatory factor 1 and not interleukin 2 is the autocrine growth factor for some helper T lymphocytes. *Proc. Natl. Acad. Sci. USA*, **84**, 824–7

96. Palacios, R., Sideras, P. and von Boehmer, H. (1987). Recombinant interleukin 4/BSF-1 promotes growth and differentiation of intrathymic T cell precursors from fetal mice *in vitro*. *EMBO J*, **6**, 91–5

97. Finkelman, F.D., Ohara, J., Goroff, D.K., Smith, J., Villacreses, N., Mond, J.J. and Paul, W.E. (1986). Production of BSF-1 during all *in vivo* T-dependent immune response. *J. Immunol.*, **137**, 2878–85

98. Schimpl, A. and Wecker, E. (1972). Replacement of T cell function by a T cell product. *Nature*, **237**, 15–17

99. Takatsu, K., Tominaga, A. and Hamaoka, T. (1980). Antigen-induced T cell-replacing factor (TRF). I. Functional characterization. *J. Immunol.*, **124**, 2414–22

100. Azuma, C., Tanabe, T., Konishi, M., Kinash, T., Noma, T., Matsuda, F., Yaoita, Y., Takatsu, K., Hammarstrom, L., Smith, C.I., Severinson, E. and Honjo, T. (1986). Cloning of cDNA for human T cell-replacing factor (interleukin 5) and comparison with the murine homologue. *Nucl. Acids Res.*, **14**, 9149–58

101. Kinashi, T., Harada, N., Severinson, E., Tanabe, T., Sideras, P., Konishi, M., Azuma, C., Tominaga, A., Bergstedt-Lindqvist, S., Takahashi, M., Matsuda, F., Yaoita, Y., Takatsu, K. and Honjo, T. (1986). Cloning of complementary DNA encoding T-cell replacing factor and identity with B-cell growth factor II. *Nature*, **324**, 70–3

102. Harada, N., Kikuchi, Y., Tominaga, A., Takaki, S. and Takatsu, K. (1985). BCGF II activity on activated B cells of a purified murine T cell-replacing factor (TRF) from a T cell hybridoma (B151K12). *J. Immunol.*, **134**, 3944–51

103. Takatsu, K., Harada, N., Hara, Y., Takahama, Y., Yamada, G., Dobashi, K. and Hamaoka, T. (1985). Purification and physiochemical characterisation of murine T cell replacing factor (TRF). *J. Immunol.*, **134**, 382–9

104. Sanderson, C.J., Warren, D.J. and Strath, M. (1985). Identification of a lymphokine that stimulates eosinophil differentiation *in vitro*. *J. Exp. Med.*, **162**, 60–79

105. Sanderson, C.J., O'Garra, A., Warren, D.J. and Klaus, G.G. (1986). Eosinophil differentiation factor also has B cell growth factor activity-proposed name interleukin 4. *Proc. Natl. Acad. Sci. USA*, **83**, 437–40

106. Swain, S.L., Kubota, E., Heistrom, H. and Dutton, R.W. (1987). Roles of antigen, direct T-B interaction and BCGF II in proliferation and differentiation of B cells. *Lymphokine Res.*, **6**, 1803A

107. Takacs, L., Berzofsky, J.A., York-Jolley, J., Akahoshi, T., Blasi, E. and Durum, S.K. (1987). IL-1 induction by murine T cell clones: detection of an IL-1 inducing lymphokine. *J. Immunol.*, **138**, 2124–31

108. Del Guercio, P., Zanetti, M., Del Guercio, M.F. and Katz, D.H. (1985). B lymphocyte regulation of the immune system. II Inhibition of Fc receptor expression of lymphocytes by BEF, a lymphokine of B cell origin. *J. Immunol.*, **134**, 3926–33

109. Billiau, A. (1987). Interferon $\beta 2$ as a promoter of growth and differentiation of B cells. *Immunol. Today*, **8**, 84–7

110. Hirano, T., Yasukawa, K., Harada, H., Taga, T., Watanabe, Y., Matsuda, T., Kashiwamura, S., Nakajima, K., Koyama, K., Iwamatsu, A., Tsunasawa, S., Sakiyama, F., Matsui, H., Takahara, Y., Taniguchi, T. and Kishimoto, T. (1986). Complementary DNA for a novel human interleukin (BSF-2) that induces B lymphocytes to produce immunoglobulin. *Nature*, **324**, 73–6

111. Zilberstein, A., Ruggieri, R., Korn, J.H. and Revel, M. (1986). Structure and expression of cDNA and genes for human interferon beta 2, a distinct species inducible by growth stimulatory cytokines. *EMBO J.*, **5**, 2529–37

# 7
# The role of IgA in the immunopathogenesis of rheumatoid arthritis

D. R. STANWORTH

## INTRODUCTION

It is now widely accepted that immunological responses play a significant role in the pathogenesis of rheumatoid arthritis.

At the cellular level, there is no doubt about the involvement of lymphoid cells, widespread infiltration by lymphocytes and plasma cells with perivascular follicle formation being a characteristic histological feature of rheumatoid arthritis synovium[1]. Moreover, immunohistochemical analysis of such tissue sections reveals evidence of substantial cellular production of IgG, IgM and IgA: as many as 15–20% of plasma cells staining with FITC-aggregated IgG, when the lymphocyte infiltration is intense[2]. On the other hand, the roles of other types of lymphocytic (K and NK cells, cytotoxic T-cells, etc.) and phagocytic cells in rheumatoid arthritis are less well defined, despite various claims as to their importance in the pathogenesis of this condition. It is, however, widely assumed that polymorphonuclear leukocytes (neutrophils) and macrophages (tissue and circulating) play important roles in the initiation of inflammatory responses in rheumatoid patients' joints as a result of involvement in free radical formation and the release of tissue-degrading lysosomal enzymes – in response to stimulation by immune complexes and other ligands (such as the C3a and C5a products of alternative complement pathway activation).

At the humoral level, both antigen–antibody complexes and anti-γ-globulins (IgM and IgG rheumatoid factors) have been implicated in the pathogenesis of rheumatoid arthritis: the binding of the latter by the former supposedly enhancing their capacity to activate the classical complement pathway, thereby increasing their deleterious properties[3,4]. Furthermore, IgG rheumatoid factor has been shown capable of self-associating to form IgG complexes[5]. Yet, despite numerous attempts, a convincing case has never been made for a central pathological role for such immune complexes in rheumatoid arthritis nor, indeed, for rheumatoid factors, despite the continued practice of employing the Waaler-Rose assay (or an equivalent latex agglutination test) as a laboratory diagnostic indicator in rheumatology departments.

The argument will be developed in this chapter that, as far as the role of humoral immunoglobulin factors in the pathogenesis of rheumatoid arthritis is concerned, too much attention has been focussed on the wrong immunoglobulins and that it is changes in IgA, and particularly the capacity of a proportion of molecules of this isotype synthesized by rheumatoid patients, to form a covalently linked complex with $\alpha_1$-antitrypsin ($\alpha_1 AT$), which is of far greater significance in this respect. For not only does the circulating level of such complexes provide a highly relevant and reliable disease marker, but they have been shown to be capable of initiating the cytolytic release of deleterious lysosomal enzymes from macrophages both *in vitro* and *in vivo* − whilst suppression of their formation by D-penicillamine and gold treatment offers a plausible explanation of the mode of action of these second line antirheumatic compounds.

## MONOMERIC IgA IN RHEUMATOID ARTHRITIS

### Changes in total IgA level

*Hypergammaglobulinaemia*
Apart from its production in neoplastic disorders involving IgA-producing cells, i.e. IgA myelomatoses[6], IgA can be produced (or lost) in large amounts secondarily to local infection or inflammation of the mucous membranes[7].

The total serum IgA levels of patients with chronic rheumatoid arthritis are quite often found to be abnormally high. For instance, seven out of 15 such patients studied in Birmingham some years ago[8] fell into this category, possessing levels in excess of $4.5\,g\,L^{-1}$. In a later study, on a larger group of 58 patients, the mean serum IgA level was found to be $4.55 \pm 3.07\,g\,L^{-1}$ and the range of serum values recorded was $0.96-12.75\,g\,L^{-1}$, the upper limit being over six times the mean normal adult serum value determined at the same time from measurement of total IgA levels in 24 healthy blood donors' sera (as will be seen from Table 7.1). In comparison, the serum IgA levels of 47 patients with 'early' rheumatoid arthritis (who had never been treated with second line antirheumatic drugs) ranged from $0.00-6.56\,gL^{-1}$, with a mean value (of $2.57 \pm 1.33\,g\,L^{-1}$), not significantly higher than that of a normal group.

Interestingly, we found the IgA levels in the joint fluids of 29 patients with chronic arthritis were comparable to those of normal adult sera; but the IgA levels of a limited number of non-rheumatoid (meniscectomy) joint fluids were lower (ranging from $0.20-0.95\,g\,L^{-1}$). These findings are consistent with the observations (referred to in the Introduction) of large numbers of IgA-producing plasma cells in rheumatoid synovium sections, the products of which comprise both major IgA isotypes although there is a slight but significant disproportionality in favour of $IgA_1$ sub-class production[9]. The finding by the same investigators of similar proportions of the two IgA sub-classes in the sera of the 28 rheumatoid arthritis patients examined in their

123

study is of considerable interest in the light of the finding[10] that non-specific polyclonal B-cell activators (e.g. pokeweed mitogen, lipopolysaccharide, etc.), in contrast to specific antigens, likewise elicit an IgA response which is equally divided between $IgA_1$ and $IgA_2$; particularly as the B-cell hyperactivity characteristic of rheumatoid arthritis appears to involve polyclonal B-cell activation by viral and bacterial products[11].

*Hypogammaglobulinaemia*
Selective IgA deficiency has been observed within the normal adult population at an incidence of 1/500 to 1/3040. This can be asymptomatic, although a most frequent complaint of IgA-deficient blood donors is recurrent infection of the upper respiratory tract and/or episodic diarrhoea[12]. There have also been reports that it can predispose to autoimmune disease in later life. IgA deficiency has been found to be associated with various disease states, such as those affecting the respiratory and gastrointestinal tracts, and, particularly, human disorders of the T-cell system, i.e. thymic dysfunction.

Not surprisingly, in view of its known marked T-cell dependency, IgA (of all the immunoglobulin isotypes) appears to be particularly prone to drug-induced deficiency. For instance, treatment of epileptics with the anti-convulsant hydantoin (2,4-imidazoline) has been observed to lead to selective IgA deficiency (i.e. $< 0.2 \, \mathrm{mg \, ml^{-1}}$) in a significant number (20–25%) of patients whose epilepsy was considered secondary to traumatic or infectious events[13]. There have also been reports (e.g. reference 14) of serum IgA deficiency in patients with Wilson's disease, where it has usually been attributed to treatment with D-penicillamine.

We observed a dramatic reduction in the serum IgA level of one of a group of 15 patients with active rheumatoid arthritis who were on an oral regimen of 1000–1250 mg per day of D-penicillamine. After 4 weeks of this treatment, her circulating IgA level had fallen from 0.9 to $0.3 \, \mathrm{g \, L^{-1}}$; no IgA at all being detectable (by quantitative immunodiffusion) in her serum after 20 weeks, and no secretory IgA being found in her saliva at 31 weeks after commencement of treatment[15]. Moreover, IgA remained undetectable in this patient's serum for several years after discontinuing penicillamine treatment, without any apparent ill effects.

Several more (i.e. four out of 45) cases of IgA deficiency have been subsequently observed in Birmingham in rheumatoid arthritis patients undergoing treatment with D-penicillamine or sodium aurothiomolate[16] and, interestingly, three of these were found to possess the haplotype HLA-A3B40 (a substantially higher incidence than the expected 1%). Moreover, subsequent examination of clinical records revealed several more patients who had unknowingly become IgA-deficient as a result of penicillamine or gold treatment (a situation which must obtain also amongst many other patients with rheumatoid arthritis who have been treated in the past with these second-line drugs). In a later study[17], on a larger group of drug-induced IgA-deficient rheumatoid patients, eight out of nine were found to possess the HLA-B12 and/or B40 marker. But of greater interest, in relation to the theme of this chapter, was the observation by these investigators that improvements in the rheumatoid activity of such patients was often associated with the development of a selective IgA deficiency (and drug toxicity). A similar observation has been made by other investigators[18], who reported a total persistent serum IgA deficiency in a rheumatoid patient showing a favourable clinical response to penicillamine treatment and who consequently suggested that the efficacy of the drug is not necessarily related to its influence on the circulating levels of IgA. Rather, as has been discussed elsewhere[19], it would seem more likely that the reason for the clinical improvement often seen in such patients can be attributable to their ability to form deleterious IgA– $\alpha_1$AT complexes; a situation which is possibly also encouraged by their production of anti-IgA antibodies, which have been found in over 70% of patients with selective IgA deficiency[20].

*IgA antibody, including rheumatoid factor, responses*

There have been few reports of specific IgA antibody responses directed against extrinsic antigens in rheumatoid arthritis, in contrast to the situation with regard to related connective tissue diseases. Thus, for instance, Gram-negative yersinia bacteria (which are facultatively intracellular, evoking largely T-cell-dependent immune responses) have been shown to be responsible for raised serum IgA levels with which inflammatory changes have been shown to be associated in patients with ankylosing spondylitis[21], and in the sera and secretions of patients with yersinia-triggered reactive arthritis[22].

In view of the increasing suspicion of the involvement of the gut in the pathology of rhematoid arthritis it might perhaps be anticipated that the exposure of patients to extrinsic (food) antigens via that route could promote specific antibody responses. And, in this context, it is interesting that the arthritic symptoms of a few rheumatoid patients have been shown to improve when a food constituent to which they have been shown to be allergic is withdrawn from their diet (see, for instance, reference 23). But, from both clinical and experimental animal (rabbit) studies[24] we have failed to obtain convincing evidence that IgE-mediated hypersensitivity reactions play a primary role in the pathogenesis of arthritis.

Of IgA antibody responses described in rheumatoid patients, those against self-IgG (i.e. rheumatoid factors) are probably the most significant. Recent studies[25] have suggested that the detection of IgA rheumatoid factor in the sera of 'early' rheumatoid patients indicates a poor prognosis, justifying a more aggressive treatment at an early stage. Of 33 patients with 'early' arthritis studied by these investigators, it was the seven who presented with raised IgA rheumatoid factor (RF) who developed erosions of their hands and wrists. Whereas, in contrast, none of the five patients who presented with isolated elevation of IgM RF developed erosive disease.

# IgA-CONTAINING COMPLEXES IN RHEUMATOID ARTHRITIS

## Immune complexes

Over the last 10–15 years, there have been many studies of the relationship between circulating complexes and clinical features in rheumatoid arthritis;

some investigators claiming to have shown that raised levels of immune complexes in serum and synovial fluid are associated with an active joint disease or with the presence of extra-articular features, whereas others have found only a weak or no association between immune complex and disease parameters.

Interestingly, relatively recent studies have reported that complexes containing both IgG and IgA, measured by polyethylene glycol precipitation assay, were most often found in the sera of rheumatoid arthritis patients at the time of a new extra-articular manifestation[26], whilst a longitudinal study of 57 patients with rheumatoid arthritis showed that the levels of such circulating complexes correlated with the occurrence of extra-articular manifestations[27] and not with changes in joint disease activity. Furthermore, it has been suggested by the latter investigators that IgA-containing immune complexes may be a good marker of the development of erosive disease and that in 'early' rheumatoid arthritis they appear to be a poor prognostic indicator, as was found for IgA RF[25] as mentioned in the previous section. This has been attributed to IgA RF being less easily cleared from the joints than IgG RF and IgM RF, 'thereby spilling over into the peripheral circulation'[25]. But it seems more likely that *complexed* IgA (e.g. IgA RF–IgG) would be subject to impaired handling – in the light of reports[28] of the relatively slow clearance by the mouse mononuclear phagocytic system of model IgA containing complexes (i.e. heat-induced IgA aggregates) compared to IgG aggregates.

## Non-immune complexes

A non-immune covalently (S-S) linked complex between IgA and $\alpha_1 AT$ is turning out to be of particular importance in the immunopathogenesis of rheumatoid arthritis, for reasons which will be discussed fully in this section. But, first, the studies which were responsible for revealing the existence of such a circulating non-immune complex in humans and for a preliminary description of its properties will be briefly outlined.

### IgA–$\alpha_1 AT$ complex in myelomatosis
Whilst searching, by means of crossed immunoelectrophoresis, for complexes between polyclonal light chains and $\alpha_1 AT$, Laurell and Thulin[29] noticed that normal human plasma contained a complex between $\alpha_1 AT$ and IgA; as well as between the anti-protease and albumin and fibrinogen. Furthermore, treatment of six rheumatoid arthritis patients with D-penicillamine for 2 weeks was observed to lead to a reduction of the amount of IgA–$\alpha_1 AT$ complex in their plasma, whereas no regular decrease in IgA occurred.

A similar complex between $\alpha_1 AT$ and IgA had been detected, by qualitative immunoelectrophoresis, by Tomasi and Hauptman[30] in the sera of 36 out of 49 patients with IgA myelomatosis, and evidence was put forward to suggest that the $\alpha_1 AT$ was linked to IgA dimers, which are frequently encountered in this condition often in addition to other polymerized forms of IgA[31]. Whilst, in a later study, Laurell and associates[32] determined the amounts of Iga-$\alpha_1 AT$ complex found in normal and IgA myeloma plasma in relation to the level of J chain (known to be involved in IgA polymer formation) as well as free IgA monomer and $\alpha_1$AT. They found that the amount of IgA–$\alpha_1$AT complexes in plasma correlated more closely with the IgA concentration than with the $\alpha_1$AT concentration; about 4% of the IgA complexing to $\alpha_1$AT in normal plasma and a variable, but smaller percentage, of the IgA in myeloma patients' sera forming such complexes. Moreover, IgA–$\alpha_1$AT complexes were found at much higher levels in those myeloma patients who secreted relatively small amounts of J chain in relation to paraprotein.

In a more recent study[33], we have confirmed and extended these observations. This included determining, by quantitative immunoelectrophoresis, the level of IgA–$\alpha_1$AT complex in the sera of 75 patients with IgA myelomatosis and, in a proportion of the sera, comparing the results with the content of polymerized forms of IgA determined by ultracentrifugal analysis. The latter measurements revealed a highly significant inverse correlation between the amount of IgA–$\alpha_1$AT complex and the amount of 10S dimer. This can be attributed to disulphide bond formation between one of the cysteine residues in the penultimate positions of the IgA heavy chains and the single cysteine residue (in position 232) of the $\alpha_1$AT polypeptide chain[34] (see Figure 7.1) thereby preventing IgA dimerization through the linking of J chain to the same cysteine in the IgA molecule. Another finding from our study was that IgA–$\alpha_1$AT complex formation in myelomatosis did not depend on the isotype of the paraprotein, the levels of complex found in the small number of sera examined which contained paraprotein of the minor allotypic form (Am2 +) of the IgA$_2$ sub-class being as high as those detected in sera containing paraprotein of the major isotypes.

The results of these investigations on the IgA–$\alpha_1$AT complex in myelomatosis are obviously highly relevant to the understanding of the nature of the complex encountered in rheumatoid arthritis patients – although we have some preliminary evidence (from gel filtration studies, etc.) that the latter complex is less heterogenous than the former, which has been reported to possess a molecular weight between 200 000 and 250 000 daltons in IgA myelomatosis[32]. Significantly, neither we nor any other laboratory (as far as I am aware) have ever detected by ultracentrifugal analysis of rheumatoid patients' sera any evidence of the polymerized forms of IgA so prevalent in IgA myeloma sera. This would seem to suggest that, like a proportion of IgA myeloma patients, sufferers from rheumatoid arthritis secrete IgA *without the accompanying J chain*, which is necessary for IgA polymerization to occur. Consequently, as in myelomatosis, such IgA molecules possess an available thiol group via which they react with $\alpha_1$-antitrypsin to form deleterious complexes capable of inducing and perpetuating inflammatory changes within patients' joints. In other words, as I have proposed elsewhere[35], rheumatoid arthritis can be considered a disease of IgA dysfunction. Most of the IgA found in normal adults' serum is in monomeric form, being synthesized in the absence of J chain, but also appearing to lack the reactive thiol group necessary for complexing (as an alternative) with $\alpha_1$AT.

*IgA–$\alpha_1$AT complexes in rheumatoid arthritis*
As was mentioned in the previous section, Laurell and Thulin[29] observed that the level of IgA–$\alpha_1$AT in the plasmas of six rheumatoid patients decreased

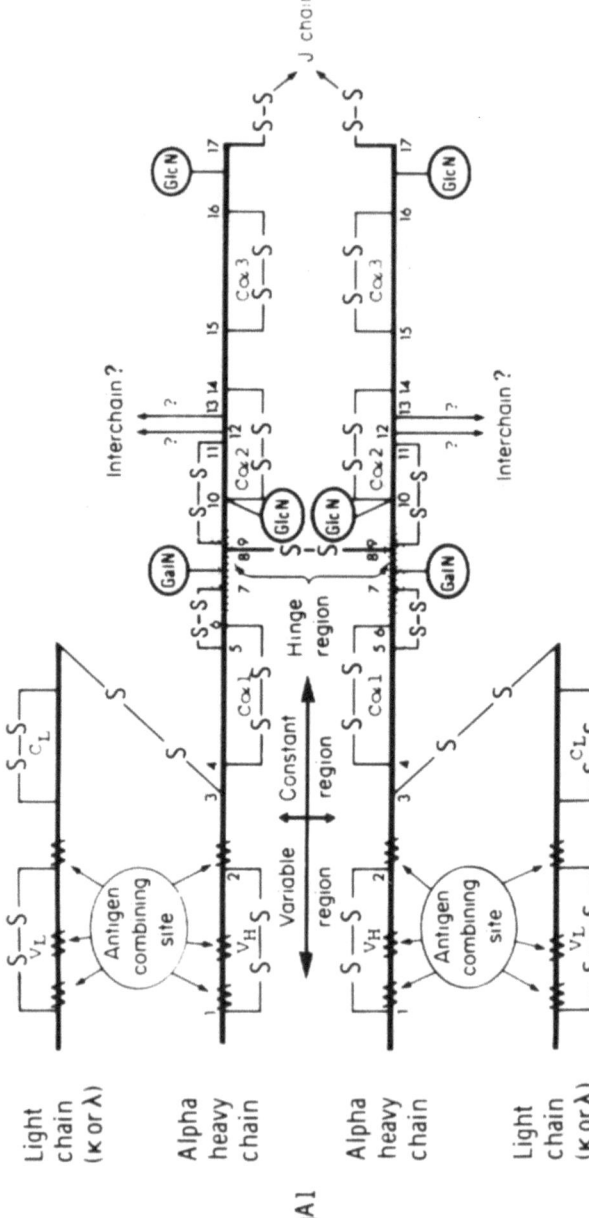

**Figure 7.1** Schematic diagram of the polypeptide structure of human IgA₁. The approximate location of galactosamine (GalN) and glucosamine (GlcN) oligosaccharides is indicated, and the possible site of interchain S–S bridges of polymeric IgA are shown. Half cysteine residues on the α-chains are numbered from the N-terminus. (Reproduced from Stanworth, D.R. and Turner, M.W. (1986). In Weir, D.M. *et al.*, *Handbook of Experimental Immunology*, Chap. 12. (Oxford: Blackwell Scientific Publications) by kind permission of authors and publisher)

as a result of their treatment with D-penicillamine. In a later study[36] on a larger group of rheumatoid patients, these findings were extended, evidence being obtained that the disappearance of the complex from the patients' circulations was paralleled by a favourable clinical response in many cases.

In the last ten years, we have obtained substantial evidence from various types of study undertaken in our laboratory that IgA–$\alpha_1$AT complex is a significant immunopathogenic factor in rheumatoid arthritis. The findings which have led us to this conclusion will now be reviewed before proposing a basis for the complex's immunopathogenicity and considering the implications of this with regard both to the future diagnosis and management of this condition.

In an initial study undertaken in Birmingham in collaboration with Dr M Shadforth and colleagues (referred to in reference 31), we found that treatment of chronic arthritis patients over an 8-month period with D-penicillamine or sodium aurothiomalate (in contrast to laevamisole) brought about a highly significant reduction in the circulating level of IgA–$\alpha_1$AT complex to within the normal range (as will be seen from Table 7.1). All (i.e. 67%) of the penicillamine-treated patients, and all but one of the gold-treated patients, who showed clinical improvement as a result of such treatment came into this category. In contrast to their marked effect on circulating IgA–$\alpha_1$AT complex levels, the gold and penicillamine treatments had a borderline significant effect (see Table 7.1) on the rheumatoid patients' serum IgA levels and no effect on their $\alpha_1$AT levels. The former observation is in line with the finding of Laurell and Thulin[29] referred to earlier, from their observations on a limited number (six) of patients treated with D-penicillamine.

**Table 7.1**  Effect of various forms of treatment on the levels of IgA–$\alpha_1$AT complex, IgA and $\alpha_1$AT in the sera of rheumatoid patients (values are means $\pm$ 1 SD)

| Group | No. | Peak area at 0 months (mg mL$^{-1}$) | Peak area at 8 months (mg mL$^{-1}$) | p-value* |
|---|---|---|---|---|
| IgA–$\alpha_1$AT complex: | | | | |
| Normal human serum | 24 | 0.30 $\pm$ 0.11 | — | — |
| Control rheumatoid | 7 | 1.54 $\pm$ 0.29 | 1.44 $\pm$ 0.34 | >0.1 |
| D-penicillamine | 9 | 1.08 $\pm$ 0.44 | 0.53 $\pm$ 0.63 | <0.01 |
| Gold | 9 | 1.47 $\pm$ 1.00 | 1.00 $\pm$ 0.46 | <0.01 |
| Levamisole | 7 | 1.40 $\pm$ 0.40 | 1.34 $\pm$ 0.39 | >0.1 |
| IgA: | | | | |
| Normal human serum | 24 | 2.00 $\pm$ 0.77 | — | — |
| Control | 7 | 4.88 $\pm$ 3.58 | 4.16 $\pm$ 4.62 | >0.1 |
| D-penicillamine | 9 | 2.93 $\pm$ 1.47 | 2.41 $\pm$ 2.22 | =0.02 |
| Gold | 9 | 4.04 $\pm$ 1.40 | 2.39 $\pm$ 1.93 | > 0.05 |
| Levamisole | 9 | 2.60 $\pm$ 1.48 | 1.66 $\pm$ 1.15 | >0.1 |
| $\alpha_1$AT: | | | | |
| Normal human serum | 24 | 2.98 $\pm$ 0.52 | — | — |
| Control rheumatoid | 7 | 4.40 $\pm$ 1.68 | 6.47 $\pm$ 4.71 | >0.1 |
| D-penicillamine | 9 | 5.59 $\pm$ 2.61 | 4.94 $\pm$ 2.28 | >0.1 |
| Gold | 9 | 5.54 $\pm$ 1.41 | 4.63 $\pm$ 0.79 | >0.1 |
| Levamisole | 7 | 3.83 $\pm$ 0.79 | 5.59 $\pm$ 2.28 | >0.1 |

*Result of paired *t*-test. Values are given in arbitrary units.
Taken from R. Haines, PhD Thesis; in preparation

129

In a later study (see Table 7.2), on a large group (58) of patients with chronic arthritis, an elevated level of circulating IgA–$\alpha_1$AT complex was confirmed (in addition to raised serum IgA and $\alpha_1$AT levels); whereas, the complex was not so frequently detected in the sera of patients with so-called 'early' rheumatoid arthritis, and the range of the serum levels of complex detected in this group did not extend to as high a value as the upper range of complex found in the sera of patients with chronic disease. Moreover, in another study on a group of 29 patients with chronic arthritis, a majority (i.e. 79%) were found (by quantitative immunoelectrophoresis) to possess high levels of IgA–$\alpha_1$AT complex in their joint fluids – in contrast to our failure to detect any complex at all in a (admittedly smaller) group of non-rheumatoid (meniscectomy) joint fluids (Table 7.2).

A comparison was made between the levels of free IgA, $\alpha_1$AT and IgA–$\alpha_1$AT complex, in 13 paired serum/joint fluid specimens from patients with active rheumatoid arthritis (see Figure 7.2). The serum levels of both IgA ($p < 0.01$) and $\alpha_1$AT ($p < 0.001$) were significantly higher than the corresponding fluid levels. While, in contrast, there was no significant difference between the serum and fluid levels of IgA–$\alpha_1$AT complex. This finding is interpreted as evidence for the local formation of the complex, from thiol-active IgA and $\alpha_1$AT within rheumatoid patients' joints.

In more recent longitudinal clinical studies, we have compared the effect of treatment of rheumatoid patients with second line antirheumatic drugs on circulating IgA–$\alpha_1$AT complex levels in relation to changes observed in commonly employed non-immunological laboratory disease markers, such as acute phase proteins and ESR. Thus, for instance, we have shown that there was not a significant ($p > 0.05$) correlation between IgA–$\alpha_1$AT complex and $\alpha_1$AT or C-reactive protein (CRP) levels in the sera of rheumatoid arthritis patients following (i.e. at 6 and 12 months) treatment with D-penicillamine or sodium aurothiomalate[37]. Whilst in another recent study[38], in which IgA–

Table 7.2  Comparison of levels of IgA, $\alpha_1$AT and IgA–$\alpha_1$AT complex in normal and rheumatoid sera and joint fluids (values are means $\pm 1$ SD, range in parentheses)

| Group | No. of specimens assayed | IgA–$\alpha_1$ -antitrypsin level (peak area cm$^{-2}$) | IgA concentration (mg mL$^{-1}$) | $\alpha_1$-antitrypsin concentration (mg mL$^{-1}$) |
|---|---|---|---|---|
| Normal human sera | 24 | 0.30 $\pm$ 0.11 (0.10 – 0.52) 1.33 $\pm$ 0.36 | 2.00 $\pm$ 0.77 (0.75 – 3.60) | 2.98 $\pm$ 0.52 (2.24 – 3.88) |
| Rheumatoid arthritis sera | 58 | 1.17 $\pm$ 0.55 (0.10 – 2.08) | 4.55 $\pm$ 3.07 (0.96 – 12.75) | 4.78 $\pm$ 1.74 (1.90 – 11.90) |
| Meniscectomy synovial fluids | 7 | 0.00 | 0.50 $\pm$ 0.27 (0.20 – 0.95) | 1.14 $\pm$ 0.50 (0.64 – 2.10) |
| Rheumatoid arthritis synovial fluids | 29 | 0.70 $\pm$ 0.50 (0.1 – 1.86) | 1.88 $\pm$ 1.30 (0.70 – 5.00) | 1.88 $\pm$ 0.90 (0.90 – 4.16) |
| 'Early' rheumatoid arthritis sera | 47 | 0.59 $\pm$ 0.37 (0.00 – 1.42) | 2.57 $\pm$ 1.33 (0.00 – 6.56) | 5.44 $\pm$ 2.03 (2.24 – 11.20) |

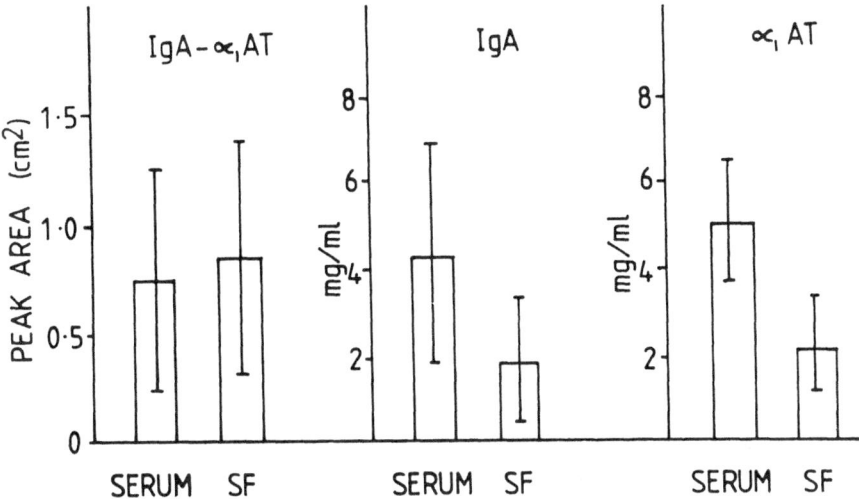

**Figure 7.2** Comparison of the levels of IgA–$\alpha_1$AT complex in paired serum/synovial fluid samples from 13 patients with active rheumatoid arthritis

$\alpha_1$AT complex was measured in paired serum and synovial fluid samples from 27 patients with an inflammatory arthritis (15 rheumatoid and 12 seronegative arthropathies) and six patients with osteoarthritis, a significant correlation was observed between either the serum or fluid complex levels and ESR. And, it was demonstrated that the level of the IgA–$\alpha_1$AT complex was higher in both the serum and joint fluid of rheumatoid compared with osteoarthritis patients, suggesting that it could be an important factor in the pathogenesis of joint inflammation. In this connection, therefore, it is interesting to note that we found a significant ($p < 0.01$) association between the level of circulating IgA–$\alpha_1$AT complex and active disease in ankylosing spondylitis patients (34% of those studied) with secondary inflammation[39].

In other recent collaborative clinical studies[40] we have monitored changes in the level of IgA–$\alpha_1$AT complex in serial serum and joint fluid samples of rheumatoid arthritis patients undergoing oral treatment with D-penicillamine in an attempt to assess objectively the value of this laboratory parameter as an index of clinical responsiveness. An attempt has been made to predict the initial clinical status of the 20 patients in the study (which included a few osteoarthritic 'controls'); and the manner in which they had responded to a period of treatment lasting up to 12 weeks, prior to breaking the number code of the specimens thus examined. A most encouraging degree of concordance was observed between the changes in the clinical status of the patients predicted in this manner and their observed clinical responses to the penicillamine treatment as determined by measurement of joint circumference (using a fixed reference point), tenderness score (Ritchie Index) and global score ('better', 'worse', 'same'). Moreover, somewhat surprisingly, the measurement of changes in the serum level of IgA–$\alpha_1$AT complex appeared to provide a much more reliable index of change in clinical status than did the changes in corresponding synovial fluid complex levels.

On the evidence of these, and our earlier findings just outlined, it is felt that the routine measurement of IgA$-\alpha_1$AT complex in the sera of patients with rheumatoid arthritis offers a more reliable guide to their clinical diagnosis and subsequent management than those serum parameters (acute phase proteins, rheumatoid factors, etc.) that are usually determined for this purpose. Towards this goal, we are in the process of developing an ELISA procedure capable of providing rapid and accurate measurement of the IgA$-\alpha_1$AT complex contents of large numbers of rheumatoid sera which should find wide application in routine clinical rheumatology laboratories.

## POSSIBLE BASIS OF THE IMMUNOPATHOGENICITY OF IgA$-\alpha_1$AT COMPLEX

It would be naive to suggest that IgA$-\alpha_1$AT complex is the only significant immunopathogenic factor in rheumatoid arthritis. Nevertheless, a substantial amount of evidence has been provided (in the previous section) to suggest that it could play a predominant role in the underlying immunopathology of many rheumatoid patients' clinical condition. We have been obtaining increasing experimental data in support of such a contention, which will now be discussed.

### In vitro studies

At the *in vitro* level, we have shown[41] that purified human IgA$-\alpha_1$AT complex is capable of eliciting the cytolytic release of lysosomal enzymes ($\beta$-glucuronidase, $\beta$-galactosidase) from isolated mouse peritoneal macrophages by a process which appears to depend on the activation of secreted C3 and the generation of a C3b ligand. Significantly, in earlier studies[42], we had observed a high degree of correlation between the capacities of several different immunological and non-immunological secretagogues to elicit acid hydrolase secretion from mouse macrophages and their abilities to activate the alternative complement pathway. These included: zymosan particles; insoluble antibody (IgG) complexes; and insoluble IgG aggregate analogues of these. In contrast, the corresponding complexes and aggregates proved ineffective when in *soluble* form. Significantly the covalently linked IgA$-\alpha_1$AT complex, which in contrast to free IgA or $\alpha_1$AT has been shown (see Figure 7.3) to be a potent activator of the C3 component of complement (provided in a fresh human serum source), is the only *soluble* complex of any of the range of those tested which has demonstrated a capacity to initiate lysosomal enzyme release from macrophages *in vitro* (as will be seen from Table 7.3). Moreover, in contrast to the acid hydrolase release effected by the insoluble immune complexes and zymosan particles referred to above, that elicited by IgA$-\alpha_1$AT complex involves *cytolysis* of the murine bone-marrow-derived macrophages (as reflected by a substantial parallel release of lactic dehydrogenase).

Clearly these findings raise the possibility that the IgA$-\alpha_1$AT complex,

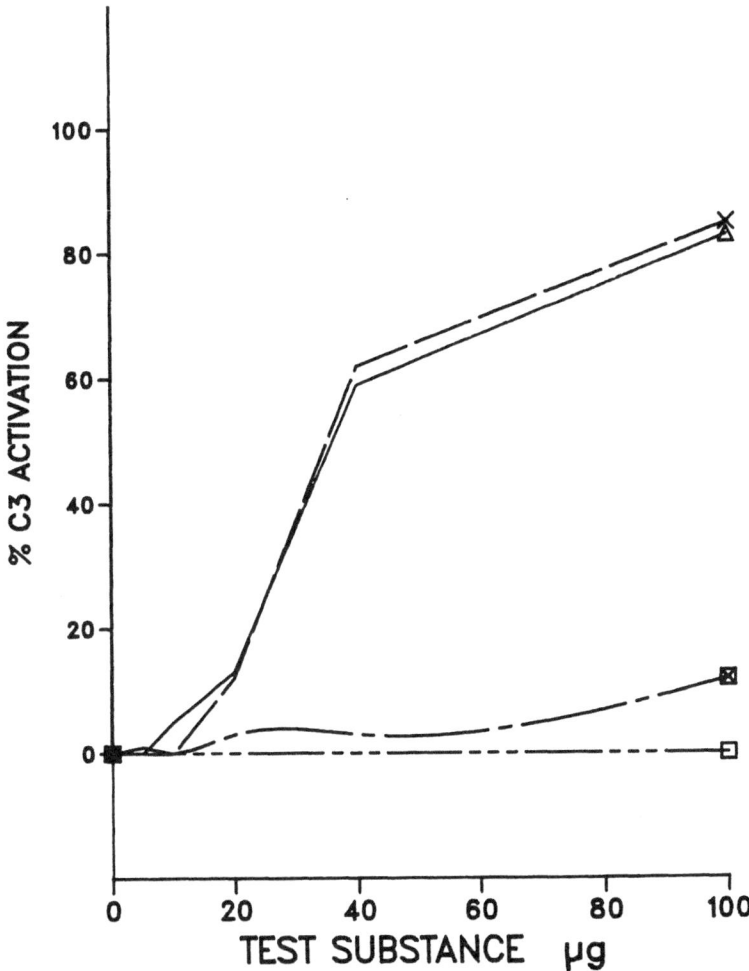

**Figure 7.3** Comparison of the capacity of purified human IgA–$\alpha_1$AT complex ($\times$) and zymosan particles ($\triangle$) to activate the alternative complement (human) pathway. Negative controls: human serum IgA ($\boxtimes$) and $\alpha_1$AT ($\square$). (Stanworth, D.R., Lewin, I.M. and Cooper, P.H.; to be published)

which our clinical studies (referred to in the previous section) showed was present at high levels in rheumatoid patients' joints and in their sera (where it serves as a highly relevant disease marker), is a major contributory factor to their arthritic lesions – particularly since we have estimated that rheumatoid patients' joint fluids can contain up to around 1 mg IgA–$\alpha_1$AT complex per ml, i.e. far in excess of the 10 $\mu$g which was needed (see Table 7.3) to effect

133

**Table 7.3** Effect of IgA–$\alpha_1$-antitrypsin, IgA and $\alpha_1$-antitrypsin on plasminogen activator (PA), $\beta$-glucuronidase (GUR) and lactate dehydrogenase (LDH) release from murine bone marrow-derived macrophages (24 h incubation period)

| Test | Control | | | +Zymosan | | |
|---|---|---|---|---|---|---|
| | PA release (U (10 μg DNA)⁻¹) | GUR (% release) | LDH (% release) | PA release (U (10 μg DNA)⁻¹) | GUR (% release) | LDH (% release) |
| Control | 0.06 | 10.7 | 10.9 | 24.62 | 15.5 | 10.7 |
| +IgA–$\alpha_1$AT (μg ml⁻¹): 10 | 0.00 | 50.0 | 90.8 | 1.40 | 45.7 | 94.9 |
| 20 | 0.00 | 44.4 | 86.9 | 0.39 | 44.5 | 95.1 |
| 30 | 0.00 | 43.3 | 93.3 | 0.29 | 42.8 | 95.6 |
| 50 | 0.00 | 37.1 | 87.8 | 0.21 | 41.6 | 95.8 |
| +IgA (μg ml⁻¹): 10 | 0.00 | 9.3 | 10.2 | 22.81 | 18.9 | 13.2 |
| 20 | 0.00 | 10.3 | 7.3 | 20.69 | 20.6 | 13.7 |
| 30 | 0.00 | 11.6 | 8.6 | 19.11 | 20.8 | 12.8 |
| 50 | 0.00 | 17.0 | 14.1 | 16.95 | 18.3 | 12.8 |
| +$\alpha_1$AT (μg ml⁻¹): 10 | 0.00 | 11.3 | 9.5 | 24.23 | 17.7 | 11.8 |
| 20 | 0.00 | 11.9 | 9.9 | 23.55 | 16.6 | 13.1 |
| 30 | 0.00 | 12.1 | 10.2 | 22.57 | 17.0 | 11.8 |
| 50 | 0.00 | 14.6 | 12.0 | 21.35 | 18.8 | 13.2 |

Taken from Stanworth et al. (1987)[41]

maximal acid hydrolase release from isolated mouse peritoneal macrophages and the amount needed to initiate maximum activation of the alternative human complement pathway *in vitro* (Figure 7.3). It can also be calculated that as much as a third of the total $\alpha_1$-antitrypsin in a rheumatoid patient's joints can be complexed to IgA, thus 'consuming' substantial amounts of this major antiprotease and presumably interfering with its capacity to neutralize degradative enzymes released into the joints. But, as just indicated, the resultant complex itself would appear to be capable of eliciting further acid hydrolase secretion. More direct evidence that such a process can indeed occur has been obtained from the measurement (in collaboration with Dr C. Elson of Bristol University) of a C3 activation product (i.e. C3d) in the joint fluids of rheumatoid patients and comparing the results with the IgA–$\alpha_1$AT complex contents of the fluids. A correlation coefficient of 0.72 was revealed by statistical analysis of the data.

It is, moreover, conceivable that the presence of relatively large amounts of IgA–$\alpha_1$AT complex in the rheumatoid patient's joints could have other deleterious effects. For instance, in this connection it was interesting to find that purified human IgA–$\alpha_1$AT complex suppressed phagocytosis of sheep erythrocytes by macrophages *in vitro*[41], because IgA polymers have been shown to inhibit IgG-dependent phagocytosis of *Candida albicans* blasto-spores[43], and uptake of IgG-coated latex particles by human polymorpho-nuclear leukocytes[44] *in vitro*. There have also been reports (e.g. reference 45) that IgA myeloma serum components (presumably the polymerized forms) suppress leukocyte chemotaxis, which is prompting us to establish whether IgA–$\alpha_1$AT complex is also capable of exhibiting such an activity. In any event, these *in vitro* observations suggest that the high levels of IgA–$\alpha_1$AT complex formed in rheumatoid patients' joints could be detrimental 'on several counts'.

## *In vivo* studies

Of the various means of inducing arthritis experimentally in animals (reviewed in reference 46) the so-called Dumonde–Glynn[47] model in rabbits shows striking histopathological similarities to the clinical condition. Furthermore, we have shown[48] that oral D-penicillamine treatment of such animals brought about (in many cases) a reduction in the severity of their inflammatory synovitis after a period of delay from the commencement of treatment which was comparable to that observed in rheumatoid patients treated with this drug. In later studies[49], by intra-articular injection of asialylated homologous IgG into pre-sensitized rabbits, we not only induced joint lesions whose main features closely resembled those seen in rheumatoid patients (i.e. the inflammatory changes were characterized by areas of extremely dense chronic inflammatory cell infiltration in which the lymphocytes were often aggregated into lymphoid follicles) but rheumatoid factor appeared in the animals' circulations, and there were signs of involvement of the contralateral control (saline-injected) knees. Interestingly, in studies employing this animal model[50], we observed the level of circulating IgA to rise abruptly, following the injection of antigen into the joints of pre-sensitized rabbits in order to induce the arthritis, an increase which was not affected by oral treatment with D-penicillamine. The concentration of IgA in the sera of such rabbits decreased markedly during the chronic phase of the experimentally induced monoarticular arthritis, falling below the lower limit of the normal range. Treatment with D-penicillamine for at least 50 days, however, restored the rabbits' serum IgA levels to the middle of the normal range, whilst having no effects on the animals' serum IgG or IgM levels, either before or after the onset of the monoarticular arthritis.

It is possibly significant that we found the kinetics of the restoration of the arthritic rabbits' serum IgA, in response to D-penicillamine treatment, correlated with the delay observed before the diminution of the monoarticular arthritis became apparent[51]. This has prompted us to speculate[50] that the decrease in circulating IgA levels observed in untreated chronic arthritic rabbits might be due to an increased rate of catabolism of the IgA possibly as a result of its binding to $\alpha_1$-antitrypsin. Yet, we have not been successful in demonstrating directly (by two dimensional immunoelectrophoresis) IgA—$\alpha_1$AT complex in the circulations of arthritic rabbits. Possibly this reflects the cellular immunological make-up of the rabbit, a species in which it has proved impossible to induce plasmacytomas experimentally.

In contrast, a high proportion of plasmacytomas induced by injecting certain chemicals (e.g. pristane) into mice (Balb/c) secrete monoclonal IgA; and a high proportion (40%) of such animals develop a peripheral arthritis and/or tenosynovitis apparently unrelated to the induction of plasmacytoma or ascites[52]. It has also proved possible to induce arthritis experimentally in most strains of mice by intra-articular injection of antigen following pre-sensitization with antigen and adjuvant[53]; susceptibility to antigen-induced arthritis in this species being thought to correlate with a high responder state, determined by T-cells. But, unlike in the immunologically-induced model of arthritis in the rabbit, daily oral treatment with D-penicillamine was found to have no significant effect on antigen-induced monoarticular arthritis in mice[54].

Returning to the rabbit system, we have recently succeeded in inducing in the joints of normal rabbits lesions which histopathologically closely resemble those seen in rheumatoid patients – merely by one injection of purified human IgA–$\alpha_1$AT complex[55]. Histological examinations of synovial sections from such animals revealed marked inflammatory changes: lining cell hypoplasia; dense cellular infiltration of predominantly mononuclear cells (plasma cells, lymphocytes, macrophages and fibroblasts can all be identified); pannus eroding the cartilage of the patella, PMN leukocytes being evident at the pannus- cartilage interface; follicular lymphoid aggregates identifiable in the suprapatellar fat pad; deposition of collagen in the subintima; and increased vascularity. It is tempting to attribute such dramatic biological changes (which were not seen in synovium sections from control rabbits, injected intra-articularly with free human serum IgA or rheumatoid joint fluid deficient in IgA–$\alpha_1$AT complex) to the ability of the IgA–$\alpha_1$AT complex to activate the alternative complement pathway, thereby eliciting the cytolytic release of lysosomal enzymes and other mediators from tissue macrophages (as discussed in the previous sub-section). Furthermore, it is conceivable that complement

C3 sub-components formed during such a process will play prominent roles in promoting the involvement of other cell types (including B lymphocytes) in the ensuing tissue changes.

## CONCLUDING COMMENTS

Evidence has been presented from studies on several different levels (clinical, experimental animal, *in vitro* cellular, etc.) which all points to the involvement of IgA in the immunopathogenesis of rheumatoid arthritis.

As dicussed above, an early rise in serum IgA rheumatoid factor (RF) during the course of rheumatoid arthritis has been found to be strongly predictive of severe disease with the early appearance of erosions[25]. Furthermore, serum levels of IgA-containing immune complexes have been found to correlate significantly with the appearance of extra-articular features, but not with changes in disease activity[27]. In contrast, determination of conventional (IgM) RF (by the Waaler-Rose agglutination assay and latex fixation) and immune complex (by the C1q binding assay) yielded no more information about the clinical state or prognosis of disease activity in rheumatoid arthritis patients than did physical examination or other common laboratory tests.

It is suggested, however (for the reasons discussed in this article) that the measurement of the non-immune IgA$-\alpha_1$AT found at high levels in rheumatoid patients' sera and joint fluids offers a much more immunopathologically relevant index of disease activity and the way that this changes in response to treatment. A scenario is envisaged as follows: a genetically susceptible individual's B lymphocytes become polyclonally activated (by viral or bacterial prodcts, etc.) with the spontaneous appearance of large numbers of IgA and IgG plaque-forming cells in both peripheral blood and synovial fluid lymphocytes, as has been reported by Al-Balaghi *et al.*[56]. The immunoglobulins secreted by the former include large numbers of molecules which are thiol-active, like many of those produced by patients with IgA myelomatosis. But, unlike the paraprotein, their secretion (by B lymphocytes) is not paralleled by J chain production. Consequently, these thiol-reactive IgA molecules do not go on to form IgA polymers, such as are seen in abundance in the circulations of patients with IgA myelomatosis. Instead, these molecules form a disulphide bond with $\gamma_1$-antitrypsin, a major acute phase anti-protease with one cysteine residue (in position 232 of its single polypeptide chain) which is also produced at heightened levels by the rheumatoid patient.

Therefore, in a sense, the $\alpha_1$AT can be regarded as playing a regulatory role in forming a mixed disulphide with the thiol-reactive IgA molecules. Unfortunately for the host, not only does this consume large amounts of a major anti-protease from within his/her joints but the resultant complex is itself capable of eliciting the release of more tissue-degrading enzymes, as a result of activation of macrophage-secreted C3 complement component.

Whether the availability of thiol-reactive IgA molecules within the rheumatoid patients' joints is sufficient to promote their interaction with $\alpha_1$AT produced there remains to be established. Possibly a change in the anti-protease molecule itself, in rheumatoid arthritis, facilitates IgA$-\alpha_1$AT disulphide bonding? Changes in the distribution of $\alpha_1$AT phenotypes (e.g. an increase in the MZ form) have been reported in rheumatoid arthritis[57]. But it is unlikely that the single amino acid substitutions involved would result in a gross change in the three-dimensional structure of the $\alpha_1$AT molecule, in which the single cysteine residue in position 232 resides in a relatively accessible position or the periphery (R.E. Carrell, personal communication). On the other hand, it is conceivable that changes in the composition of $\alpha_1$AT-bound oligosaccharide, analogous to those which we have found in rheumatoid IgG molecules[58], could render this cysteine residue more accessible for interaction with a penultimate cysteine in one of the $\alpha$-chains of the IgA molecule – a possibility which we are now investigating.

There is considerable controversy about the mode of action of antirheumatic drugs; symposia are being held on whether they influence the underlying disease process in rheumatoid arthritis and whether any are capable of bringing about true disease remission. D-penicillamine and gold (disodium aurothiomalate) are thought to come into the latter category, although the evidence for this has been scanty. It is now suggested that the crucial feature in the efficacy of such second-line drugs is their thiol activity as a result of which they form mixed disulphides with the thiol-active IgA molecules produced by rheumatoid patients, which are then harmlessly excreted. It is also possible that such compounds prevent deleterious IgA–$\alpha_1$AT complex formation within patients' joints by suppressing the catalytic activity of the B lymphocyte sulphydryl oxidase which has been implicated in the linking of IgM and, supposedly, IgA 7s sub-units to J chain in the polymerization of immunoglobulins of these classes[59], which is assumed also to be involved in catalysing the linking of IgA to $\alpha_1$AT.

It is interesting to note that as long as 24 years ago it was postulated by Lorber and associates[60] that impaired sulphydryl group reactivity in rheumatoid arthritis may be due to the acceleration of disulphide bonding which could result in 'macroglobulin formation, protein denaturation and autoimmunity'. Later, sulphydryl–disulphide interchange between rat serum SH groups and dithiobis-nitrobenzoic acid was used in an attempt to measure the relative efficacy of various antirheumatic drugs[61]. More recently, measurement of total serum SH has been employed to assess the effects of treatment of rheumatoid patients with D-penicillamine and other forms of antirheumatic drugs[62]. Interestingly, it was noted in this study that serum SH reactivity increased in rheumatoid patients receiving treatment with non-SH-containing drugs like fenclofenac and benoxaprofen, as well as in patients on D-penicillamine or sodium aurothiomalate. It was suggested that the former exert their effect by inducing a conformational change in serum albumin, thereby increasing the reactivity of its free sulphydryl group. In a preliminary study in collaboration with Dr M. Shadford (and colleagues at the North Staffs Rheumatology Centre), we found that the abnormally high levels of IgA–$\alpha_1$AT complex in the sera of rheumatoid patients who responded well to treatment with benoxaprofen and fenclofenac (like those of 'good' responders to penicillamine and gold) fell to well within the normal limits. In contrast, the level of the complex tended to remain abnormally high in the circulations of 'poor' responders to these drugs over the 8-month treatment period studied.

The presence of a free thiol group in many second-line antirheumatic drugs has been previously recognized, but an explanation as to how this influences the efficacy of such compounds has not been forthcoming. Nevertheless, it has been suggested that their further study could throw light on the pathogenesis of rheumatoid arthritis, besides facilitating the development of more effective and less toxic second-line agents[63]. In this chapter, an explanation has now been provided as to how compounds like D-penicillamine and disodium aurothiomalate exert their effect, based on a central immunopathogenic role for IgA–$\alpha_1$AT complex in rheumatoid arthritis. The implications of this claim are far reaching with regard both to the introduction into clinical rheumatology laboratories of more relevant diagnostic and monitoring laboratory techniques, and to the development of more effective and less toxic antirheumatic drugs.

## Acknowledgements

I am grateful for help over the years from many of my co-workers: in particular, Ian Hunneyball (now Head of Biology at Boots Research); Robert Haines (now passing on his scientific knowledge to school children); and Ian Lewin (my incomparable research assistant). I am pleased also to acknowledge generous financial support from The Arthritis and Rheumatism Council.

## References

1. Geiler, G. (1976). Proliferative and exudative features of the rheumatoid synovium. In Dumonde, D.C. (ed.). *Infection and Immunology in the Rheumatic Diseases.* Chapter 50, pp. 413–16. (Oxford: Blackwell)
2. Geiler, G. (1971). The antibody synthesis of the synovial membrane in rheumatoid arthritis. In Mullen, W., Harweth, H.G. and Fehr, K. (eds.). *Rheumatoid Arthritis.* pp. 317–23. (New York, London: Academic Press)
3. Winchester, R.J., Agnello, V. and Kunkel, H.G. (1970). Gammaglobulin complexes in synovial fluids of patients with rheumatoid arthritis. *Clin. Exp. Immunol.,* **6,** 689–706
4. Winchester, R.J., Kunkel, H.G. and Agnello, V. (1971). Occurrence of γ-globulin complexes in serum and joint fluid of rheumatoid patients; use of monoclonal rheumatoid factors in reagents for their demonstration. *J. Exp. Med.,* **134,** 286s–295s
5. Pope, R.M., Teller, D.C. and Mannik, M. (1971). Association of antibodies to IgG (rheumatoid factors) in rheumatoid arthritis. *Proc. Natl. Acad. Sci. USA,* **71,** 517–21
6. Stanworth, D.R. (1985). Immunoglobulinopathies. In Gynn, L.E. and Steward, M.W. (eds.). *Antibody Production.* pp. 183–231. (New York, Chichester: John Wiley)
7. Lamm, M.E. (1976). Cellular aspects of immunoglobulin A. *Adv. Immunol.,* **22,** 223–90
8. Stanworth, D.R., Johns, P., Felix-Davis, D.D. and Wilkinson, B.R. (1976). The effect of long term D-penicillamine treatment on serum immunoglobulin and antibody levels in rheumatoid arthritis. In Munthe, E. (ed.). *Penicillamine Research in Rheumatoid Disease.* (Proceedings Symposium at Spåtind, Norway). pp. 132–45. (Oslo: Fabritius & Sønner)
9. Hrnčiř, Z. and Tichý, M. (1978). Subclasses IgA1 and IgA2 in serum and synovial fluid in rheumatoid arthritis and reactive synovitis of local origin. *Ann. Rheum. Dis.,* **37,** 518–22
10. Conley, M.E., Chan, M.A. and Sigal, N.H. (1987). *In vitro* regulation of IgA sub-class production. III Selective transformation of IgA1 producing cells by Epstein-Barr virus. *J. Immunol.,* **138,** 1403–7
11. Moller, F., Strom, H. and Al-Balaghi, S. (1980). Role of polyclonal activation in specific immune responses. Relevance for findings of antibody activity in various diseases (editorial). *Scand. J. Immunol.,* **12,** 177–82

12. Dammacco, F., Tursi, A., Luciuero, G. and Bonomo, L. (1976). Selective IgA deficiency: a heterogenous immunodeficiency syndrome. *Ric. Clin. Lab.* **6** (Suppl. 3), 45–55
13. Fontana, A., Sauter, R., Grob, P.J. and Joller, H. (1976). IgA deficiency, epilepsy and hydantoin medication. *Lancet*, **ii**, 228–30
14. Strickland, G.T. and Leu, M.L. (1975). Wilson's disease. Clinical and laboratory manifestations in 40 patients. *Medicine*, **54**, 113–37
15. Stanworth, D.R., Johns, P., Williamson, N., Shadforth, M., Felix-Davis, D. and Thompson, R. (1977). Drug-induced IgA deficiency in rheumatoid arthritis. *Lancet*, **1**, 1001–2
16. Johns, P., Felix-Davies, D.D., Hawkins, L.F., Mackintosh, P., Shadforth, M.F., Stanworth, D.R., Thompson, R.A. and Williamson, N. (1978). IgA deficiency in patients with rheumatoid arthritis treated with D-penicillamine or gold. *Ann. Rheum. Dis.*, **37**, 289. (Abstract)
17. Delamere, J.P., Grindulis, K. and Farr, M. (1983). Effects on rheumatoid activity of drug-induced changes in serum immunoglobulins: particularly selective IgA deficiency. *Arthr. Rheum. Dis.*, **42**, 231 (Abstract)
18. Mbuyi-Muamba, W., Stevens, E. and Dequeker, J. (1981). Good response to D-penicillamine in a IgA-deficient rheumatoid patient. *Scand. J. Rheumatol.*, **10**, 31–2
19. Stanworth, D.R. (1982). D-penicillamine-induced immunodeficiency. In Dawkins, R.L., Christiansen, F.Z. and Zilko, P.J. (eds.) *Immunogenetics in Rheumatology: Musculoskeletal Disease and D-pencillamine*. Chapter 8–20, pp. 358–61. (Amsterdam: Excerpta Medica Congress Series 602)
20. Petty, R.E., Palmer, N.R. and Cassidy, Y.J.T. (1979). The association of auto-immune diseases and anti-IgA antibodies in patients with selective IgA deficiency. *Clin. Exp. Immunol.*, **37**, 83–8
21. Cowling, P., Ebringer, R. and Ebringer, A. (1984). Association of inflammation with raised serum IgA in ankylosing spondylitis. *Ann. Rheum. Dis.*, **39**, 545–9
22. Grandfors, K. and Toivanen, A. (1986). IgA anti-yersinia antibodies in Yersinia triggered reactive arthritis. *Ann. Rheum. Dis.*, **45**, 561–5
23. Parke, A.L. and Hughes, G.R.V. (1981). Rheumatoid arthritis and food: a case study. *Br. Med. J.*, **282**, 2027–29
24. Stanworth, D.R. (1985). The role of IgE and IgA in rheumatoid arthritis. *Hungarian Rheumatol. Suppl., Proc. EULAR Symp. on Current Immunological Concepts in Rheumatology - Immunopathology, Genetics and Therapy*, Budapest, Sept. 1984, pp. 9–16
25. Withrington, R.H., Teitsson, I., Valdimarsson, H. and Seifert, M.H. (1984). Prospective study of eary rheumatoid arthritis. 2. Association of rheumatoid factor isotypes with fluctuations in disease activity. *Ann. Rheum. Dis.*, **43**, 678–85
26. Jans, H., Halberg, P. and Lorenzen, I. (1983). Circulating immune complexes in rheumatoid arthritis with extra-articular manifestations. *Scand. J. Rheumatol.*, **12**, 215–18
27. Westedt, M.L., Daha, M.R, Baldwin, W.M., Stijnen, T. and Cats, A. (1986). Serum immune complexes containing IgA appear to predict erosive arthritis in a longitudinal study in rheumatoid arthritis. *Ann. Rheum. Dis.*, **45**, 809–15
28. Egido, J., Sancho, J., Rivera, F. and Sanchez-Cresdo, M. (1982). Handling of soluble IgA aggregates by the mononuclear phagocytic system in mice. A comparison with IgG aggregates. *Immunology*, **46**, 1–7
29. Laurell, C.B. and Thulin, E. (1975). Complexes in human plasma between $\alpha_1$-antitrypsin and IgA$_1$ and $\alpha_1$-antitrypsin and fibrinogen. *Scand. J. Immunol.*, **4**, (Suppl. 2), 7–12
30. Tomasi, T. and Hauptman, S. (1974). The binding of trypsin to human IgA. *J. Immunol.*, **112**, 2274–7
31. Stanworth, D.R. (1981). The effect of D-penicillamine treatment on humoral immunological factors in clinical and experimental arthritis. In Maini, R.N. and Berry, H. (eds.). *Modulation of Autoimmunity and Disease: the Penicillamine Experience.* pp. 31–35 (New York: Praeger)
32. Laurell, C.B., Grubb, A. and Thulin, E. (1976). J Chain and $\alpha_1$-antitrypsin – IgA complexes in sera with polyclonal and monoclonal IgA. *Ric. Clin. Lab.*, **6** (Suppl. 3), 57–67
33. Stanworth, D.R., Lewin, I. and Crockson, R.A. (1985). Measurement of IgA–$\alpha_1$-antitrypsin ($\alpha_1$AT) complex in the sera of patients with IgA myelomatosis. *Immunol. Lett.*, **11**, 277–80
34. Carrell, R.W., Jeppsson, J.V., Laurell, C.B., Brennon, S.W., Owen, M.C., Vaughan, L. and Boswell, D.R. (1982). Structure and variation of human $\alpha_1$-antitrypsin. *Nature*, **298**, 329–33

35. Stanworth, D.R.(1985). IgA dysfunction in rheumatoid arthritis. *Immunol. Today,* **6**, 43–5
36. Wolheim, F.A., Jeppson, J.O. and Laurell, C.B. (1976). Plasma $\alpha_1$antitrypsin–IgA complexes, plasma cysteine and urinary cysteine penicillamine disulphide excretion: correlation with responsiveness to penicillamine in rheumatoid arthritis. In Munthe, F. (ed.). *Pencillamine in Rheumatic Diseases: Mode of Action. A Key to Pathogenesis.* pp. 152–60. (Oslo: Fabritius & Sónner)
37. Dawes, P.T., Jackson, R., Shadforth, M.F., Lewin, I. and Stanworth, D.R. (1987). The relationship between the complex of immunoglobulin A and alpha-1-anti-trypsin; its constituent components and the acute phase response as measured by C-reactive protein in rheumatoid arthritis treated with gold or D-penicillamine. *Br. J. Rheumatol,* **26**, 351–3
38. Dawes, P.T., Lewin, I. and Stanworth, D.R. (1987). The relationship between the serum and synovial fluid levels of IgA-$\alpha_1$ anti-trypsin (AT) complex with ESR in patients with rheumatoid arthritis. (In preparation)
39. Struthers, G.R., Lewin, I., Bacon, P.A. and Struthers, G.R. (1987). IgA–$\alpha_1$ antitrypsin complexes in ankylosing spondylitis. (In preparation)
40. Stanworth, D.R., Lewin, I.V., Bell, A.L., Boyd, M.W.J. and Haire, M. (1987). A study of the value of measurement of IgA–$\alpha_1$-antitrypsin complex as an index of response to treatment in rheumatoid arthritis. (In preparation)
41. Stanworth, D.R., Lewin, I.V. and Cooper, P. H. (1987). Preliminary observations on a simplified rabbit model of arthritis. (In preparation)
42. Riches, D.W.H. and Stanworth, D.R. (1981). Studies on the possible involvement of complement component C3 in the initiation of acid hydrolase secretion by macrophages. 1. Correlation between enzyme-releasing and complement-activating capacities of several secretagogues. *Immunology,* **44**, 29–39
43. Wilton, J.M.A. (1978). Suppression by IgA of IgG-mediated phagocytosis by human polymorphonuclear leucocytes. *Clin. Exp. Immunol.,* **74**, 423–8
44. Van Epps, D.E., Reed, K. and Williams, R.C. (1978). Suppression of human PMN bactericidal activity by human IgA paraproteins. *Cell. Immunol.,* **36**, 363–76
45. Van Epps, D.E. and Williams, R.C. (1977). Suppression of leukocyte chemotaxis by human IgA myeloma components. *J. Exp. Med.,* **144**, 1227–42
46. Hunneyball, I.M. and Stanworth, D.R. (1981). Immunological models of rheumatoid arthritis with particular reference to the rabbit. *IRCS J. Med. Sci.,* **9**, 1–4
47. Dumonde, D.C. and Glynn, L.E. (1962). The production of arthritis in rabbits by an immunological reaction to fibrin. *Br. J. Exp. Pathol.,* **43**, 373–83
48. Hunneyball, I.M., Stewart, C.A. and Stanworth, D.R. (1979). Effect of oral D-penicillamine treatment in experimental arthritis and associated immune responses in rabbits. III Reduction of the monoarticular arthritis. *Ann. Rheum. Dis.,* **38**, 271–8
49. Hunneyball I.M. and Stanworth, D.R. (1983). The successful use of asialylated IgG as an immunogen and arthritogen in the rabbit. *Immunology,* **49**, 511–18
50. Hunneyball, I.M., Stewart, G.A. and Stanworth, D.R. (1978). The effects of oral D-penicillamine in experimental arthritis and the related response in rabbits. I. The effect on humoral parameters. *Immunology,* **34**, 1053–61
51 Hunneyball, I.M., Stewart, G.A. and Stanworth, D.R. (1977). Effect of D-penicillamine on chronic experimental arthritis in rabbits. *Ann. Rheum. Dis.,* **36**, 378–80
52. Hopkins, S.J., Freemont, A.J. and Jayson, M.I.V. (1984). Pristane-induced arthritis in Balb/c mice. I. Clinical and histological features of the arthropathy. *Rheumatol. Int.,* **5**, 21–8
53. Brackertz, D.M., Tchell, G.F., Vadas, M.A., Mackay, I.R. and Miller, J.F.A.P. (1977). Studies on antigen-induced arthritis in mice. II Immunological correlates of arthritis susceptibility in mice. *J. Immunol.,* **118**, 1639–44
54. Hunneyball, I.M., Crossley, M.J. and Spowace, M. (1986). Studies on the effects of pharmacological agents on antigen-induced arthritis in Balb/c mice. *Proc. Int. Symp. on Anti-rheumatics, analgesics and immunomodulators.* Monte Carlo, March 1986. Abstract 267
55. Stanworth, D.R., Lewin, I.V. and Hunneyball, I.M. (1987). Studies of the effect of IgA–$\alpha_1$AT complex on biochemical and functional parameters of bone marrow-derived mouse macrophages *in vitro.* (In preparation)
56. Al-Balaghi, S., Strom, H. and Moller, E. (1985). Effect of drug therapy on circulating and synovial fluid Ig-secreting cells in rheumatoid arthritis. *Ann. Rheum. Dis.,* **44**, 232–8
57. Fagerhol, M.K. and Cox, D.W. (1981). The Pi polymorphism: genetic, biochemical and clinical aspects of human $\alpha_1$-antitrypsin. *Adv. Hum. Genet.,* **6**, 1–62

58. Parekh, R.B., Dwek, R.P., Sutton, R.J., Fernandes, D.L., Leung, A., Stanworth, D.R., Rademacher, T.W., Mizuochi, T., Taniguchi, T., Matsuta, K., Takeuchi, T., Nagano, Y., Miyamoto, T. and Kobata, A. (1985). Association of rheumatoid arthritis and primary osteoarthritis with changes in the glycosylation pattern of total serum IgG. *Nature,* **316,** 452–7

59. Roth, A.R. and Koshland, M.E. (1981). Identification of a lymphocyte enzyme that catalyses pentamer immunoglobulin M assembly. *J. Biol. Chem.,* **256,** 4633–9

60. Lorber, A., Pearson, C.M., Meredith, W.L. and Granta-Mandell, L.F. (1964). Serum sulphydryl determination and significance in connective tissue diseases. *Ann. Intern. Med.,* **61,** 423–34

61. Walz, D.T. and Dimartino, M.J. (1972). Effect of anti-arthritic drugs in sulphydryl reactivity in rat serum. *Proc. Soc. Exp. Biol. Med.,* **140,** 263–8

62. Hall, N.D., Blake, D.R. and Bacon, P.A. (1981). The significance of serum sulphydryl measurements in patients with rheumatoid arthritis treated with D-penicillamine. In Maini, R.N. and Berry, H. (eds.). *Modulation of Autoimmunity and Disease: the Pencillamine Experience.* pp. 143–9 (Praeger)

63. Drury, P.L., Rudge, S.R. and Perrett, D. (1984). Structural requirements for activity of certain 'specific'; anti-rheumatic drugs: more than a simple thiol group? *Br. J. Rheumatol.,* **23,** 100–06

# 8
# Immune reactions in the rheumatoid synovial tissue

## L. KLARESKOG and H. WIGZELL

## INTRODUCTION

For the understanding of the immunopathogenic process in the rheumatoid synovial tissue, there are two issues that are of particular interest: (i) which regulatory and effector mechanisms are involved in the formation of the rheumatic lesions and, most importantly, (ii) what is the specificity (specificities) of the immune reactions responsible for the subsequent development of the multiple immunological and inflammatory events that can be observed in the joints of individuals with advanced rheumatoid arthritis (RA).

Concerning the first of these issues, considerable progress has been made during the last few years which has permitted the knowledge of basic immunology to be directly applicable to the arthritic process; the major part of this review will be devoted to the description of how different immunocompetent cells are involved in the formation of synovial inflammation in RA. Concerning the question of the specificity of arthritogenic immune reactions, the relatively scarce information available will be discussed under the prejudice that new immunological techniques will permit major advances in this area during the next few years. Finally, we will briefly consider the experience available from a few experimental model systems for arthritis where the same types of cells as in human RA appear to be responsible for the development of arthritic lesions. It is conceivable that basic studies of immunoregulation as well as new approaches for therapy made in these models will also be of relevance for human disease.

## GENERAL FEATURES OF IMMUNOPATHOLOGICAL EVENTS IN THE RHEUMATOID JOINT

A characteristic feature of rheumatoid synovial tissue is the accumulation of large amounts of lymphocytes – and sometimes plasma cells – within the synovial tissue and a proliferation of synovial lining cells (for a review, see

Ref. 1). Evidence was early provided for the involvement of both antibody-producing cells and T lymphocytes in the synovial inflammation; active immunoglobulin production was demonstrated within biopsies of *in vitro* cultured rheumatoid synovial tissue[2], whereas the majority of lymphocytes eluted from rheumatoid synovium were found to carry T-cell markers, i.e. form rosettes with sheep red blood cells[3,4].

It was, however, with the introduction of antibodies specific for molecules with defined functions in the interactions between lymphoid cells that it was first possible more systematically to apply the knowledge of basic cellular immunology to the study of synovial inflammation. Moreover, the synovial tissue was – in being easily accessible for investigation – one of the tissues that were first investigated with these techniques. It has subsequently been shown that many features first recognized in synovial inflammation in RA are common to other inflammatory conditions such as the tuberculin reaction in the skin[5,6], thyroiditis[7,8], myositis[9] and keratoconjunctivitis[10,11].

The feature that was first recognized as a potential prerequisite for a local immune activation in the synovial tissue was the dramatically increased number of class II transplantation antigen-expressing cells in the rheumatoid synovium. Thus, whereas only a subpopulation of the cells within the normal thin synovial lining layer are class II antigen-positive[12,13], a large number of cells both within the thickened lining layer and deeper in the synovial tissue were found, in active RA, to express class II transplantation antigens when investigated with the help of immunofluorescence microscopy on frozen sections of synovial tissue[12,13]. Later, it was shown that a similarly pronounced expression of class II antigens is present among the cells of the pannus penetrating cartilage and bone at the site where the synovial inflammation is most active and where erosion of cartilage and bone takes place[14,15]. Studies on cells eluted from the rheumatoid synovial tissue by means of enzymatic digestion showed that cells with different morphology including 'dendritic', macrophage-like and fibroblastoid cells expressed class II antigens[12,16–18]. They also demonstrated that a mixture of these cells could mediate a class II antigen-dependent T-lymphocyte activation[12,17] in a similar way as was earlier shown for other class II expressing cells such as 'dendritic' cells from lymphoid organs[19], macrophages[20] and epidermal Langerhans cells[21]. The simultaneous demonstration of class II expression on a high proportion of synovial T lymphocytes eluted from synovial tissue of RA patients[12,22,23], indicated that T-cell activation indeed takes place in the rheumatoid synovium *in vivo*. This notion was further substantiated by the immunomorphological demonstration that many of the synovial T lymphocytes that could be identified *in situ* with the help of monoclonal anti-T-cell antibodies were accumulated in clusters in close association with class II expressing cells with a dendritic morphology[5,13,24,25]. Most of the cells in these clusters were CD4-positive cells known to have the capacity for activation in cell to cell contact with class II expressing accessory cells (see Ref. 26).

A basic hypothesis was consequently formulated proposing that a local class II antigen-dependent T lymphocyte activation takes place within the rheumatoid synovial tissue. Such activated T lymphocytes producing interleukins, for example $\gamma$-interferon, would induce class II antigen expression on previously class II negative cells, which in turn increases the capacity for a local T-cell activation[5,12,13]. As a consequence of this potentially vicious circle, we will see a subsequent B lymphocyte activation as well as activation and proliferation of a multitude of inflammatory effector cells such as macrophages and granulocytes. The obvious implication of this hypothesis for further research has been to emphasize studies on how the local T-cell activation is regulated in more detail; considering the fluctuating character of rheumatoid arthritis it should be possible to identify mechanisms contributing both to up- and down-regulation of T-cell reactions of importance for arthritis development. In order to obtain a comprehensive picture of these issues, we would obviously need to know the specificity of the most critical synovial immune reactions. Lacking much of this knowledge (see later sections in this review) important knowledge can still be gained from *in situ* immunomorpho- logical studies on synovial tissue as well as from further *in vitro* studies on suspended cells obtained from inflamed synovial tissues.

## IMMUNOMORPHOLOGICAL CHARACTERIZATION OF SYNOVIAL TISSUE IN DIFFERENT KINDS OF SYNOVITIS

Immunomorphological investigation of synovial tissue requires either that biopsies are taken in association with orthopaedic surgery, i.e. the materials represent late stages of RA or osteoarthritis (OA), or are taken at arthroscopy from patients where no indication for orthopaedic surgery exists. In the latter case it is possible to obtain biopsies also from mild cases of synovitis and at different stages of a given disease. By these means one may hope not only to get a more detailed picture of the immunological events that take place during the development of early synovitis into a chronic RA, but also to obtain better diagnostic criteria than we have today to determine whether an acute synovitis is likely to develop into a chronic disease or not.

From the studies on biopsies obtained by arthroscopy, it first turned out that the cell pattern with many CD4-positive T lymphocytes present in close association with class II expressing non-lymphocytic cells was by no means unique for the synovial inflammation in RA. Instead, a marked infiltration of CD4-positive T-cells was seen in all types of synovitis investigated, irrespective of whether the synovitis was part of the disease process in RA, juvenile chronic arthritis (JCA), ankylosing spondylitis or simply traumatic synovitis[27]. Particularly from the findings in traumatic synovitis, it was assumed that infiltration of CD4-positive T-cells into a particular tissue and a preferential location of these cells close to class II expressing, potentially antigen- presenting cells, constitutes a general reaction pattern secondary to multiple stimuli. Similar reaction patterns have also later been observed in the skin in conjunction with irritant as well as with immunological stimuli[28]. This cellular pattern should confer a high degree of 'alertness' for T-cell reactivity to any endogenous or exogenous antigen that is present within the actual tissue. It thus appears that the difference between an immunological disease such as RA and other types of more unspecific synovial inflammation is that in RA the 'alertness' indeed leads to an activation of the synovial T lymphocytes, whereas in traumatic synovitis or in OA no such activation is normally taking place. As a logical consequence of the differences between the states of T-cell activation in the respective diseases, there are also marked differences in numbers of class II expressing synovial lining cells in RA compared to OA/traumatic synovitis, respectively[29,30].

The investigations on arthroscopically obtained biopsies revealed two additional points of interest, namely that a marked T-cell infiltration can be seen in early cases of synovitis before any synovial cell proliferation has taken place[27] and, secondly, that the cell patterns may vary considerably between different parts of the synovium of a particular joint[31]. These data suggest that T-cell infiltration may precede the synovial lining layer proliferation. The data also emphasize that the stimuli that drive the synovial inflammation are able to act very locally.

A number of detailed immunomorphological studies on orthopaedic surgery specimens have, during recent years, further expanded our knowledge of the synovial process in advanced stages of RA. Thus immuno-electron microscopy has led to the clarification that macrophage-like type A[32] cells and, to a limited extent, fibroblast-like type B[32] synovial lining cells may express class II transplantation antigens in RA[33,34]. Using combinations of histochemical and immunomorphological methods as well as immuno-electron microscopy, it has further been shown that class II transplantation antigen expression is seen on conventional macrophages that contain unspecific esterases[35] and express other macrophage cell-surface markers[25,27,36]. Class II antigens are also found on non-macrophage cells with dendritic morphology, among them the cells denoted interdigitating cells that stain with a monoclonal antibody specific for a particular determinant of class II antigens[37]. The pannus region where the earliest and most active inflammatory response occur, has been studied in some detail using sections encompassing both bone, cartilage and soft tissue. It was demonstrated that virtually all cells close to the cartilage and bone expressed class II transplantation antigens using staining with monoclonal antibodies specific for DR, DQ and DP antigens, respectively. DR antigens showed the broadest distribution, DP was found on a slightly lower number of cells and DQ was expressed only on relatively few of the cells in immediate contact with the cartilage[14] (also L. Klareskog, *Br. J. Rheumatol.*, (in press)). Subsequent double staining with rabbit anti-class II antigen antibodies and monoclonal antibodies towards macrophage markers revealed that class II expressing cells with macrophage or fibroblastoid characteristics are present in parallel in the cartilage-pannus region (L. Klareskog, *Br. J. Rheumatol.*, (in press)).

The distribution of T lymphocytes belonging to different phenotypically distinct subpopulations has also been studied in detail. Thus, electron microscopic studies have provided a comprehensive picture of the cell-to-cell contacts that are present between CD4-positive cells and dendritic class II expressing cells in certain cell-rich areas of the rheumatoid synovium, whereas CD8-positive cells are preferentially located in other parts of the synovium, termed 'transitional' areas[34,38]. As will be discussed further below, there exists at present no evidence that the relative proportions of cells with CD4 or CD8 markers mirror degrees of activation or suppression of immune reactions of relevance for arthritis development (see also discussion in Ref. 5).

## FUNCTIONAL CHARACTERIZATION OF CELLS ELUTED FROM RHEUMATOID SYNOVIAL TISSUE

Normal synovial lining cells can be obtained at autopsy by means of instillation of trypsin into knee joints of individuals without previous joint disease (for methodological description, see Ref. 39). Most cells eluted by this protocol display characteristics of type 'A' cells earlier described in situ[32], i.e. they express macrophage cell surface markers, contain non-specific esterases and express class II transplantation antigens as well as Fc receptors[17]. A further link between conventional macrophages and these synovial lining cells was provided from experiments with mouse bone-marrow chimaeras where Ia-expressing normal synovial lining cells were shown to be derived from the bone-marrow[40]. More importantly, suspended human normal synovial lining cells also display a capacity to mediate a class II antigen-dependent activation of allogeneic T lymphocytes[17] showing that normal lining cells without previous stimulation can function as accessory cells in T-cell activation in early stages of synovitis.

Concerning cells eluted from rheumatoid synovial tissue by means of enzymatic digestion, it was shown earlier that unseparated adherent cells could activate both allogeneic T-cells or autologous T-cells after co-incubation with relevant antigens such as PPD[12,17]. These studies did not, however, establish which cell type(s) in the rheumatoid joint is preferentially responsible for the T-cell activation, nor did they answer the equally interesting question whether certain synovial cells exert suppressor influence on T-cell activation. Consequently, efforts have been made to fractionate the non-lymphocytic, largely class II positive synovial cells in order further to investigate their immunoregulatory functions in vitro. Using density gradients and ligands specific for different cell surface markers to fractionate synovial cells, it has been possible to obtain fractions of class II expressing cells that are more efficient in T-cell activation than are unfractionated synovial non-lymphocytic cells[5,41-43]. In these fractions there is an enrichment of cells with a dendritic morphology which show similarities to those efficient antigen-presenting cells previously isolated from murine lymphoid organs[19] as well as from human peripheral blood[44]. Some cells within these fractions also stained with an antibody that preferentially binds to cells denoted 'interdigitating' cells[37,41]. Although these studies suggested that dendritic cells within the actual fractions are important in synovial T-cell activation, it is plausible that other types of class II expressing synovial cells such as macrophages, fibroblastoid cells or endothelial cells[20,45,46], also contribute to local T-cell activation.

The studies on subfractions of adherent rheumatoid synovial cells indicated a suppressive effect on T lymphocyte activation by some of these cells. Thus, addition of large numbers of adherent cells to allogeneic as well as to autologous T lymphocyte cultures inhibited rather than stimulated T-cell proliferation[24,41]. After fractionation of the adherent cells on Percoll density gradients it was shown that cells within the lightest fractions exerted a strong inhibitory action on T-cell proliferation when added to the cultures. Most of the inhibitory adherent cells displayed macrophage markers and a very intense staining for class II antigens which indicated their activated state. In analysing

147

the mechanisms responsible for the suppression it was shown that cells within this Percoll fraction (but not within the others) produced prostaglandin type $E_2$ ($PGE_2$) in sufficient amounts to explain some of the observed suppression, but also that other molecules secreted by activated macrophages probably contribute to the suppression[41].

It is thus feasible that during the activation of T lymphocytes in the synovial tissue, lymphokines released from these T-cells are contributing not only to a more efficient antigen presentation from cells induced to express class II antigens as discussed above. If we assume that there is in rheumatoid synovial inflammation an over-reaction of T lymphocytes due to as yet unknown mechanisms, the activated T-cells will also be prone to trigger non-specific negative feedback systems, such as activated macrophages producing prostaglandins, peroxides, etc.[47]. It is possible that such physiological events will have a particularly adverse effect when they occur in the vicinity of the joint. They may here contribute to the pathogenetic process of arthritis whereas similar reactions occurring for example in the skin would not give rise to such damaging long-term effects.

Concerning the more fundamental questions of what perpetuates T-cell activation in RA and why it is not appropriately controlled by means of specific immunoregulatory mechanisms, our knowledge is still very scarce. Major advances will here have to await more data about the specificity of the immune reactions in the rheumatoid joint. Some indirect evidence concerning the regulatory roles of different subpopulations of T-cells obtained from experimental animal systems will be provided in the following sections of this chapter, whereas available evidence on functions of human synovial T-cell populations will be covered in other chapters of this book.

## SPECIFICITY OF IMMUNE REACTIONS WITHIN THE RHEUMATOID SYNOVIAL TISSUE

The evidence that specific immune reactions are essential in the development of RA is so far mainly indirect but is supported by studies on RA–class II MHC gene associations. Thus, the first noted moderate associations between susceptibility to RA/JCA and HLA-Dw4/HLA-DRw4[48,49] have suggested that the tendency to acquire RA/JCA might be due to differences in immune responsiveness to some as yet unknown antigen under control by major histocompatibility complex (MHC)-linked immune response genes[50,51]. This argument has since been substantiated and strengthened by further detailed genetic studies that have taken advantage of both molecular analysis of relevant class II antigen genes[52] and the possibility of analysing class II antigens with the help of alloreactive human T-cell clones[53]. Both of these studies have indicated a stronger association between certain defined structures on class II antigen molecules and susceptibility for RA/JCA than was found in earlier studies using serological typing systems. They have also more definitely identified the class II transplantation antigens as being responsible for the varied immune responsiveness towards certain antigens[50]. Both from these considerations and from the above-mentioned evidence for a crucial role of activated synovial T-cells in RA, there is an urgent need to study the specificity of rheumatoid synovial T-cells that have been activated *in vivo* against potential arthritogenic molecules. Of particular interest is the study of immune reactivity against antigens that may be under appropriate MHC-linked immune response gene control. As it is possible that T lymphocytes activated within the rheumatoid synovial tissue will only leave the actual inflammatory lesion to a limited extent (compare the tendency for local inflammatory lesions discussed above), these studies should preferentially be performed on cells eluted from synovial tissue where an active inflammation currently takes place. So far, only limited studies have been carried out using this approach; one such study from our own laboratory demonstrated that T lymphocytes eluted from rheumatoid synovial tissue of three out of four investigated patients with active RA displayed reactivity against cartilage-derived collagen type II[5]. In subsequent experiments similar results have been obtained in three out of six additional investigated RA patients (L. Klareskog, unpublished observation). Another recent study demonstrated high reactivity of synovial fluid lymphocytes against a *Mycobacterium tuberculosis* antigen, which displays an immunological cross-reactivity with cartilage proteogly-cans[54]. The anti-mycobacterium reactivity was interestingly restricted to synovial fluid lymphocytes in patients with RA of recent onset, whereas peripheral blood lymphocytes also showed an increased anti-mycobacterium reactivity in cases where the RA had been present for more than 1 year. It is not known, however, to what extent similar types of reactions can be demonstrated in other types of synovial inflammation, and to what extent T-cell reactivity towards still other types of exogenous or endogenous antigens can be demonstrated in RA.

Knowledge concerning the specificity of antibody-producing synovial cells in RA is also limited. Using the same arguments as discussed for local T-cell responsiveness, circulating antibodies as well as circulating B-cells/plasma cells may only in part mirror the occurrence of antibody-producing cells in the synovial tissue. Thus antibodies, particularly auto-antibodies that are produced within the inflamed synovium, may easily be complexed either with exposed autoantigens, for example in the cartilage[15,55], with rheumatoid factors, or with anti-idiotypic antibodies. The most logical way to avoid these difficulties should be to study the antibody-producing cells either *in situ* or after elution of cells from the synovial tissue. The first technique was used by Munthe and Natvig[56] who incubated frozen sections of rheumatoid synovial tissue with fluorescein-coupled heat-aggregated IgG. A high proportion of the plasma cells within the investigated synovial tissue bound the FITC-coupled IgG, which was interpreted to mean that these cells produced rheumatoid factors. This notion has since been strengthened by further *in situ* studies by other groups[57] and from analysis of the specificities of antibody-producing synovial cells with the help of haemolytic plaque techniques[58]. Using a similar *in situ* approach but a slightly different technique, where frozen synovial sections are incubated with biotin-labelled antigens followed by detection of bound molecules by means of avidin-biotin-peroxidase complexes (ABC technique), we have obtained very similar results to those of Munthe and Natvig concerning the numbers of synovial B-cells/plasma

149

cells in RA that bind aggregated IgG. We could, in addition, show that biotin-labelled native collagen type II bound to a substantial but more limited number of cells than the RF containing cells in five out of six investigated synovial specimens from RA patients[59]. These data would suggest that autoantibodies present in the relevant inflamed tissue will only occasionally reach the circulation, as anti-collagen II antibodies are known to occur in serum in only a low percentage of patients with RA[60-62].

Further analysis at the single cell level using the hybridoma or Epstein-Barr virus (EBV)-transformation technology now available should permit us to get an even more comprehensive picture of which antibodies are actually produced locally in the synovial tissue in RA. With this knowledge as a background it should then be possible to attack the more fundamental questions of how these reactions are triggered, which of them may contribute to development of arthritic lesions and which, in contrast are 'innocent' bystanders in the arthritic process.

## COMPARATIVE STUDIES ON SYNOVIAL INFLAMMATION IN EXPERIMENTAL AUTOIMMUNE ARTHRITIS IN RODENTS

In trying to understand how immune reactions in the rheumatoid synovial tissue are regulated, there is an obvious need for experimental animal systems with similar types of synovial immune reactions as those present in the human situation. We have recently demonstrated sizeable similarities between the cell patterns described for human RA and those seen in the inflamed joints in both collagen II induced arthritis (CIA)[63,64] and adjuvant arthritis (AA)[65] in the rat. Large numbers of class II expressing cells are seen penetrating the cartilage and bone and many T lymphocytes, with the majority carrying the CD4 marker, are seen in the inflamed synovium. As is clearly shown by double staining experiments in the rat CIA model, the CD4 positive T-cells are preferentially located close to class II antigen expressing non-lymphocytic synovial cells[63]. In analogy with the human situation, these cell patterns could consequently be used to hypothesize that T lymphocytes constitute the cells primarily responsible for development of arthritis with the proliferation of synovial lining and other features of synovitis occurring secondarily to T-cell activation. In contrast to the human situation, however, this hypothesis can in the animal models be tested experimentally. Three types of experiments have demonstrated that activated T lymphocytes are indeed necessary and sufficient to cause development of such arthritic lesions:

(1)  Neither adjuvant arthritis nor collagen-induced arthritis can be induced in nude, thymus deficient rats[63,66];

(2)  *In vivo* treatment of mice and rats with monoclonal anti-T lymphocyte antibodies prevents the onset of both adjuvant arthritis and collagen arthritis[65,67];

(3)  Both arthritic forms can be induced in previously healthy animals after injection of *in vitro* cultured lines and clones of autoreactive clones of T-helper cells that react specifically either to collagen type II[68] or to *Mycobacterium tuberculosum* and to cartilage proteoglycan[69,70].

In collagen arthritis there is in addition evidence for a pathogenetic role of anti-collagen II antibodies, possibly acting in synergy with autoreactive T lymphocytes[71,72].

The situation in these two kinds of experimental arthritis is thus in several respects similar to the one assumed to exist in human RA. However, the specificities of the immune reactions in the two animal models are different and we do not know whether the specificity patterns of arthritogenic immune reactions in human RA will turn out to be similar to those seen in any of the animal models. Nevertheless, it is feasible that the human and animal systems may have similar immunoregulatory mechanisms; the animal systems may consequently be used to provide clues concerning questions that are particularly difficult to study in humans. One such question that has repeatedly been asked concerning human disease (among them RA) is to what extent CD8-positive T lymphocytes exert a suppressive influence on the development of inflammatory autoimmune disease. Taking advantage of the possibility of experimentally eliminating all CD8-positive cells from peripheral lymphoid organs and from the circulation in rats by means of in vivo treatment with Ox8 (anti-CD8) antibodies[73], the role of CD8-positive cells was investigated in different phases of experimental arthritis. It appeared that the elimination of CD8-positive cells both from the circulation and from the inflamed joint failed to affect the development of adjuvant arthritis when the Ox8 antibodies were given simultaneously with the arthritogenic Mycobacterium tuberculosum bacteria[65]. A uniform direct influence on CD8-positive T-cells is therefore unlikely to be responsible for the enhanced development of AA seen in animals treated with low doses of cyclophosphamide or low dose irradiation[65,74]. A subsequent experiment where anti-CD8 antibodies were given to animals which had been experimentally made resistant to adjuvant arthritis by injections of subarthritogenic doses of mycobacteria, showed that elimination of all CD8-positive cells only partially eliminated the specific resistance to the disease (P. Larsson, L. Klareskog et al., in preparation). It can be concluded, consequently, that both in the induction phase as well as in a refractory phase of the disease, CD8-positive T lymphocytes may not be the only or perhaps not even the major T lymphocyte group that counteracts the development of inflammatory arthritis. The search for specific suppressor mechanisms in these diseases must thus also be directed to other aspects of T-cell regulation, for example towards network regulation within the CD4-positive T-cell population. Evidence that the search for specific suppressor mechanisms in autoimmune disease and methods for inducing such suppression may be very rewarding have been presented by a series of studies by Holoshitz, Cohen and associates. They demonstrated that 'attenuated' mycobacterium-specific T-helper cell clones could, after injection into rats, confer a specific unresponsiveness to further development of adjuvant arthritis[75]. These and similar experiments carried out in other systems[76] indicate that once we have identified the specificity of arthritogenic immune reactions in human arthritis, the experimental animal systems will provide us not only with good aetiopathogenic hypotheses but also with models for specific treatment of human disease.

151

## CONCLUDING REMARKS

The data reviewed in this chapter emphasize that the basic cellular features of the immune reactions that take place in the rheumatoid synovial tissue are not unique to RA. They are present also in other types of synovitis as well as in other tissues during various forms of inflammatory disease. Thus the process by which synovial T-cell activation is influenced by an increased local expression of class II transplantation antigens and gives rise to a delayed type hypersensitivity (DTH)-like reaction may constitute a prototype for several forms of human inflammatory disease. Concerning the question why such inflammatory disease is particularly prone to affect the joints, we have to search for unique features of inflammatory joint disease, especially in RA. Apart from a possibly unique MHC-class II gene association, there are two main such features of interest: (i) inflammatory joint disease occurs close to cartilage and often wanes when cartilage is removed and substituted, for example, by a mechanical joint device, and (ii) the pronounced production of rheumatoid factors (RF) in RA. The hypotheses most often forwarded to explain the common occurrence of inflammation in joints either suggest that microbial agents such as EB virus or *Mycobacterium tuberculosum* display immunological cross-reactivity with structures of the joint[77,70], or that autoimmunity towards cartilage structures is easily triggered due to the normally immunologically privileged status of cartilage compounds[78]. As suggested from the data on immunological cross-reactivity between *Mycobacterium tuberculosum* and cartilage proteoglycans[54,70], these two possibilities may well coincide. There is an obvious need, however, to incorporate not only the localization to the joint but also the tendency for RF production into a working hypothesis for the development of RA. One such hypothesis might be formulated from a recent proposal that a specific connection may exist between autoimmunity to cartilage-derived collagen type II and RF production. Thus increased levels of RF have been found in both guineapigs[79] and mice[80] immunized with native collagen type II. Furthermore, a monoclonal anti-idiotypic antibody specific for autoanticollagen II antibodies in the mouse also displayed RF activity[80,81]. By means of modern techniques for analysis of the specificity of synovial lymphocytes, it should now be possible to investigate empirically the value of this and other working hypotheses which try to encompass the various features of RA.

### References

1. Soren, A. (1978). *Histodiagnosis and Clinical Correlations of Rheumatoid and other Synovitis.* (Stuttgart: George Thieme Publishers)
2. Smiley, J.O., Sachs, C. and Ziff, M. (1968). *In vitro* synthesis of immunoglobulins by rheumatoid synovial membrane. *J. Clin. Invest.*, **47**, 624–32
3. Abrahamsen, T.G., Fröland, S.S., Natvig, J.B. and Pahle, J. (1975). Elution and characterization of lymphocytes from rheumatoid inflammatory tissue. *Scand. J. Immunol.*, **4**, 823–30
4. VanBoxel, J.A. and Paget, V.A. (1975). Predominantly T-cell infiltrate in rheumatoid synovial membranes. *N. Engl. J. Med.*, **293**, 517–21

5. Klareskog, L., Forsum, U., Scheynius, A., Kabelitz, D. and Wigzell, H. (1982). Evidence in support of a self-perpetuated HLA-DR dependent delayed type cell reaction in rheumatoid arthritis. *Proc. Natl. Acad. Sci. USA*, **79**, 3632—6
6. Scheynius, A., Klareskog, L. and Forsum, U. (1982). In situ identification of T lymphocyte subsets and HLA-DR expressing cells in the human skin tuberculin reaction. *Clin. Exp. Immunol.*, **49**, 325—30
7. Hanafusa, T., Pujol-Borrell, P., Ciovato, L., Russell, R.C.G., Doniach, D. and Bottazzo, G.F. (1983). Aberrant expression of HLA-DR antigen on thyrocytes in Graves disease: relevance for autoimmunity. *Lancet*, **ii**, 1111—15
8. Jansson, R., Karlsson, A. and Forsum, U. (1984). Intrathyroidal HLA-DR expression and T lymphocyte phenotypes in Graves thyreotoxicosis, Hashimoto's thyreoiditis and nodular colloid goitre. *Clin. Exp. Immunol.*, **58**, 264—72
9. Olsson, T., Henriksson, K.G., Klareskog, L. and Forsum, U. (1985). HLA-DR expression, T lymphocyte phenotypes, OKM1 and OKT9 reactive cells in inflammatory myopathy. *Muscle Nerve*, **8**, 419—25
10. Lindahl, G., Hedfors, E., Klareskog, L. and Forsum, U. (1985). Epithelial HLA-DR expression and T lymphocyte subsets in salivary glands in Sjögren's syndrome. *Clin. Exp. Immunol.*, **61**, 475—82
11. Adamson, T., Fox, R., Frisman, D. and Howell, F. (1983). Immunohistological analysis of lymphoid infiltrates in primary Sjögren's syndrome using monoclonal antibodies. *J. Immunol.*, **130**, 203—8
12. Klareskog, L., Forsum, U., Malmnäs-Tjernlund, U., Kabelitz, D. and Wigren, A. (1981). Appearance of anti-HLA-DR reactive cells in normal and rheumatoid synovium. *Scand. J. Immunol.*, **14**, 183—92
13. Janossy, G., Panayi, G., Duke, O., Bofill, M., Poulter, L.W. and Goldstein, G. (1981). Rheumatoid arthritis: a disease of T lymphocyte macrophage immunoregulation. *Lancet*, **ii**, 839—43
14. Klareskog, L., Johnell, O. and Hulth, A. (1984). Expression of HLA-DR and HLA-DQ antigens on cells within the cartilage-pannus junction in rheumatoid arthritis. *Rheumatol. Int.*, **4** (Suppl.), 11—15
15. Klareskog, L., Johnell, O., Hulth, A., Holmdahl, R. and Rubin, K. (1986). Reactivity of monoclonal anti-collagen II antibodies with cartilage and synovial tissue in rheumatoid arthritis and osteoarthritis. *Arthr. Rheum.*, **29**, 730—40
16. Winchester, R.J. and Burmester, G. (1981). Demonstration of Ia antigens on certain dendritic cells and on a novel elongated cell found in human synovial tissues. *Scand. J. Immunol.*, **14**, 441—7
17. Klareskog, L., Forsum, U., Kabelitz, D., Plöen, L., Sundström, C., Nilsson, K., Wigren, A. and Wigzell, H. (1982). Immune functions of human synovial cells: phenotypic and T-cell regulatory properties of macrophage-like cells that express HLA-DR. *Arthr. Rheum.*, **25**, 488—501
18. Burmester, G.R., Dimitriu-Bona, A., Watares, S.J. and Winchester, R.J. (1983). Identification of three major synovial cell populations by monoclonal antibodies directed to Ia antigens and antigens associated with monocytes/macrophages and fibroblasts. *Scand. J. Immunol.*, **17**, 69—82
19. Steinman, R.M. and Nussenzweig, M.C. (1980). Dendritic cells: features and functions. *Immunol. Rev.*, **53**, 125—48
20. Unanue, E.R. (1984). Antigen-presenting function of the macrophage. *Annu. Rev. Immunol.*, **2**, 395—428
21. Stingl, G., Tamaki, K., Katz, S.I. (1980). Origin and function of epidermal Langerhans cells. *Immunol. Rev.*, **53**, 149—74
22. Burmester, G.R., Yu, D.T.Y., Irani, A.M., Kunkel, H.G. and Winchester, R.J. (1982). Ia + T-cells in synovial fluid and tissue of patients with rheumatoid arthritis. *Arthr. Rheum.*, **24**, 1370—6
23. Förre, Ö., Egeland, T.G., Dobloug, J.H., Kvien, T.K. and Natvig, J.B. (1982). Autologous mixed lymphocyte reactions in patients with rheumatoid arthritis and juvenile rheumatoid arthritis: both non-T and in vivo activated T cells can act as stimulator cells. *Scand. J. Immunol.*, **16**, 173—9
24. Klareskog, L., Forsum, U., Wigren, A. and Wigzell, H. (1982). Relationships between HLA-DR expressing cells and T lymphocytes of different subsets in rheumatoid synovial tissue. *Scand. J. Immunol.*, **15**, 501—7

25. Förre, Ö., Thoen, J., Lea, T., Dobloug, J.H., Mellbye, O.J., Natvig, J.B., Pahle, J. and Solheim, B.G. (1982). In situ characterization of mononuclear cells in rheumatoid tissues using monoclonal antibodies. Scand. J. Immunol., 16, 315–19

26. Engleman, E.G., Benike, C.J., Grumet, F.C. and Evans, R.L. (1981). Activation of human T lymphocyte subsets: Helper and suppressor/cytotoxic T-cells recognize and respond to distinct histocompatibility antigens. J. Immunol., 127, 2124–9

27. Lindblad, S., Klareskog, L., Hedfors, E., Forsum, U. and Sundström, C. (1983). Phenotypic characterization of synovial tissue in situ in different types of synovitis. Arthr. Rheum., 26, 1321–32

28. Scheynius, A., Fischer, T., Forsum, U. and Klareskog, L. (1984). Phenotypic characterization in situ of inflammatory cells in allergic and irritant contact dermatitis in man. Clin. Exp. Immunol., 55, 81–90

29. Johnell, O., Hulth, A. and Henriksson, A. (1986). T-lymphocyte subsets and HLA-DR expressing cells in the osteoarthritic synovialis. Scand. J. Rheumatol. (In press)

30. Malone, D.G., Wahl, S.M., Tsokos, M., Cattell, H., Decker, J.L. and Wilder, R.L. (1984). Immune function in severe active rheumatoid arthritis: a relationship between peripheral blood mononuclear cell proliferation to soluble antigens and synovial tissue immunohisto-logic characteristics. J. Clin. Invest., 74, 1173–85

31. Lindblad, S. and Hedfors, E. (1985). Intra-articular variation in synovitis. Local macroscopic and microscopic signs of inflammatory activity are significantly correlated. Arthr. Rheum., 28, 977–86

32. Barland, P., Novikoff, A.B. and Hamerman, D. (1962). Electron microscopy of the human synovial membrane. J. Cell Biol., 14, 207–30

33. Shiozawa, S., Shiozawa, K. and Fujita, T. (1983). Presence of HLA-DR antigen on synovial type A and B cells: an immuno-electron microscopic study in rheumatoid arthritis, osteoarthritis and normal traumatic joints. Immunology, 50, 587–94

34. Iguchi, T., Kurosaka, M. and Ziff, M. (1986). Electron microscopic study of HLA-DR and monocyte/macrophage staining cells in the rheumatoid synovial membrane. Arthr. Rheum., 29, 600–13

35. Poulter, L.W., Duke, O., Hobbs, S., Janossy, G. and Panai, G. (1982). Histochemical discrimination of HLA-DR positive cell populations in the normal and arthritic synovial lining. Clin. Exp. Immunol., 48, 381–8

36. Burmester, G.R., Locher, P., Koch, B., Winchester, R.J., Dimitriu-Bona, A., Kalden, J.R. and Mohr, W. (1983). The tissue architecture of synovial membranes in inflammatory and non-inflammatory joint diseases. Rheumatol. Int., 3, 173–81

37. Poulter, L.W., Duke, O., Hobbs, S., Janossy, G., Panayi, G. and Seymour, G. (1983). The involvement of interdigitating (antigen-presenting) cells in the pathogenesis of rheumatoid arthritis. Clin. Exp. Immunol., 51, 247–54

38. Kurosaka, M. and Ziff, M. (1983). Immunoelectron microscopic study of the distribution of T cell subsets in rheumatoid synovium. J. Exp. Med., 158, 1191–210

39. Fraser, J.R.E. and McCall, J.F. (1965). Culture of synovial cells in vitro. Notes on isolation and propagation. Ann. Rheum. Dis., 24, 351–9

40. Klareskog, L., Forsum, U. and Wigzell, H. (1982). Murine synovial intima contains I-A, I-E/C positive bone-marrow derived cells. Scand. J. Immunol., 15, 508–13

41. Klareskog, L., Holmdahl, R., Rubin, K., Victorin, A. and Lindgren, J.A. (1985). Different populations of rheumatoid adherent cells mediate activation versus suppression of T lymphocyte proliferation. Arthr. Rheum., 28, 863–72

42. Waalen, K., Thoen, J., Förre, Ö., Hovig, T., Teigland, J. and Natvig, J.B. (1986). Rheumatoid synovial dendritic cells as stimulators in allogeneic and autologous mixed leucocyte reactions – comparisons with autologous monocytes as stimulator cells. Scand. J. Immunol., 23, 233–41

43. Zvaifler, N.J., Steinman, R.M., Kaplan, G., Lau, L.L. and Rivelis, M. (1985). Identification of immunostimulatory dendritic cells in the synovial effusions of patients with rheumatoid arthritis. J. Clin. Invest., 76, 789–800

44. Van Voorhis, W.C., Hair, L.S., Steinman, R.M. and Kaplan, G. (1982). Human dendritic cells: enrichment and characterization from peripheral blood. J. Exp. Med., 155, 1172–87

45. Hirschberg, H., Braathen, L. and Thorsby, E. (1982). Antigen presentation by vascular endothelial cells and epidermal Langerhans cells: the role of HLA-DR. Immunol. Rev., 66, 57–77

46. Geppert, T.D. and Lipsky, P.E. (1985). Antigen presentation by interferon-gamma-treated endothelial cells and fibroblasts: differential ability to function as antigen-presenting cells despite comparable Ia expression. *J. Immunol.*, **135**, 3750–62

47. Metzger, Z., Hoffeld, J.T. and Oppenheim, J.J. (1980). Macrophage-mediated suppression I. Evidence for participation of both hydrogen peroxide and prostaglandins in suppression of murine lymphocyte proliferation. *J. Immunol.*, **124**, 983–8

48. Stastny, P. (1976). Mixed lymphocyte cultures in rheumatoid arthritis. *J. Clin. Invest.*, **57**, 1148–57

49. Stastny, P. (1978). Association of the B-cell alloantigen DRw4 with rheumatoid arthritis. *N. Engl. J. Med.*, **298**, 869–71

50. Peterson, P.A. and Rask, L. (1986). Genes and antigens of the HLA-D region. In Solheim, B.G., Möller, E. and Ferrone, S. (eds.) *HLA class II Antigens. A Comprehensive Review of Structure and Function.* pp. 1–14. (Berlin, Heidelberg: Springer-Verlag)

51. Jeannet, M. (1986). Class II HLA antigens in autoimmune and immune-mediated diseases. In Solheim, B.G., Möller, E. and Ferrone, S. (eds.) *HLA class II Antigens. A Comprehensive Review of Structure and Function.* pp. 489–514. (Berlin, Heidelberg: Springer-Verlag)

52. Nepom, B.S., Palmer, J., Kim, S.J., Hansen, J.A., Holbeck, S.L. and Nepom, G.T. (1986). Specific genomic markers for the HLA-DQ subregion discriminate between DR4+ insulin-dependent diabetes mellitus and DR4+ seropositive juvenile rheumatoid arthritis. *J. Exp. Med.*, **164**, 345–50

53. Goronzy, J., Weyand, C.M. and Garrison Fathman, C. (1986). Shared T cell recognition sites on human histocompatibility leucocyte antigen class II molecules of patients with seropositive rheumatoid arthritis. *J. Clin. Invest.*, **77**, 1042–9

54. Holoshitz, J., Klajman, A., Drucker, I., Lapidot, Z., Yaretzky, A., van Eden, W. and Cohen, I.R. (1986). T lymphocytes of rheumatoid arthritis patients show augmented reactivity to a fraction of mycobacteria cross-reactive with cartilage. *Lancet*, **ii**, 305–9

55. Jasin, H.E. (1985). Autoantibody specificities of immune complexes sequestered in articular cartilage of patients with rheumatoid arthritis and osteoarthritis. *Arthr. Rheum.*, **28**, 241–8

56. Munthe, E. and Natvig, J.B. (1972). Immunoglobulin classes, subclasses and complexes of IgG rheumatoid factor in rheumatoid plasma cells. *Clin. Exp. Immunol.*, **12**, 55–70

57. Fehr, K., Velvart, M., Rauber, M., Knöpfel, M., Baici, A., Salgam and Böni, A. (1981). Production of agglutinators and rheumatoid factors in plasma cells of rheumatoid and non-rheumatoid synovial tissue. *Arthr. Rheum.*, **24**, 510–19

58. Egeland, T., Lea, T., Saari, G., Mellbye, O.J. and Natvig, J.B. (1982). Quantitation of cells secreting rheumatoid factors of IgG, IgA and IgM class after elution from rheumatoid synovial tissue. *Arthr. Rheum.*, **25**, 1445–53

59. Klareskog, L., Rubin, K. and Holmdahl, R. (1986). Binding of collagen type II to rheumatoid synovial cells. *Scand. J. Immunol.*, **24**, 705–14

60. Andrioupolos, N.A., Mestecky, J., Wright, G.P. and Miller, E.J. (1976). Antibodies to native and denatured collagens in sera of patients with rheumatoid arthritis. *Arthr. Rheum.*, **19**, 613–17

61. Clague, R.B., Firth, S.A., Lennox Holt, P.J., Skingle, J., Greenbury, C.L. and Webley, M. (1983). Serum antibodies to type II collagen in rheumatoid arthritis: comparison of 6 immunological methods and clinical features. *Ann. Rheum. Dis.*, **42**, 537–44

62. Pereira, R.S., Black, C.M., Duance, V.C., Jones, V.E., Jacoby, R.K. and Welsh, K.I. (1985). Disappearing collagen antibodies in rheumatoid arthritis. *Lancet*, **ii**, 501–2

63. Klareskog, L., Holmdahl, R., Larsson, E. and Wigzell, H. (1983). Role of T lymphocytes in collagen II induced arthritis in rats. *Clin. Exp. Immunol.*, **51**, 117–25

64. Holmdahl, R., Rubin, K., Klareskog, L., Dencker, L., Gustafson, G. and Larsson, E. (1985). Appearance of different lymphoid cells in synovial tissue and in peripheral blood during the course of collagen II induced arthritis in rats. *Scand. J. Immunol.*, **21**, 197–204

65. Larsson, P., Holmdahl, R., Dencker, L. and Klareskog, L. (1985). In vivo treatment with W3/13 (anti-pan T) but not with Ox8 (anti-suppressor/cytotoxic T) monoclonal antibodies impedes the development of adjuvant arthritis in rats. *Immunology*, **56**, 383–91

66. Kohashi, O., Pearson, C.M., Tamaoki, N., Tanaka, A., Shimamura, K., Ozawa, A., Kotani, S., Saito, M. and Hioki, K. (1981). Role of thymus for N-acetyl-muramyl-L-alanyl-D-isoglutamin-induced polyarthritis and granuloma formation in euthymic and athymic nude rats or in neonatally thymectomized rats. *Infect. Immunol.*, **31**, 758–66

67. Ranges, G.E., Sriram, S. and Cooper, S.M. (1985). Prevention of type II collagen-induced arthritis by *in vivo* treatment with anti-L3T4. *J. Exp. Med.*, **162**, 1105–10
68. Holmdahl, R., Klareskog, L., Rubin, K., Larsson, E. and Wigzell, H. (1985). T lymphocytes in collagen II induced arthritis in mice. Characterization of arthritogenic collagen II specific T cells lines and clones. *Scand. J. Immunol.*, **22**, 295–306
69. Holoshitz, J., Naparstek, Y., Ben-Nun, A. and Cohen, I.R. (1984). Arthritis induced in rats by cloned T lymphocytes responsive to mycobacteria but not to collagen type II. *J. Clin. Invest.*, **73**, 211–15
70. Van Eden, W., Holoshitz J., Nevo, Z., Frenkel, A., Klajman, A. and Cohen, I.R. (1985). Arthritis induced by a T lymphocyte clone that responds to mycobacterium tuberculosis and to cartilage proteoglycans. *Proc. Natl. Acad. Sci. USA*, **82**, 5117–20
71. Stuart, J.M. and Dixon, F.J. (1982). Serum transfer of collagen-induced arthritis in mice. *J. Exp. Med.*, **158**, 378–92
72. Taurog, J.D., Kerwar, S.S., McReynolds, R.A., Sandberg, G.P., Leary, S.L. and Mahowald, M.L. (1985). Synergy between adjuvant arthritis and collagen-induced arthritis in rats. *J. Exp. Med.*, **162**, 962–78
73. Holmdahl, R., Olsson, T., Moran, T. and Klareskog, L. (1985). *In vivo* treatment of rats with monoclonal anti T cell antibodies. Immunohistochemical and functional analysis in normal rats and in experimental allergic neuritis (EAN). *Scand. J. Immunol.*, **22**, 157–69
74. Lennon, V.A. and Byrd, W.J. (1973). Experimental arthritis in thymectomized rats with an impaired humoral immune response. *Nature*, **244**, 38–40
75. Holoshitz, J., Naparstek, Y., Ben-Nun, A. and Cohen, I.R. (1983). Lines of T lymphocytes induce or vaccinate against autoimmune arthritis. *Science*, **219**, 56–8
76. Cohen, I.R., Ben-Nun, A., Holoshitz, J., Maron, R. and Zerubavel, R.L. (1984). Vaccination against autoimmune disease using lines of autoimmune T lymphocytes. *Immunol. Today*, **4**, 227–30
77. Fox, R., Sportsman, R., Rhodes, G., Luka, J., Pearson, G. and Vaughan, J. (1986). Rheumatoid arthritis synovial membrane contains a 62 000 molecular weight protein that shares an antigeni epitope with the Epstein-Barr virus-encoded associated nuclear antigen. *J. Clin. Invest.*, **77**, 1539–47
78. Steffen, C. (1970). Consideration of pathogenesis of rheumatoid arthritis as collagen autoimmunity. *Z. Immunol. Forsch.*, **139**, 219–27
79. Wolf, B., Bashey, R.I., Newton, C.D. and Jimenez, S.A. (1986). Development of rheumatoid factors and anti-F(ab)$_2$ antibodies in guineapigs immunized with type II bovine collagen. *Int. Arch. Appl. Immunol.*, **80**, 214–20
80. Holmdahl, R., Tarkowski, A., Nordling, C., Rubin, K. and Klareskog, L. (1987). Connection between autoimmunity to cartilage collagen type II and rheumatoid factor production. In Bona, C. and Zanetti, M. (eds.) *Idiotypes in Health and Disease*. (In press)
81. Holmdahl, R., Nordling, C., Rubin, K., Tarkowski, A. and Klareskog, L. (1986). Generation of monoclonal rheumatoid factors (RF) after immunization with collagen II-anti-collagen II immune complexes. An anti-idiotypic antibody to anti-collagen II is simultaneously a rheumatoid factor. *Scand. J. Immunol.*, **24**, 197–203

# 9
# Experimental animal models of chronic arthritis

R. L. WILDER

Current theories of pathogenesis of rheumatoid arthritis and related arthritides hypothesize that the joint disease reflects a genetically regulated immunological reaction directed at either: (i) an exogenous agent that localizes to the joints or (ii) an articular autoantigen. These concepts, as suggested by studies of arthritis in animals, will almost certainly be modified in the future since immunological reactions directed at exogenous or host antigens may overlap, i.e. the responses are not necessarily mutually exclusive. With the view that animal models may provide insights into pathogenetic mechanisms of arthritis in humans, I will summarize our current understanding of the major experimentally-induced animal models of chronic erosive arthritis.

The models that will be reviewed include adjuvant and related arthritides in the rat, collagen arthritis in the rat and mouse, antigen-induced arthritis in the rabbit and mouse, and streptococcal and lactobacillus cell wall-induced arthritis in the rat and mouse. Particular emphasis will be given to significant data regarding (i) causative mechanisms and stimuli, (ii) pathogenesis and the role of the immune system, and (iii) regulatory factors. For more detailed discussion of the older literature the reader is referred to previous reviews[1,2]. The spontaneously developing MRL-1pr/1pr mouse model, although important and widely studied, will not be covered.

## ADJUVANT ARTHRITIS AND RELATED ARTHRITIDES

Adjuvant arthritis, historically, is a model of erosive arthritis in rats that is induced by intradermal administration (footpad or base of tail) of Freund's complete adjuvant, which is an oil and water emulsion containing heat killed *Mycobacteria tuberculosis* or *Mycobacteria butyricum*. After a latent period of 9–14 days, swelling develops primarily in distal extremities (wrists, ankles and paws) and persists for several weeks and ultimately results in joint destruction. The caudal vertebrae may also be involved resulting in spondylitis. Histologically, the earliest phases of disease exhibit an exudative inflammatory reaction in the stroma of the synovial membrane, in periarticular tissue, about tendons/tendon sheaths, along periosteum and between muscle bundles. The joint spaces contain primarily polymorphonuclear leukocytes while the tissues contain primarily mononuclear cells. Subsynovial oedema and fibrin deposition are also prominent features. As the disease progresses, hypertrophy of synovial villi, hyperplasia of synovial lining cells and active periosteal new bone formation become prominent[3]. The later stages are marked by growth of granulation tissue with mainly a residual mononuclear cell infiltrate. Progressively fewer acute inflammatory cells and less intense vascular congestion are noted.

Other tissues that also frequently show abnormalities include spleen/lymph nodes (hyperplasia and granulomas), liver (granulomas) and bone marrow (increased cellularity). Other occasionally observed abnormalities include balanitis, conjunctivitis and auricular chondritis. The heart, lungs, kidneys and brain are usually normal.

The clinical picture thus has some features in common with rheumatoid arthritis in humans but more closely resembles Reiter's syndrome. In parallel with this concept, most investigators have reported that rheumatoid factors are not produced, although highly sensitive techniques have generally not been employed.

## Characteristics of the arthritogenic stimulus

Although Freund's complete adjuvant is the classic and most commonly used inducer of the model disease, considerable effort has been expended to define the essential components in the mixture. Clearly, the volume, type of oil, and composition of the emulsion are important variables[4,5]. Moreover, many types of bacteria in a water and oil emulsion are adjuvant active and may also induce arthritis. The active component in the bacteria is clearly the cell wall peptidoglycan but additional variability results from differences in particle size and hydrophilic-hydrophobic properties. The minimum structure which retains at least measurable biologic activity is the peptidoglycan fragment, muramyl dipeptide[6-11]. Available data suggest that the oil emulsion prolongs the *in vivo* clearance of the peptidoglycan. For example, muramyl dipeptide injected in saline is eliminated *in vivo* with a half-life of about 2 h and requires repeated injections to induce even mild transient arthritis, whereas when administered as a water and oil emulsion, it induces chronic, although mild, disease after a single injection[10,12]. A complicating aspect of current understanding is that not all adjuvant active materials are derived from bacteria. In fact at least one oil, CP 20961, is adjuvant active itself and induces arthritis indistinguishable from the classic disease[13]. Presumably tissue persistence and appropriate hydrophilic–hydrophobic properties are essential characteristics.

The primary effect of adjuvants is on macrophages[14,15]. Depending on dose, type of macrophage and other factors, adjuvants induce a spectrum of cellular phenotypic changes reflecting minimal activation to the death of the cell. Activated macrophages may produce increased levels of a variety of mediators, such as interleukin-1 and prostaglandins. Although the direct effect of adjuvant active materials is on macrophages, they may indirectly have profound effects on other cell types including T and B lymphocytes, as well as various types of mesenchymal cells.

Considerable controversy has existed as to whether the induction of arthritis by adjuvants is a direct (adjuvant localized in the joints) or indirect (adjuvant localized remotely outside the joint) effect. Data, as discussed further below, for both points of view can be cited, although the strongest evidence supports an indirect autoimmune aetiology secondary to structural mimicry between adjuvant and articular antigens. Nevertheless, small quantities of adjuvant do localize in the joints and are slowly eliminated[16].

### Pathogenetic mechanisms and role of the immune system

A large body of data support the view that adjuvant arthritis is dependent upon the immune system, particularly the thymus and thymus-dependent lymphocytes (T-cells). After a lag period of 9–14 days, a T-helper/inducer mononuclear cell-rich infiltrate appears in the joints in parallel with development of joint swelling. This infiltrate and chronic disease are not observed in congenitally immunodeficient athymic rats or in rats with induced immunodeficiency (e.g., cyclosporin A, high dose cyclophosphamide or irradiation treatment, or in vivo treatment with anti-T-cell antibodies)[9,11,17,18].

The strongest argument for T-cells and an autoimmune process is that arthritis can be induced, although often with variable results, in naive recipients by administration of T-cells from diseased animals[19]. The transferred disease process has been further characterized by the use of T-cell lines and clones reactive with M. tuberculosis. Transfer of various lines or clones into naive recipients may either induce arthritis or render the animal resistant to disease induction. Interestingly, a highly arthritogenic clone reactive to M. tuberculosis also displayed cross-reactivity with proteoglycan purified from cartilage[20–24]. This observation suggested that the disease may, in fact, be an autoimmune process triggered by structural mimicry between antigens in the environment and host antigens. This observation does not, however, exclude an important role for a direct response to adjuvant-related substances that localize to the joint during the induction of the response. Moreover, the structural mimicry hypothesis does not readily explain the disease produced by non-immunogenic muramyl dipeptide in oil or adjuvant active oils alone (e.g. CP20961), nor does it fully explain the granulomas in the spleen, lymph nodes and liver that clearly develop around oil droplets. The latter lesions probably reflect a direct response to the oil-based adjuvant that localizes to these sites. Most likely, adjuvant-induced pathology reflects responses directed at both the adjuvant and host antigens.

Adjuvant-injected animals also develop a number of lymphoid abnormalities including depressed mitogen responsiveness, autologous mixed lymphocyte reaction, interleukin-2 production and localized response to inflammatory agents[25-30]. The significance of these observations, many of which have also been observed in chronic diseases in man, remain largely undefined.

### Factors influencing susceptibility

Adjuvant arthritis is relatively specific for rats, although mice and hamsters may develop mild, transient inflammatory oedema[31]. Among inbred rat strains, large differences in susceptibility are observed. Susceptibility appears to be a dominant or codominant trait, influenced by multiple gene loci, distinct from the major histocompatibility complex[10,32-34]. The mechanisms underlying these species and strain susceptibility differences are not understood.

An interesting observation that apparently has not been pursued is the apparent linkage of adjuvant arthritis with dextran sensitivity[35]. Because of the increasing interest in the role of mast cells in immunologically mediated disease, this area needs further investigation.

A number of other factors have been shown to influence disease susceptibility. For example, joints innervated with neurons containing high density substance P develop more severe disease than those with low density innervation supporting a role for neurogenic factors in the disease process[36,37].

Microbial factors other than administered adjuvant are also important. Mycoplasma infection decreases the severity of adjuvant arthritis in LEW rats[38]. Pathogen-free or conventionally bred F344 rats are generally resistant to adjuvant arthritis, whereas germ-free F344 rats, which are immunologically underdeveloped, are highly susceptible. Colonization of the germ-free rats with gram positive bacteria enhances susceptibility, whereas colonization with gram negatives suppresses disease susceptibility[39,40]. It seems likely that uncontrolled infectious or other microbial factors may explain many of the differences in reported results between various laboratories.

## COLLAGEN-INDUCED ARTHRITIS

Collagen-induced arthritis (CIA) is an experimentally induced autoimmune model of chronic, erosive arthritis in rats and mice. It is produced by sensitization to native type 2 collagen, a major component of articular cartilage. Denatured type 2 collagen and collagen types 1, 3 or 4 are not arthritogenic[41,42].

The disease process is biphasic. About 5 days after subcutaneous administration of the collagen (emulsified in incomplete Freund's adjuvant), fibrin deposits appear in the joint space and synovial tissues simultaneously with development of oedema. By 12 days, hyperplasia of synovial lining cells is noted. The later phase of the disease overlaps with the early phase and exhibits a granulocyte-rich infiltrate in the joint space and a mononuclear cell-rich infiltrate in the sublining synovial tissues. The lining cell layer shows continued hypertrophy and granulation tissue develops. Marginal erosions and periostitis with prominent new bone growth are also characteristic features[3,42-44].

Clinically, the model resembles adjuvant arthritis in its articular features but otherwise, despite some claims otherwise, appears to utilize distinct pathogenetic pathways for production of arthritis, at least for the initiation of arthritis[3,18,45-49]. It has certain similarities to rheumatoid arthritis and seronegative polyarthropathies in humans.

## Pathogenetic mechanisms and role of the immune system

A very large amount of research effort in the last several years has been devoted to studying immune mechanisms in CIA. Clearly, the arthritic process is dependent upon anti-type 2 collagen autoimmunity[41,42] with both humoral and cellular immune processes playing important roles. Initiation of the disease process requires the production of IgG antibody in sufficient amounts, with an appropriate subclass, that is capable of binding certain arthritogenic epitopes on type 2 collagen and is also capable of activating the complement system[50-64]. Some authors have stated, based upon studies of passive anti-collagen antibody transfer, that antibody and complement alone are sufficient to produce the major manifestations of arthritis such as synovial proliferation, pannus formation, marginal erosions and destruction of cartilage.

Other studies indicate that thymus-dependent lymphocytes also play an important role. For example, T-helper/inducer lymphocytes are major components of the chronic synovial cellular infiltrate. Arthritis does not develop in immunodeficient athymic nude or cyclosporin A-treated rats[65-68]. Arthritis does not develop in animals treated prophylactically with total body irradiation, or with anti-T cell, or anti-class II major histocompatibility complex antibodies[69-71]. Moreover, passive transfer of T-cells or T-cell lines or clones reactive with type 2 collagen may induce or inhibit the disease process[72-75]. Finally, type 2 collagen specific T-cell lines have been reported to produce a cytokine that induces arthritis when injected intra-articularly in naive recipients[76].

In addition to T and B lymphocytes, their products and other non-specific inflammatory mediators, important functions for macrophages and neutrophils are also apparent[77-79]. Thus, data support the view that multiple host mechanisms interact to generate the pathologic process in this autoimmune arthritis model.

## Host factors regulating susceptibility

Not surprisingly, host genetic factors play an instrumental role in the development of CIA. In both rats and mice, wide variation in susceptibility is observed between inbred rat strains. Major histocompatibility complex (MHC)-linked genes appear to exert primary control of the immune response to type 2 collagen, but non-MHC genes are also important[50,59,80-83]. Moreover, in some inbred strains, sex-related factors are important modulators of disease development[83,84]. The value of identifying genetically-controlled differences in susceptibility is that they provide an opportunity to define critical pathogenetic mechanisms in the disease process. The CIA model is especially important in this context.

## ANTIGEN-INDUCED ARTHRITIS

Antigen-induced arthritis is an experimental model of chronic arthritis in mice and rabbits that is produced by intra-articular injection of antigen into a recipient previously immunized with the antigen. In the original description by Dumonde and Glynn, rabbits were given a single intradermal injection of fibrin in complete Freund's adjuvant, followed 2 to 3 weeks later by an intra-articular injection of fibrin[85]. Subsequent studies have used a variety of antigens and have tended to utilize mice as the host species.

The nature of the induced lesion varies depending on type, dose and frequency of antigen injection[86], and also depends on a variety of host factors as discussed below, but hyperplasia and hypertrophy of synovial lining cells are a prominent component. In the most severe forms, the arthritis is arthus-like initially but is followed within a few days by infiltration of mononuclear cells[85]. Granulocytes are prominent components in the synovial fluid but are sparse in synovial tissue[87]. Depending on the chronicity of the process, variable degrees of bony erosion and cartilage loss ultimately develop. Periosteal new bone growth is another prominent feature[88].

### Role of the antigen in the disease process

Considerable research effort has been devoted to defining the role of the antigen in the model. The effects of a variety of antigens (fibrin, ferritin, horseradish peroxidase, albumin, ovalbumin, catalase) have been studied and results establish that the disease is clearly antigen-specific. Intra-articular injection of irrelevant antigen does not produce the full blown monoarthritis.

The multiple studies have shown that the persistence of free antigen in the joint space is short because the antigen is rapidly bound by antibody. The binding of the antigen by antibody leads to its persistence in the joint[89–91].

Impressive evidence indicates that electrical charge on the antigen determines both the site and amount of the antigen that is retained in the joint. Negatively charged antigen appears to have no affinity for cartilage and large amounts of antibody are required for its retention in the joint, primarily in loose collagenous connective tissue but not in hyaline cartilage. In contrast, positively charged antigen complexes are retained in substantially greater amounts and are noted in both collagenous connective tissue and hyaline cartilage. In addition, the amount of antigen retained in the joint determines the severity of the chronic arthritis[91–93].

Of potential relevance to the understanding of flare-up phenomena in human arthritides is the observation that an involved joint develops an exacerbation of inflammation after oral or intravenous antigen challenge. Doses of antigen as small as 10 nanograms are sufficient to induce a measurable

162

change in the inflammatory process[94–96]. Clearly, such a mechanism could lead to chronic arthritis if the source of antigen was present in the gastrointestinal tract.

## Pathogenetic mechanisms and role of the immune system

The original investigators postulated that the model represented a delayed hypersensitivity reaction to persistent antigen[85]. This concept is clearly correct. The immunized animals demonstrate a typical delayed type hypersensitivity reaction at usual test sites[97]. The arthritis does not develop in nude mice and can be inhibited by treatment of susceptible animals with antithymocyte antibodies or irradiation and, of course, the mode of induction suggests immunological hypersensitivity[98].

B lymphocytes and antibodies are also important. There is a marked increase in synthesis by inflamed synovium of immunoglobulin that specifically binds the antigen. As noted above, the antibody prolongs the clearance of the antigen from the joint and partly determines its localization, i.e. cartilage surface[91,92].

The antigen–antibody complexes undoubtedly play a role in the initial arthus-like reaction, but the importance of complement system is unclear. Complement depletion with cobra venom apparently has no effect in mice, whereas rabbits treated with cobra venom or deficient in C6 have delayed onset of the arthus-type reaction[99,100].

Recent studies have addressed the detailed mechanisms by which the immune system produces joint destruction. Data indicate that the immune system enhances the new bone formation and contributes to the decreases in chondrocyte proteoglycan synthesis and even chrondrocyte death. Additional evidence indicates that peroxides may be directly responsible for these effects[88,93,101].

## Regulatory mechanisms

In mice, antigen-induced arthritis is clearly regulated by host genetic mechanisms. Surveys of inbred strains of mice have identified resistant and susceptible strains. The work indicated that the response is controlled by a limited number of autosomally dominant and unlinked genes, one of which was loosely linked to the major histocompatibility complex[102–104]. The genetic control in this model, undoubtedly, is inter-related to regulation of the immune response to the antigen.

## STREPTOCOCCAL CELL WALL-INDUCED ARTHRITIS

Streptococcal cell wall-induced arthritis is an experimentally induced animal model of arthritis that is induced by systemic administration of cell wall fragments in aqueous solution which are relatively resistant to biodegra-dation[105–124]. The rat is the principal experimental animal utilized, guinea-pigs

163

also develop similar disease but have been studied in much more limited manner. Mice are generally resistant to disease although a recent report described acute erythema and swelling of peripheral joints after intravenous injection of cell walls to certain inbred mouse strains[125].

Within 24 h of administration of group A streptococcal cell wall fragments to LEW/N rats, acute erythema and swelling develop in peripheral joints coincident with the localization of cell wall fragments in the blood vessels of the synovium and in the subchrondral bone marrow. Histologically, this early-onset phase of disease is characterized by oedema, fibrin deposition and infiltration by phagocytic cells of granulocytic and monocytic lineage. This initial phase peaks in severity at 3 days and subsides over the next week. About 3 weeks after cell wall administration a second phase of swelling develops and, although it waxes and wanes in severity, persists for months. Histologically, it is characterized by exuberant synovial lining and sublining cell proliferation, infiltration by T-helper/inducer lymphocytes and macrophages, and marginal erosion of bone and cartilage. It ultimately destroys the more severely affected joints. In contrast to adjuvant, collagen- and antigen-induced arthritis, periosteal new bone formation is absent or generally a very late development. The axial skeleton is not involved. Thus, the clinical, histological and radiological features of the experimental joint disease closely resemble those observed in adult and juvenile rheumatoid arthritis in humans.

Other pathologic abnormalities that may develop include hepatic granulomas[106,109,110,126,127], splenic and lymph node hypertrophy/hyperplasia[109] and occasional eye inflammation.

### Characteristics of the arthritogenic stimulus

Cell wall fragments (peptidoglycan with its associated group-specific polysaccharide heteropolymer) from group A, B or C streptococci induce severe acute and chronic arthritis but group D streptococci induces a milder and more transient erosive arthritis[128]. Arthritogenicity is associated with lysozyme resistance and apparently high rhamnose content in the group specific polysaccharide heteropolymer[109,110,114–116,129], which appears to protect the peptidoglycan from degradation. This property allows the cell wall fragments to persist *in vivo* for months in the joints. Rendering the cell walls susceptible to lysozyme cleavage by acetylation or degrading the cell walls *in vitro* or *in vivo* with the enzyme mutanolysin, inhibits the development of chronic arthritis[117,118].

Since streptococcal cell wall fragments contain peptidoglycan, the active moiety in adjuvants, it would be expected that these substances would also be adjuvant active. Although this is highly likely to be the case, this point has not, to my knowledge, been adequately documented in the published literature. Like other adjuvants, it probably acts directly on macrophages to induce their activation and indirectly activates other cellular elements involved in immune and inflammatory reactions. In addition to its direct effects on cells, streptococcal cell walls also directly activate the complement system[130].

## Pathogenetic mechanisms and role of the immune system

Cogent evidence now exists demonstrating that both thymus-independent and thymus-dependent processes play a role in the development of the experimental arthritis[110,111]. All LEW rats (euthymic and immunodeficient athymic and cyclosporin A-treated rats) develop the rapid onset, early phase exudative arthritis, but only euthymic rats with intact T lymphocyte function develop the chronic proliferative and erosive disease. The chronic phase disease is associated with synovial infiltration of T-helper/inducer lymphocytes. Further evidence supporting a critical role for T-lymphocytes in the chronic disease is the observation that reconstitution of athymic rats with T-lymphocytes permits development of the chronic disease[121]. On the other hand, the rapid onset acute disease can be inhibited by systemic administration of cobra venom which inactivates the complement system. This treatment, however, does not affect the development of the chronic proliferative and erosive disease[119,120].

Explants of diseased synovial tissue spontaneously secrete a number of products during *in vitro* culture, these products include collagenase, prostaglandin $E_2$ and several cytokines (further characterization in progress) which modulate synovial cell growth and function[112,122]. These observations are important because bone and cartilage erosion appear to be mediated directly by synovial fibroblast-like cells with a 'transformed' appearance[122]. The abnormal proliferation and invasive properties of these cells are apparently induced by and dependent upon T-lymphocyte and macrophage products. Thus, the pathogenetic process appears to resemble a localized synovial neoplasm that is regulated and driven by products from immune cells. The initiating factor, as stated previously, is deposition of the cell walls in the joints.

Like adjuvant-injected rats, streptococcal cell wall injected rats develop several immunological defects including anergy, depressed splenic mononuclear cell proliferative responses to mitogens[109,131] and defective production of interleukin-2[131]. As is the case with adjuvant arthritis, the significance of these abnormalities is unknown, but they are reminiscent of similar defects in patients with rheumatoid arthritis and other chronic inflammatory diseases.

## Factors influencing susceptibility

Susceptibility to the development of chronic arthritis is markedly dependent on genetic background. For example, LEW/N, or M520/N inbred rats develop severe arthritis approaching 100% incidence, while F344/N, CAR/N or WKY/N rats are relatively resistant[106,108,109]. These differences are not due to a failure to deposit cell walls in synovial tissues. Cell walls appear to distribute similarly but chronic disease does not develop. Since F344/N, CAR/N and LEW/N rats possess a similar major histocompatibility complex (MHC) haplotype, non-MHC gene loci probably play important roles in the regulation of the disease process[123,124]. The MHC, particularly the Ia region, does play an important role since it has been demonstrated that class II MHC antigen expression in the synovium is markedly increased in diseased tissues, i.e. class

II antigen expression parallels disease incidence and severity (R. Wilder *et al.*, submitted for publication). These observations provide potential molecular level insights into the mechanisms regulating disease susceptibility.

Sex-related factors are also a major factor in certain rat strains. For example, LEW/N female rats are highly susceptible to chronic disease but LEW/N male rats are not. The sex-linked effects appear to be mediated by sex hormones. Castration or oestrogen administration to males markedly exacerbates the disease process[113].

## LACTOBACILLUS CELL WALL-INDUCED ARTHRITIS

Lactobacillus cell wall-induced arthritis is an experimental model in rats closely resembling the streptococcal cell wall model[129,132,133] except that cell walls from *Lactobacillus casei* are utilized. However, it has been studied far less extensively than the streptococcal cell wall model. The major difference between this model and the streptococcal cell wall model, thus far, has been absence of hepatic granulomas in lactobacillus cell wall injected rats. Disease, like that in the streptococcal cell wall model, is dependent upon localization and persistence of the cell walls in the joints. The model is particularly interesting, with respect to human disease, because lactobacillus is a component of the normal gastrointestinal flora, implying that an enormous load of potential arthritogenic stimuli are present in the normal gastrointestinal tract.

## CONCLUDING REMARKS

Although none of the animal models can be equated with a specific form of arthritis in humans, the data from animal models clearly provide new insights regarding the immunopathogenesis of chronic arthritis. From the information reviewed here, many important concepts are evident. A listing of the major concepts would include:

(1) Joint pathology, resembling that in human disease, can be induced in animals by a variety of aetiological agents. This observation suggests that human conditions, like rheumatoid arthritis, may be syndromes with common endpoints that may be induced by a variety of aetiological agents.

(2) Microbial components, particularly cell wall components derived from enteric organisms, are potential aetiological agents in humans. In addition to their ability to induce disease by direct localization to synovium, they may also induce disease remotely as a result of structural mimicry between host structures in the joint and a microbial structure.

(3) The immune system, particularly T lymphocytes, plays an essential role in the disease process. It appears to regulate the growth and differentiation of connective tissue cells in the joint.

166

(4)   Host genetic factors (in addition to the MHC) and sex-related factors also play a major role in determining the type, incidence and severity of disease in response to a particular aetiological gent.

This listing can be extended indefinitely but, in any event, it is clear that animal models provide an indispensible investigative approach for unravelling fundamental aspects of arthritis in humans.

## References

1.  Gardner, D.L. (1960). The experimental production of arthritis. *Ann. Rheum. Dis.*, **19**, 297–317
2.  Sokoloff, L. (1984). Animal models of rheumatoid arthritis. *Int. Rev. Exp. Pathol.*, **26**, 108–45
3.  Carlson, R.P., Datko, L.J., O'Neill-David, L., Blazek, E.M., DeLustro, F., Beideman, R. and Lewis, A.J. (1985). Comparison of inflammatory changes in established type II collagen- and adjuvant-induced arthritis using outbred Wistar rats. *Int. J. Immunopharmacol.*, **7**, 811–26
4.  Lussier, A., De Medicis, R. and Tetreault, L. (1984). Adjuvant arthritis: influence of the adjuvant volume and composition on the established arthritis. *Int. J. Tissue React.*, **6**, 105–10
5.  Best, R., Christian, R. and Lewis, D.A. (1984). Effect of particle size of dried mycobacteria on adjuvant induced arthritis in the rat. *Agents Actions*, **14**, 265–8
6.  Kohashi, O., Tanaka, A., Kotani, S., Shiba, T., Kusumoto, K., Ykogawa, K. and Ozawa, A. (1980). Arthritis inducing ability of a synthetic adjuvant, MDP and bacterial dissacharide peptides related to different oil vehicles and their composition. *Infect. Immun.*, **29**, 70–75
7.  Nagao, S. and Tanaka, A. (1980). Muramyl depeptide induced adjuvant arthritis. *Infect. Immun.*, **28**, 624–6
8.  Chang, Y., Pearson, C. and Chedid, L. (1981). Adjuvant polyarthritis: induction by MDP, the smallest peptide subunit of bacterial peptidoglycan. *J. Exp. Med.*, **153**, 1021–6
9.  Kohashi, O., Aikara, K., Ozawa, A., Kotani, S. and Azuma, I. (1981). Role of thymus for MDP-induced arthritis and granuloma formation in euthymic and athymic nude rats or neonatally thymectomized rats. *Infect. Immun.*, **31**, 758–66
10. Zidek, Z., Masik, K. and Jiricka, Z. (1982). Arthritogenic activity of a synthetic immunoadjuvant, muramyl dipeptide. *Infect. Immun.*, **35**, 674–9
11. Kohashi, O., Aikara, K., Ozawa, A., Kotani, S. and Azuma, I. (1982). New model of a synthetic adjuvant, MDP, induced arthritis: clinical and histologic studies in athymic nude and euthymic rats. *Lab. Invest.*, **47**, 27–36
12. Parant, M., Parant, L., Chedid, A., Yapo, J., Petit, J. and Lederer, B. (1979). Muramyl dipeptide (14-C labelled) in the mouse. *Int. J. Immunopharmacol.*, **1**, 35–41
13. Chang, Y.H., Pearson, C. and Abe, C. (1980). Adjuvant polyarthritis IV. Induction by a synthetic adjuvant: Immunologic, histopathologic and other studies. *Arthr. Rheum.*, **23**, 62–71
14. Takada, H., Tsujimotoń, M., Kata, K., Kotani, S., Kusumoto, S., Inage, M., Shiba, T., Tano, I., Kawata, S. and Yokogawa, K. (1979). Macrophage activation by bacterial cell walls and related synthetic compounds. *Infect. Immun.*, **25**, 48–53
15. Wahl, L., Wahl, S. and McCarthy, S. (1980). Adjuvant activation of macrophage functions. In Unanue, E.R. and Rosenthal, A.S. (eds.) *Macrophage Regulation of Immunity*. pp. 491–504. (New York: Academic Press)
16. Glenn, E., Bowman, B., Rohloff, N. and Seely, R. (1977). A major contributory cause of arthritis in adjuvant-inoculated rats: Granulocytes. *Agents Actions*, **7**, 265–82
17. Larsson, P., Holmdahl, R., Dencker, L. and Klareskog, L. (1985). *In vivo* treatment with W3/13 (anti-pan T) but not with OX8 (anti-suppressor/cytotoxic T) monoclonal antibodies impedes the development of adjuvant arthritis in rats. *Immunology*, **56**, 383–91

18. Kaibara, N., Hotokebuchi, T., Takagishi, K., Katsuki, I., Morinaga, M., Arita, C. and Jingushi, S. (1984). Pathogenetic difference between collagen arthritis and adjuvant arthritis. *J. Exp. Med.*, **1**, 1388–96
19. Taurog, J., Sandberg, G. and Mahowald, M. (1983). The cellular basis of adjuvant arthritis. I. Enhancement of cell-mediated passive transfer by concanavalin A and by immunosuppressive pre-treatment of the recipient. *Cell Immunol.*, **75**, 271–82
20. Holoshitz, J., Matitiau, A. and Cohen, I.R. (1984). Arthritis induced in rats by cloned T lymphocytes responsive to mycobacteria but not to collagen type II. *J. Clin. Invest.*, **73**, 211–5
21. Holoshitz, J., Matitiau, A. and Cohen, I.R. (1985). Role of the thymus in induction and transfer of vaccination against adjuvant arthritis with a T lymphocyte line in rats. *J. Clin. Invest.*, **75**, 472–7
22. Holoshitz, J. Naparstek, Y., Ben-Nun, A., Marquardt, P. and Cohen, I.R. (1984). T lymphocyte lines induce autoimmune encephalomyelitis, delayed hypersensitivity and bystander encephalitis or arthritis. *Eur. J. Immunol.*, **14**, 729–34
23. van Eden, W., Holoshitz, J., Nevo, Z., Frenkel, A., Klajman, A. and Cohen, I.R. (1985). Arthritis induced by a T-lymphocyte clone that responds to Mycobacterium tuberculosis and to cartilage proteoglycans. *Proc. Natl. Acad. Sci. USA*, **82**, 5117–20
24. Cohen, I.R., Holoshitz, J., van Eden, W. and Frenkel, A. (1985). Current comment: T lymphocyte clones illuminate and affect therapy of experimental arthritis. *Arthr. Rheum.*, **28**, 841–5
25. Gilman, S.C., Daniels, J.F., Wilson, R.E., Carlson, R.P. and Lewis, A.J. (1984). Lymphoid abnormalities in rats with adjuvant-induced arthritis. I. Mitogen responsiveness and lymphokine synthesis. *Ann. Rheum. Dis.*, **43**, 847–55
26. Pasternak, R.D., Maks, R.L., Hubbs, S.J. and DiPasquale, G. (1985). Effect of antirheumatic agents on the mitogen response of arthritic rat spleen cells. *Res. Commun. Chem. Pathol. Pharmacol.*, **48**, 353–67
27. Lee, J.C., Rebar, L., Demuth, S. and Hanna, N. (1985). Suppressed IL-2 production and response in AA rats: role of suppressor cells and the effect of auranofin treatment. *J. Rheumatol.*, **12**, 885–91
28. Crowe, W.E., Battisto, J.R. and Smith, R.N. (1985). The autologous mixed lymphocyte reaction is decreased in Freund's adjuvant-injected rats of arthritis-susceptible and -insusceptible strains. *Arthr. Rheum.*, **28**, 537–41
29. Binderup, L. (1985). Effects of isoprinosine in animal models of depressed T-cell function. *Int. J. Immunopharmacol.*, **7**, 93–101
30. Mangan, F.R., Rager, J.P. and Thomson, M.J. (1985). The effect of adjuvant arthritis on the subsequent local inflammatory response in rats. *Br. J. Exp. Pathol.*, **66**, 1–5
31. Gerler, V., Kertel, W. and Franke, A. (1974–1975). Vergleicherde Histologie der Adjuvans-Arthritis bei Ratten, Mausen und Hansterm. *Allerg. Immunol.*, **20/21**, 251–2
32. Battisto, J., Smith, R., Beckman K., Steintichl, M. and Willis, W. (1982). Susceptibility to adjuvant arthritis in DA and F344 rats. A dominant trait controlled by an autosomal gene locus linked to MHC. *Arthr. Rheum.*, **25**, 1194–200
33. Mackenzie, A., Sibley, P. and White, B. (1979). Resistance and susceptibility to the induction of rat adjuvant disease. Diverging susceptibility and severity achieved by selective breeding. *Br. J. Exp. Pathol.*, **60**, 507–12
34. Tonneau, D., Mach, P., Kihan, A. and Pelbaue, F. (1982). T suppressor lymphocytes regulation of adjuvant arthritis in two inbred strains of rats. *Clin. Exp. .Immunol.*, **49**, 645–51
35: Eisen, V., Freeman, P., Laveday, C. and West, G. (1973). Blood changes in experimental arthritis in two types of genetically different rats. *Br. J. Pharmacol.*, **49**, 688–95
36. Levine, J.D., Clark, R., Devor, M., Helms, C., Moskowitz, M.A. and Basbaum, A.I. (1984). Intraneuronal substance P contributes to the severity of experimental arthritis. *Science*, **226**, 547–9
37. Levine, J.D., Moskowitz, M.A. and Basbaum, A.I. (1985). The contribution of neurogenic inflammation in experimental arthritis. *J. Immunol.*, **135**, (2 Suppl.), 843s–847s
38. Taurog, J.D., Leary, S.I., Cremer, M.A., Mahowald, M.L., Sandberg, G.P. and Manning, P.J. (1984). Infection with *Mycoplasma pulmonis* modulates adjuvant- and collagen-induced arthritis in Lewis rats. *Arthr. Rheum.*, **27**, 943–6

39. Kohashi, O., Kohashi, Y., Takahashi, T., Ozawa, A. and Shigematsu, N. (1985). Reverse effect of gram-positive bacteria vs. gram-negative bacteria on adjuvant-induced arthritis in germfree rats. *Microbiol. Immunol.*, **29**, 487–97
40. Kohashi, O., Kohashi, Y., Takahashi, T., Ozawa, A. and Shigematsu, N. (1986). Suppressive effect of *Escherichia coli* on adjuvant-induced arthritis in germ-free rats. *Arthr. Rheum.*, **29**, 547–53
41. Stuart, J., Townes, A. and Kang, A. (1984). Collagen autoimmune arthritis. *Annu. Rev. Immunol.*, **2**, 199–218
42. Trentham, D.E. (1982). Collagen arthritis as relevant model for rheumatoid arthritis. Evidence pro and con. *Arthr. Rheum.*, **25**, 911–16
43. Jamieson, T.W., De Smet, A.A., Cremer, M.A., Kage, K.L. and Lindsley, H.B. (1985). Collagen-induced arthritis in rats. Assessment by serial magnification radiography. *Invest. Radiol.*, **20**, 324–30
44. Caulfield, J.P., Hein, A., Dynesius-Trentham, R. and Trentham, D.E. (1982). Morphologic demonstration of two stages in the development of type II collagen-induced arthritis. *Lab. Invest.*, **46**, 321–43
45. Trentham, D., McCune, W., Susman, P. and David, J. (1980). Autoimmunity to collagen in adjuvant arthritis. *J. Clin. Invest.*, **66**, 1109–17
46. DeLustro, F., Carlson, R.P., Datko, L.J., DeLustro, B. and Lewis, A.J. (1984). The absence of antibodies to type II collagen in established adjuvant arthritis in rats. *Agents Actions*, **14**, 673–9
47. Chang, Y.H. and Iizuka, Y. (1984). Adjuvant polyarthritis. VIII. Differences in immuno-pathogenesis between type II collagen arthritis and adjuvant arthritis. *Agents Actions*, **15**, 529–34
48. Cremer, M., Stuart, J., Townes, A. and Kang, A. (1980). Collagen induced arthritis in rats: A study of type II collagen for adjuvant activity. *J. Immunol.*, **124**, 2912–8
49. Taurog, J.D., Kerwar, S.S., McReynolds, R.A., Sandberg, G.P., Leary, S.L. and Mahowald, M.L. (1985). Synergy between adjuvant arthritis and collagen-induced arthritis in rats. *J. Exp. Med.*, **162**, 962–78
50. Wooley, P., Luthra, H., Stuart, J. and David, C. (1981). Type II collagen induced arthritis in mice I. MHC (I region) linkage and antibody correlates. *J. Exp. Med.*, **154**, 688–700
51. Stuart, J., Cremer, M., Townes, A. and Kang, A. (1982). Type II collagen induced arthritis in rats. Passive transfer with serum and evidence that IgG anticollagen antibodies can cause arthritis. *J. Exp. Med.*, **155**, 1–16
52. Kerwar, S., Bauman, N., Oronsky, A. and Soboda, J. (1981–82). Studies of type II collagen induced polyarthritis in rats. Effect of complement depletion. *J. Immunopharmacol.*, **3**, 323–37
53. Kakimoto, K., Hirofuji, T. and Koga, T. (1984). Specificity of anti-type II collagen antibody response in rats. *Clin. Exp. Immunol.*, **57**, 57–62
54. Ridge, S.C., McReynolds, R.A., Mitcho, Y.L., Bauman, N., Oronsky, A.L., Kerwar, S.S. (1984). Passive transfer of collagen arthritis: studies with affinity-purified anticollagen IgG prepared in rabbits. *Clin. Immunol. Immunopathol.*, **33**, 402–11
55. Helfott, S.M., Bazin, H., Dessein, A. and Trentham, D.E. (1984). Suppressive effects of anti-μ-serum on the development of collagen arthritis in rats. *Clin. Immunol. Immnopathol.*, **31**, 403–11
56. Ridge, S.C., Oronsky, A.L. and Kerwar, S.S. (1984). *In vitro* synthesis of anticollagen IgG by sensitized lymph node cells derived from type II collagen-induced polyarthritic rats. *Immunopharmacology*, **7**, 195–9
57. Firth, S.A., Morgan, K., Evans, H.B. and Holt, P.J. (1984). IgG subclasses in collagen-induced arthritis in the rat. *Immunol. Lett.*, **7**, 243–7
58. Wooley, P.H., Luthra, H.S., Griffiths, M.M., Stuart, J.M., Huse, A. and David, C.S. (1985). Type II collagen-induced arthritis in mice. IV. Variations in immunogenetic regulation provide evidence for multiple arthritogenic epitopes on the collagen molecule. *J. Immunol.*, **135**, 2443–51
59. Watson, W.C. and Townes, A.S. (1985). Genetic susceptibility to murine collagen II autoimmune arthritis. Proposed relationship to the $IgG_2$ autoantibody subclass response, complement C5, major histocompatibility complex (MHC) and non-MHC loci. *J. Exp. Med.*, **162**, 1878–91

60. Wooley, P.H., Luthra H.S., Griffiths, M.M., Stuart, J.M., Huse, A. and David, C.S. (1985). Type II collagen-induced arthritis in mice. IV. Variations in immunogenetic regulation provide evidence for multiple arthritogenic epitopes on the collagen molecule. *J. Immunol.*, **135**, 2443–51

61. Englert, M., McReynolds, R.A., Landes, M.J., Oronsky, A.L. and Kerwar, S.S. (1985). Pretreatment of rats with anticollagen IgG renders them resistant to active type II collagen arthritis. *Cell Immunol.*, **90**, 258–66

62. Terato, K., Hasty, K.A., Cremer, M.A., Stuart, J.M., Townes, A.S. and Kang, A.H. (1985). Collagen-induced arthritis in mice. Localization of an arthritogenic determinant to a fragment of the type II collagen molecule. *J. Exp. Med.*, **162**, 637–46

63. Hirofuji, T., Kakimoto, K., Hori, H., Nagai, Y., Saisho, K., Sumiyoshi, A. and Koga, T. (1985). Characterization of monoclonal antibody specific for human type II collagen: possible implication in collagen-induced arthritis. *Clin. Exp. Immunol.*, **62**, 159–66

64. Holmdahl, R., Rubin, K., Klareskog, L., Larsson, E. and Wigzell, H. (1986). Characterization of the antibody response in mice with type II collagen-induced arthritis, using monoclonal anti-type II collagen antibodies. *Arthr. Rheum.*, **29**, 400–10

65. Takagishi, K., Kaibara, N., Hotokebuchi, T., Arita, C., Morinaga, M. and Arai, K. (1985). Serum transfer of collagen arthritis in congenitally athymic nude rats. *J. Immunol.*, **134**, 3864–7

66. Holmdahl, R., Rubin, K., Klareskog, L., Dencker, L., Gustafson, G. and Larsson, E. (1985). Appearance of different lymphoid cells in synovial tissue and in peripheral blood during the course of collagen II-induced arthritis in rats. *Scand. J. Immunol.*, **21**, 197–204

67. Henderson, B., Staines, N.A., Burrai, I. and Cox, J.H. (1984). The anti-arthritic and immunosuppressive effects of cyclosporine on arthritis induced in the rat by type II collagen. *Clin. Exp. Immunol.*, **57**, 51–6

68. Kaibara, N., Morinaga, M., Arita, C., Hotokebuchi, T. and Takagishi, K. (1985). Serum transfer of collagen arthritis to cyclosporin-treated, type II collagen-tolerant rats. *Clin. Immunol. Immunopathol.*, **35**, 252–60

69. Ranges, G.E., Spiram, S. and Cooper, S.M. (1985). Prevention of type II collagen-induced arthritis by *in vivo* treatment with anti-L3T4. *J. Exp. Med.*, **162**, 1105–10

70. Brahn, E. and Trentham, D.E. (1984). Effect of antithymocyte serum on collagen arthritis in rats: evidence that T cells are involved in its pathogenesis. *Cell Immunol.*, **86**, 421–8

71. Wooley, P.H., Luthra, H.S., Lafuse, W.P., Huse, A., Stuart, J.M. and David, C.S. (1985). Type II collagen-induced arthritis in mice. III. Suppression of arthritis by using monoclonal and polyclonal anti-Ia antisera. *J. Immunol.*, **134**, 2366–74

72. Holmdahl, R., Klareskog, L., Rubin, K., Larsson, E. and Wigzell, H. (1985). T lymphocytes in collagen II-induced arthritis in mice. Characterization of arthritogenic collagen II-specific T-cell lines and clones. *Scand. J. Immunol.*, **22**, 295–306

73. Burrai, I., Henderson, B., Knight, S.C. and Staines, N.A. (1985). Suppression of collagen type II-induced arthritis by transfer of lymphoid cells from rats immunized with collagen. *Clin. Exp. Immunol.*, **61**, 368–72

74. Brahn, E., Trentham, D.E. (1984). Antigen-specific suppression of collagen arthritis by adoptive transfer of spleen cells. *Clin. Immunol. Immunopathol.*, **31**, 124–31

75. Kresina, T.F. and Moskowitz, R.W. (1985). Adoptive transfer of suppression of arthritis in the mouse model of collagen-induced arthritis. Evidence for a type II collagen-specific suppressor T cell. *J. Clin. Invest.*, **75**, 1990–8

76. Helfgott, S.M., Dynesius-Trentham, R., Brahn, E. and Trentham, D.E. (1985). An arthritogenic lymphokine in the rat. *J. Exp. Med.*, **162**, 1531–45

77. Lelie, C.A., Gonnerman, W.A., Ullman, M.D., Hayes, K.C., Franzblau, C. and Cathcart, E.S. (1985). Dietary fish oil modulates macrophage fatty acids and decreases arthritis susceptibility in mice. *J. Exp. Med.*, **162**, 1336–49

78. Prickett, J.D., Trentham, D.E. and Robinson, D.R. (1984). Dietary fish oil augments the induction of arthritis in rats immunized with type II collagen. *J. Immunol.*, **132**, 725–9

79. Schrier, D., Gilbertsen, R.B., Lesch, M. and Fantone, J. (1984). The role of neutrophils in type II collagen-induced arthritis in rats. *Am. J. Pathol.*, **117**, 26–9

80. Griffiths, M.M. and DeWitt, C.W. (1981). Immunogenetic control of experimental collagen-induced arthritis in rats. II. ECIA susceptibility and immune response to type II collagen (Calf) are linked to RT1. *J. Immunogenet.*, **8**, 463–70

81. Griffiths, M.M. and DeWitt, C.W. (1984). Genetic control of collagen-induced arthritis in rat: the immune response to type II collagen among susceptible and resistant strains and evidence for multiple gene control. *J. Immunol.*, **132**, 2830−6

82. Griffiths, M.M., Eichwald, E.J., Martin, J.H., Smith, C.B. and DeWitt, C. (1981). Immunogenetic control of experimental type II collagen-induced arthritis: I. Susceptibility and resistance among inbred strains of rats. *Arthr. Rheum.*, **24**, 781−9

83. Griffiths, M.M., DeWitt, C.W. (1985). Multiple gene control of collagen arthritis in rats. *Transplant Proc.*, **17**, 1879−82

84. Holmdahl, R., Jansson, L., Gullberg, D., Rubin, K., Forsberg, P.O. and Klareskog, L. (1985). Incidence of arthritis and autoreactivity of anti-collagen antibodies after immunization of DBA/1 mice with heterologous and autologous collagen II. *Clin. Exp. Immunol.*, **62**, 638−46

85. Dumonde, D. and Glynn, L. (1967). The production of arthritis in rabbits by an immunological reaction to fibrin. *Br. J. Exp. Pathol.*, **43**, 373−83

86. Goldlust, M., Rich, K. and Brown, W. (1978). Immune synovitis in rabbits. Effects of differing schedules for intra-articular challenge with antigen. *Am. J. Pathol.*, **91**, 329−44

87. Graham, R.C., Jr and Shannon, S. (1972). Peroxidase arthritis. I. An immunologically mediated inflammatory response with ultrastructural cytochemical localization of antigen and specific antibody. *Am. J. Pathol.*, **67**, 69−94

88. Schalkwijk, J., van den Berg, W.B., van de Putte, L.B., Joosten, L. and van der Sluis, M. (1985). Effects of experimental joint inflammation on bone marrow and periarticular bone. A study of two types of arthritis, using variable degrees of inflammation. *Br. J. Exp. Pathol.*, **66**, 435−44

89. Hollister, J. and Mannik, M. (1974). Antigen retention in joint tissues in antigen-induced arthritis. *Clin. Exp. Immunol.*, **16**, 615−27

90. Jasin, H. and Cooke, T. (1978). The inflammatory role of immune complexes trapped in joint collagenous tissues. *Clin. Exp. Immunol.*, **33**, 416−24

91. van den Berg, W. and van de Putte, L. (1985). Electrical charge of the antigen determines its localization in the mouse knee joint. Deep penetration of cationic BSA in hyaline articular cartilage. *Am. J. Pathol.*, **121**, 224−34

92. van den Berg, W., van de Putte, L., Zwarts, W. and Joosten, L. (1984). Electrical charge of the antigen determines intraarticular antigen handling and chronicity of arthritis in mice. *J. Clin. Invest.*, **74**, 1850-9

93. Kruijsen, M., van den Berg, W. and van de Putte, L. (1985). Influence of the severity and duration of murine antigen-induced arthritis on cartilage proteoglycan synthesis and chondrocyte death. *Arthr. Rheum.*, **28**, 813−9

94. Lens, J., van den Berg, W. and van de Putte, L. (1984). Flare-up of antigen-induced arthritis in mice after challenge with intravenous antigen: studies on the characteristics of and mechanisms involved in the reaction. *Clin. Exp. Immunol.*, **55**, 287−94

95. Lens, J., van den Berg, W., van de Putte, L., Berden, J. and Lems, S. (1984). Flare-up of antigen-induced arthritis in mice after challenge with intravenous antigen: effects of pre-treatment with cobra venom factor and anti-lymphocyte serum. *Clin. Exp. Immunol.*, **57**, 520−8

96. Lens, J., van den Berg, W., van de Putte, L. and van den Bersselaar, L. (1984). Flare-up of antigen-induced arthritis in mice after challenge with oral antigen. *Clin. Exp. Immunol.*, **58**, 364−71

97. Goldberg, V., Lance, E. and Davis, P. (1974). Experimental immune synovitis in the rabbit. Relative roles of cell mediated and humoral immunity. *Arthr. Rheum.*, **17**, 993−1005

98. Steffen, C., Muller, C., Stellamor, K. and Zeithlhofer, J. (1982). Influence of X-ray treatment on antigen-induced arthritis. *Ann. Rheum. Dis.*, **41**, 532−7

99. Stenzler, S. and Miller, F. (1977). Failure of cobra venom to inhibit antigen-induced arthritis. *Arthr. Rheum.*, **20**, 1567

100. DeShayo, C. and DeShayo, M. (1975). Arthritis in the rabbit joint: A quantitated model. *Rheumatology*, **6**, 268−82

101. Schalkwijk, J., van den Berg, W., van de Putte, L., Joosten, L. and van den Bersselaar, L. (1985). Cationization of catalase, peroxidase, and superoxide dismutase. Effect of improved intra-articular retention on experimental arthritis in mice. *J. Clin. Invest.*, **76**, 198−205

102. Brackertz, D., Mitchell, G. and Mackay, I. (1977). Antigen-induced arthritis in mice. II. Induction of arthritis in various strains of mice. *Arthr. Rheum.*, **20**, 841–50

103. Brakertz, D., Mitchell, G., Vadas, M., Mackay, I. and Miller, J. (1977). Studies on antigen-induced arthritis in mice II. Immunologic correlates of arthritis in mice. *J. Immunol.*, **118**, 1639–44

104. Brackertz, D., Mitchell, G., Vadas, M. and Mackay, I. (1977). Studies on antigen-induced arthritis in mice III. Cell and serum transfer experiments. *J. Immunol.*, **118**, 1645–8

105. Cromartie, W.J., Craddock, J.C., Schwab, J.H., Anderle, S.K. and Yang, C.H. (1977). Arthritis in rats after systemic injection of streptococcal cells or cell walls. *J. Exp. Med.*, **146**, 1585–602

106. Wilder, R.L., Calandra, G.B., Garvin, A.J., Wright, K.D. and Hansen, C.T. (1982). Strain and sex variation in the susceptibility of streptococcal cell wall-induced polyarthritis in the rat. *Arthr. Rheum.*, **25**, 1064–72

107. Clark, R.L., Cuttino, J.T., Anderle, S.K., Cromartie, W.J. and Schwab, J.H. (1979). Radiologic analysis of arthritis in rats after systemic injection of streptococcal cell walls. *Arthr. Rheum.*, **22**, 25–35

108. Calandra, G.B., Wilder, R., Garvin, J., Hansen, C. and Wright, K. (1982). Genetic analysis of the development of group A streptococcal cell wall mediated arthritis in rats. In Holm, S.E. and Christensen, P. (eds.) *Basic Concepts of Streptotocci and Streptococcal Diseases.* pp. 313–314. (Surrey, England: Reedbooks Ltd)

109. Wilder, R.L., Allen, J.B., Wahl, L.M., Calandra, G.B. and Wahl, S.M. (1983). The pathogenesis of Group A streptococcal cell wall-induced polyarthritis in the rat: Comparative studies in arthritis resistant and susceptible inbred rat strains. *Arthr. Rheum.*, **26**, 1442–51

110. Allen, J.B., Malone, D.G., Wahl, S.M., Calandra, G.B. and Wilder, R.L. (1985). The role of the thymus in streptococcal cell wall-induced arthritis and hepatic granuloma formation. Comparative studies of pathology and cell wall distribution in athymic and euthymic rats. *J. Clin. Invest.*, **76**, 1042–56

111. Yocum, D.E., Allen, J.B., Wahl, S.M., Calandra, G.B. and Wilder, R.L. (1986). Inhibition by cyclosporin A of streptococcal cell wall-induced arthritis and hepatic granulomas in rats. *Arthr. Rheum.*, **29**, 262–73

112. Haraoui, B., Wilder, R.L., Allen, J.B., Sporn, M.D., Helfgott, K.K. and Brinckerhoff, C.E. (1985). Dose-dependent suppression by the synthetic retinoid, 4-hydroxyphenyl retinamide, of streptococcal cell-induced arthritis in rats. *Int. J. Immunopharmacol.*, **7**, 903–16

113. Allen, J.B., Blatter, D., Calandra, G.B. and Wilder, R.L. (1983). Sex hormonal effects on the severity of streptococcal cell-induced polyarthritis in the rat. *Arthr. Rheum.*, **26**, 560–3

114. Schwab, J.H. and Ohanian, S.H. (1967). Degradation of streptococcal cell wall antigens in vivo. *J. Bacteriol.*, **94**, 1346–52

115. Smialowicz, R.J. and Schwab, J.H. (1977). Processing of streptococcal cell walls by rat macrophages and human monocytes in vitro. *Infect. Immun.*, **17**, 591–8

116. Eisenberg, R., Fox, A., Greenblatt, J.J., Anderle, S.K., Cromartie, W.J. and Schwab, J.H. (1982). Measurement of bacterial cell wall in tissues by solid phase radioimmunoasssay: Correlation of distribution and persistence with experimental arthritis in rats. *Infect. Immun.*, **38**, 127–35

117. Stimpson, S.A., Lerch, R.A., Cleland, D.R., Yarnall, D.P., Clark, R.L., Cromartie, W.J. and Schwab, J.H. (1986). Effect of acetylation on arthropathic activity of group A streptococcal cell walls. *Arthr. Rheum.*, **29**, S101

118. Janusz, M.J., Chetty, C., Eisenberg, R.A., Cromartie, W.J. and Schwab, J.H. (1984). Treatment of experimental erosive arthritis in rats by injection of muralytic enzyme mutanolysin. *J. Exp. Med.*, **160**, 1360–74

119. Lambris, J.D., Allen, J.B. and Schwab, J.H. (1980). In vivo changes in complement induced with peptidoglycan–polysaccharide polymers from streptococcal cell walls. *Infect. Immun.*, **35**, 377–80

120. Schwab, J.H., Allen, J.B., Anderle, S.K., Daldorf, F., Eisenberg, R. and Cromartie, W.J. (1982). Relationship of complement to experimental arthritis induced in rats with streptococcal cell walls. *Immunology*, **46**, 83–8

121. Ridge, S.C., Zabriskie, J.B., Oronsky, A.L. and Kerwar, S.S. (1985). Streptococcal cell wall arthritis: Studies with nude (athymic) inbred LEW rats. *Cell. Immunol.*, **96**, 231–4

122. Yocum, D.E., Allen, J.B., Wahl, S.M. and Wilder, R.L. (1986). Mononuclear cell dependent mechanisms of bone and cartilage destruction in streptococcal cell wall-induced arthritis in rats. *Arthr. Rheum.*, **29**, S11
123. Allen, J.B. and Wilder, R.L. (1985). Regulation of susceptibility to streptococcal cell wall induced arthritis in rats. *Arthr. Rheum.*, **28**, 1318–9
124. Anderle, S.K., Allen, J.B., Wilder, R.L., Eisenberg, R.A., Cromartie, W.J. and Schwab, J.H. (1985). Measurement of streptococcal cell wall in tissue of rats resistant or susceptible to cell wall-induced chronic erosive arthritis. *Infect. Immun.*, **49**, 836–7
125. Koga, T., Kakimoto, K., Hirofuji, T., Kotani, S., Ohkuni, H., Watanabe, K., Okada, N., Okada, H., Suniyoshi, A. and Saisho, K. (1985). Acute joint inflammation in mice after systemic injection of the cell wall, its peptidoglycan, and chemically defined peptidoglycan subunits from various bacteria. *Infect. Immun.*, **50**, 27–34
126. Wahl, S.M., Hunt, D.A., Allen, J.B., Wilder, R.L., Paglia, L. and Hand, A.R. (1986). Bacterial cell wall-induced hepatic granulomas. An *in vivo* model of T cell dependent fibrosis. *J. Exp. Med.*, **163**, 884–902
127. Wahl, S.M., Allen, J.B., Dougherty, S., Evequox, V., Pluznik, D., Wilder, R.L., Hand, A.R. and Wahl, L.M. (1986). T lymphocyte dependent evaluation of bacterial cell wall induced hepatic granulomas. *J. Immunol.*, **137**, 2199–209
128. Stimpson, S.A., Brown, R.R., Anderle, S.K., Klapper, D.G., Clark, R.L., Cromartie, W.J. and Schwab, J.H. (1986). Arthropathic properties of cell wall polymers from normal flora bacteria. *Infect. Immun.*, **51**, 240–9
129. Lehman, T.J., Allen, J.B., Plotz, P.H. and Wilder, R.L. (1985). Bacterial cell wall composition, lysozyme resistance, and the induction of chronic arthritis in rats. *Rheumatol. Int.*, **5**, 163–7
130. Greenblatt, J.R., Boackle, R.J. and Schwab, J.H. (1978). Activation of the alternate complement pathway by peptidoglycan from streptococcal cell wall. *Infect. Immun.*, **91**, 296–303
131. Ridge, S.C., Zabriskie, J.B., Osawa, H., Diamanstein, T., Oronsky, A. and Kerwar, S.S. (1986). Administration of group A streptococcal cell walls to rats induces an interleukin 2 deficiency. *J. Exp. Med.*, **164**, 327–32
132. Lehman, T.J.A., Allen, J.B., Plotz, P.H. and Wilder, R.L. (1983). Polyarthritis in rats following the systemic injection of Lactobacillus casei cell walls in aqueous suspension. *Arthr. Rheum.*, **26**, 1259–65
133. Lehman, T.J.A., Allen, J.B., Plotz, P.H. and Wilder, R.L. (1984). *Lactobacillus casei* cell wall-induced arthritis in rats: Cell wall fragment distribution and persistence in chronic arthritis-susceptible LEW/N and resistant F344/N rats. *Arthr. Rheum.*, **27**, 939–42

# 10
# B lymphocyte activation and differentiation

C. J. M. MELIEF

## INTRODUCTION

Dysregulation of antibody production by cells of the B-cell lineage is an important feature in rheumatoid arthritis and allied disorders, as argued elsewhere in this volume. In order better to understand the pathophysiology of the immune abnormalities associated with the rheumatic disorders, insight into the normal B-cell response and its regulation is crucial. To begin with the intricate connections of the humoral immune response with antigen-presenting cells (APC) and T-cells, the carriers of cell-mediated immunity, should be noted. Remarkable progress has been made in recent years in understanding the B-cell response and its regulation in genetic and molecular terms. Much is now known concerning the elegant process of genetic recombination that allows the creation of individually distinct receptor (immunoglobulin) molecules on B-cells.

Antigen presentation by dendritic cells/macrophages to T- and B-cells and the role of products of the major histocompatibility complex (MHC) and soluble products of these APC (complement factors, cytokines such as interleukin-1) has been scrutinized in detail. A wealth of data has challenged the absorptive capacity of immunologists' brains concerning soluble products (lymphokines) of T-helper cells and other cytokines, with stimulatory action on B-cell maturation and/or proliferation. Although many mechanisms and models have been described with respect to APC function and lymphokine (cytokine) action in the B-cell response – down to molecular detail – a synthesis in which the relative importance of each mechanism is given its appropriate weight in the grand total of events is still lacking. In this chapter I shall not attempt such a synthesis but I shall review some major facts as they stand now.

## IMMUNOGLOBULIN ASSEMBLY AND B-CELL REPERTOIRE FORMATION

A key feature of B-cell biology is that the B-cell repertoire (the capacity to recognize a myriad of different antigens) is formed in an antigen-independent fashion. Thus long before encounter with antigen individually distinct immunoglobulin molecules are assembled in developing B-cells and finally expressed at the cell surface of mature B-cells as complete membrane-bound immunoglobulin molecules.

The assembly of immunoglobulin (Ig) genes, like that of T-cell receptor genes involves a finely tuned process of recombination between genes encoding the variable and constant portions of the receptor molecule. The molecular details of immunoglobulin gene rearrangement have been reviewed in Refs. 1–3. The variable region of the heavy (H) chain of the Ig molecule is encoded by three germline DNA segments; a $V_H$ segment encoding most of the gene, which is hooked up to a D (diversity) segment, which in turn is linked to a $J_H$ (joining) segment. The V, D and J segments are encoded in three separate clusters on the Ig locus on chromosome 14 of man. The variable region of the $\kappa$ or $\lambda$ light chains is encoded by two germline DNA segments: $V_L$ and $J_L$. The human $\kappa$ and $\lambda$ light chain regions are located on chromosomes 2 and 22, respectively. These different germline elements are separated by non-coding regions of variable length. The different elements are hooked up to each other during B-cell differentiation by a controlled recombination process in which recombination recognition sequences are utilized, consisting of characteristic heptamer and nonamer base sequences, separated by a spacer of 12 or 23 base pairs (reviewed in Ref. 3 for the mouse).

The utilization of alternative V, D, J segments creates a large number of different possibilities. Additional variability of antigen-binding regions is created by imprecision in the joining process leading to loss or gain of nucleotides (reviewed in Ref. 3). The exact number of VDJ heavy and VJ light chain segments in the human genome is not known at present, but the situation is likely to be closely analogous to that in the mouse. In this species there are 500 $V_H$, 15 $D_H$ and four $J_H$ segments in addition to 200 $V_L$ $\kappa$ and four $V_J \kappa$ segments[4]. In the mouse, in contrast to man, $\lambda$ light chains contribute only little to the repertoire. Assembled variable region genes are transcribed and eventually fused to a constant region-encoding sequence to form the complete heavy or light chain messenger RNA. The first constant region gene available to the heavy chain variable gene transcript is the $C\mu$ gene. The complete mRNA for the $\mu$ chain of IgM is thus generated and the $\mu$ chain synthesis can be started. By recombination of $V_H$ transcripts to constant H chain genes further downstream (class switching) other classes of immunoglobulin heavy chain are produced in the following sequence: $\mu$, $\delta$, $\gamma3$, $\gamma1$, $\alpha1$, $\gamma2$, $\gamma4$, $\varepsilon$, $\alpha2$.

## MATURATION OF HUMAN B LYMPHOCYTES IN RELATION TO CELL SURFACE MARKER EXPRESSION

As indicated in the previous section the hallmark of B-cell maturation is immunoglobulin gene assembly, eventually followed by immunoglobulin

175

protein expression. Intracytoplasmic $\mu$ chain is the first Ig gene product to become expressed during B-cell maturation and the cell at this stage is termed a pre-B-cell. Several reviews on human B lymphocyte markers other than immunoglobulin are available[5-7]. Pre-B-cells express the CD10 surface marker (common ALL antigen, CALLA) in addition to the CD19 B-cell specific differentiation marker. In addition, pre-B-cells express HLA class II antigens at the cell surface and cytoplasmatically terminal transferase (TdT) activity. The CD19 and HLA class II surface markers remain expressed throughout maturation to surface immunoglobulin positive B-cells and upon activation of B-cells to Ig-secreting plasma cells. Plasma cells themselves are negative for these markers. Upon maturation of pre-B-cells to B-cells Ig light chains are synthesized allowing cell surface expression of IgM (and IgD). In addition the CD20 pan-B-cell marker is expressed on surface Ig (Ig) positive B-cells. Like the CD19 marker CD20 remains expressed up to the plasma cell stage when both B-cell specific markers are lost. TdT activity is only expressed in early B-cells, probably because the enzyme is involved in the process of Ig gene assembly[3]. CD10 expression is lost slightly later than TdT positivity. The functional significance of surface markers such as CD10, CD19 and CD20 is yet to be elucidated. However, some interesting observations have been made. For example, anti-CD19 and CD20 monoclonal antibodies (MoAb) have been observed to inhibit differentiation of normal B-cells and/or B-cell lines[7-10]. One particular anti-CD20 MoAb in addition stimulated resting B-cells from the G0 to the G1 phase of the cell cycle[8,9]. The two different effects of this MoAb remain to be explained[7].

Another functionally interesting surface structure is the receptor for the C3d fragment of complement (CR2). This receptor is B-cell specific and also known as the CD21 antigen of B-cells. Polyclonal and monoclonal anti-CR2 antibodies stimulate B-cells to proliferate and differentiate in the presence of T-cells or T-derived soluble factors[11-13]. CR2 also serves as the receptor for Epstein Barr virus (EBV) on human B-cells[14]. Binding of EBV to the receptor may be one of the signals causing B-cell proliferation by EBV, but clearly not the only one[7,13]. The complement receptor CR1, the C3b receptor, may also be involved in human B-cell triggering[15]. In the mouse C3b or C3d, either aggregated or Sepharose-bound can replace accessory cell factors in the B-cell cycle[13].

Receptors for lymphokines and other cytokines are clearly of major significance in the B-cell response, but they will be discussed in the next two sections.

## CELLULAR INTERACTIONS IN ANTIBODY PRODUCTION

Antibody production and its regulation is the result of interactions between three main cell types: antigen-presenting accessory cells (dendritic cells, macrophages/monocytes), T lymphocytes and B lymphocytes[13]. Only a few antigens are capable of eliciting antibody production without help from helper

T lymphocytes. Such T-cell signals are necessary for B-cell activation next to the binding of antigen to surface immunoglobulin[13]. The sequence of events in the more typical T-cell-dependent antibody response can be described as follows[13,16-21]. Antigen (Ag) is presented in the context of class II HLA molecules on the surface of APC to CD4$^+$ CD8$^-$ helper T lymphocytes. The T-cell receptor (TCR) $\alpha,\beta$ complex on these T-cells recognizes the complex Ag/HLA class II (HLA-DP, DQ or DR) and transduces a triggering signal to the interior of the T-cell via the TCR-associated CD3 series of polypeptides. T-cell triggering is facilitated by certain cytokines liberated by the APC, the best characterized of which is interleukin-1 (IL-1).

Subsequently the activated helper T-cells start the production of lymphokines such as interleukin-2 (IL-2), interferon-$\gamma$ (IFN-$\gamma$), interleukin 4 (IL-4) and several others. The mode of operation of these various factors will be discussed in the next paragraph. Suffice it to state here that some of them, e.g. IL-2, act in an autocrine fashion on the helper cells themselves to upregulate receptor expression, as well as on the B-cells. Other lymphokines liberated by helper T-cells may act more or less on the B-cells only. The lymphokines, together with factors secreted by antigen-presenting cells, all contribute to optimal growth and differentiation of antigen-triggered B-cells. B-cells characteristically and in contrast to T lymphocytes see free antigen in the body fluids and do not need presentation of antigen in the context of HLA molecules. However, since B-cells, like APC, express class II HLA molecules, T helper cells can also recognize antigen on the surface of B lymphocytes, e.g. when antigen is specifically bound to surface Ig. This latter mechanism of HLA restricted antigen recognition on the surface of B-cells may facilitate close interaction between Ag-binding B-cells on one hand and Ag-binding T-cells and APC on the other hand, thus allowing optimal conditions for antibody production.

Indeed a fair body of evidence indicates that B-cells can serve as APC to T-helper cells, probably more on the basis of non-specific adsorption or processing of antigen at the B-cell surface, rather than specific binding of antigen to Ig receptors[22-25]. However if HLA class II recognition on the surface of B-cells were a prerequisite for B-cell-activation by helper T lymphocytes, all forms of T–B collaboration involved in antibody production would be MHC class II restricted. While there is evidence that MHC class II antigens play an important role in the excitation reaction, there is also evidence for MHC non-restricted activation (reviewed in Ref. 13). Recent data from our laboratory showed that inhibition of T-cell-dependent B-cell differentiation by anti-HLA class II monoclonal antibodies was due to interference with (a) function(s) of accessory cells other than B-cells essential for B-cell differentiation[26].

In summary, antibody production is the result of complex interactions between HLA class II positive APC, antigen-stimulated (HLA class II restricted) helper T-cells and antigen-stimulated B-cells. The helper T-cells deliver their helper signals to the antigen-activated B-cells at least partially by lymphokines which are non-MHC restricted in action, although their secretion by T-helper cells (induction) depends on MHC class II restricted APC–T-helper cell interaction.

## CYTOKINES IN THE REGULATION OF ANTIBODY PRODUCTION

Various reviews deal with the regulation by cytokines of B-cell growth and differentiation necessary for antibody production[13,18,27-30]. Until recently a rather sharp distinction was made between cytokines causing B-cell growth/proliferation (without differentiation) and those causing B-cell differentiation only (without proliferation). However, various recombinant cytokines have now unequivocally been shown to possess both activities. In this review we shall only discuss those cytokines that are undisputed single biochemical entities with proven biological effects. For practical purposes we shall limit the discussion therefore to the cytokines proven to be single gene products, the genes for which have been cloned and characterized. These cytokines are interleukin-1 (IL-1), interleukin-2 (IL-2), interleukin-4 (IL-4), interferon-$\gamma$ (IFN-$\gamma$), and B-cell stimulatory factor-2 (BSF-2).

### Interleukin-1

It is now clear that IL-1-like activity can be produced by almost every cell type tested. In addition IL-1 has pleiotropic effects on the growth and differentiation of numerous cell types of both lymphoid and non-lymphoid origin[30]. With respect to stimulation of B-cell growth and differentiation it is convenient to make a distinction between direct effects on B-cell(s) (precursors) and an indirect effect via stimulation of helper T-cells. There are two forms of IL-1, IL-1$\alpha$ with an isoelectric point (pI) of 5.0 and IL-1$\beta$ with a pI of 7.0. Both forms have a molecular weight of 17 000 daltons. Human EBV-transformed B lymphocytes possess receptors for both IL-1$\alpha$ and IL-1$\beta$[31]. It therefore seems likely that IL-1 can have a direct effect on B-cells. Indeed IL-1 has been shown to induce maturation of pre-B-cells and to act as a cofactor in clonal expansion of B-cells in the mouse[30]. A similar direct action of IL-1 may occur on human B-cells[30]. The possible physiological relevance of these findings is further strengthened by the finding that not only antigen presenting cells produce IL-1, but also human B-cells themselves[32,33]. Indirectly IL-1 may augment B-cell responses by stimulating helper T-cells. This may occur by at least two mechanisms: (i) direct comitogenic action of IL-1 on helper T-cells together with antigen and class II HLA molecules, (ii) increased IL-1 receptor expression. The result of this is increased release by the T-helper cells of lymphokines causing B-cell growth and differentiation, including IL-2, IFN-$\gamma$ and IL-4[30].

### Interleukin-2

Like IL-1, IL-2 can promote B-cell growth and differentiation both directly and indirectly by stimulation of the release of B-cell reactive lymphokines by helper T-cells. Direct stimulation of B-cell growth/differentiation only occurs with activated and not resting B-cells[18,34-36]. However, resting B lymphocytes can be induced to produce Ig if normal CD4$^+$ CD8$^-$ T-cells are also present[34].

178

The mechanism of this appears to be the production, upon incubation with IL-2, by the CD4$^+$ CD8$^-$ helper T-cells, of lymphokines other than IL-2 which then stimulate the B-cells to secrete Ig[34]. This point was further elaborated by the identification of a neoplastic CD4$^+$ lymphocyte, which was incapable of IL-2 production, but when given exogenous IL-2 induced Ig production in resting B-cells, presumably by release of helper factors[37]. Depending on the stage of activation of B-cells, IL-2 is capable of causing both B-cell proliferation and differentiation. Proliferation was found both early and late following B-cell activation by *Staphylococcus aureus* Cowan I (SAC), whereas differentiation by IL-2 occurred only early after activation[35]. Differentiation late after activation was however promoted by BSF-2 (BCDF) (see below). Thus, IL-2 has a key role in the regulation of immunoglobulin production by B-cells[18]. On one hand it acts in an autocrine fashion on CD4$^+$ CD8$^-$ helper cells (which themselves are the major source of IL-2 following triggering by antigen and MHC) to release other B-cell growth and differentiation factors in a two-step lymphokine cascade. Secondly, IL-2 in its own right supports the growth and differentiation of B-cells, once activated, especially early after activation.

**Interleukin-4**

IL-4, previously called B-cell stimulatory factor-1 (BSF-1), is a more recently isolated lymphokine, which again, like IL-1 and IL-2, has pleiotropic effects on a variety of cells, including B-cells. Most published reports deal with the activity of murine IL-2 on murine cells, but the human IL-4 gene has now also been cloned[38], almost simultaneously with the murine gene[39,40]. Because studies concerning the effect of IL-4 on the human B-cell response have only just started and no general picture is available yet, the murine data will mainly be reviewed here. It is likely, however, that just as for IL-1 and IL-2 many of the data can be extrapolated to the human immune system.

The first reported activity of murine IL-4 is its ability to synergize with anti-IgM antibody to induce proliferation of B-cells[41]. Later it was found that IL-4 prepares resting B-cells more promptly to enter S-phase in response to various stimuli[42]. IL-4 also increases class II MHC antigen expression on resting B-cells[43,44] and stimulates the secretion of IgG$_1$ and IgE by lipopolysaccharide-stimulated B-cells[45,46]. IL-4 can thus be considered both a B-cell growth and differentiation factor. Interestingly interferon-$\gamma$ (a lymphokine with B-cell stimulatory activity in its own right) inhibits the action of IL-4 on resting B-cells[47]. IL-4 is released by helper T lymphocytes following triggering by antigen and MHC presented on APC The importance of IL-4 for the induction of antibody production was recently illustrated by the finding that only those cloned CD4$^+$ T-cells which produce IL-4 following appropriate stimulation by antigen and MHC were capable to induce specific antibody production by B-cells[21]. Apart from resting B-cells[42,48], IL-4 also acts on resting T-cells, which proliferate in response to IL-4 plus phorbol myristate acetate. Both CD4$^+$ and CD8$^+$ T-cells show this response[49].

More physiologically, IL-4, like IL-2, mediates autocrine growth of helper T-cells after antigenic stimulation[50]. Finally, it should be mentioned that IL-4 increases the proliferative rate of certain mast cell lines co-stimulated with interleukin-3 (IL-3)[51]. IL-3 has not been reported to act on B-cells.

The first report dealing with the function of human recombinant IL-4 shows that, like murine IL-4, it stimulates proliferation of anti-IgM activated human B-cells and stimulates proliferation of human helper T-cell clones[38].

## Interferon-$\gamma$

IFN-$\gamma$ is primarily known as a lymphokine capable of inhibiting virus replication. However it can apparently also stimulate human B-cells to proliferate or differentiate under certain conditions (reviewed in Ref. 29). In one study IFN-$\gamma$ together with IL-2 was capable of inducing IgM and IgG secretion in SAC-stimulated human B-cells[52]. In this case IL-2 was considered to cause proliferation of the activated B-cells and IFN-$\gamma$ maturation of B-cells to Ig-secreting cells. Other researchers, however, have denied a differentiation-inducing effect of IFN-$\gamma$ and have noted a proliferation-inducing effect of IFN-$\gamma$ on suboptimally anti-IgM-stimulated B-cells[53].

## B-cell stimulatory factor-2

B-cell stimulatory factor-2 (BSF-2), also known under the name B-cell differentiation factor (BCDF), is a lymphokine functionally characterized by its capacity to cause immunoglobulin production by SAC-activated human B-cells or B-cell lines[54–57]. It appears to be a late acting factor inducing differentiation of antigen-activated B-cells to immunoglobulin-secreting cells. The gene encoding human BSF-2 has been recently cloned[58]. The primary sequence of BSF-2 deduced from the cDNA showed that BSF-2 is a novel interleukin different from all other known cytokines[58].

## SUMMARY

Antibody production is the result of close interaction between class II HLA positive antigen-presenting cells (APC), helper T lymphocytes and B lymphocytes. Antigen is presented by the APC in the context of class II HLA on their surface to specific T-helper lymphocytes which recognize the antigen/HLA class II complex and proliferate in response. IL-1 produced by the APC (as well as by other cells) facilitates activation of the helper T lymphocytes. The activated T-cells produce a variety of lymphokines, of which the best characterized are IL-2, IL-4 (BSF-1), IFN-$\gamma$ and BSF-2. Together these lymphokines, mostly operating at close range, stimulate antigen-triggered B lymphocytes to produce immunoglobulin of the same specificity as the original B-cell surface immunoglobulin that interacted with antigen. Antibody production may be further stimulated by T-helper cells directly recognizing the antigen/class II MHC complex at the surface of the B lymphocytes.

# References

1. Tonegawa, S. (1983). Somatic generation of antibody diversity. *Nature*, **302**, 575–81
2. Hood, L., Kronenberg, M. and Hunkapillar, T. (1985). T-cell antigen receptor and the immunoglobulin supergene family. *Cell*, **40**, 225–9
3. Alt, F.W., Blackwell, T.K., DePinho, R.A., Reth, M.G. and Yancopoulos, G.D. (1986). *Immunol. Rev.*, **89**, 5–30
4. Goverman, J., Hunkapillar, T. and Hood, L. (1986). A speculative view of the multicomponent nature of T cell antigen recognition. *Cell*, **45**, 475–84
5. Nadler, L.M. (1986). B Cell/Leukemia Panel Workshop. Summary and comments. In Reinherz, E.L., Haynes, B.F., Nadler, L.M. and Bernstein, I.D. (eds.) *Leukocyte Typing II* p. 3. (Berlin: Springer Verlag)
6. Shaw, S. (1987). Characterization of human leukocyte differentiation antigens. *Immunol. Today*, **8**, 1–3
7. Golay, F.T. (1986). Functional B-lymphocyte surface antigens. *Immunology*, **59**, 1–5
8. Clark, E.A., Shu, G. and Ledbetter, J.A. (1985). Role of the Bp35 cell surface polypeptide in human B-cell activation. *Proc. Natl. Acad. Sci. USA*, **82**, 1766–70
9. Golay, J.T., Clark, E.A. and Beverley, P.C.L. (1985). The CD20 (Bp35) antigen is involved in activation of B cells from the G0 to the G1 phase of the cell cycle. *J. Immunol.*, **135**, 3795–801
10. Golay, J., Rawle, F. and Beverley, P. (1986). B lymphocyte surface antigens involved in the regulation of immunoglobulin secretion. In Reinherz, E.L., Haynes, B.F., Nadler, L.M. and Bernstein, I.D. (eds.). *Leukocyte Typing II.* p. 463. (Berlin: Springer Verlag)
11. Frade, R., Crevon, M.C., Marel, M., Vazquez, A., Krikorian, L., Charriaut, C. and Galavant, P. (1985). Enhancement of human B cell proliferation by antibody to the C3d receptor, the gp 140 molecule. *Eur. J. Immunol.*, **15**, 73–6
12. Wilson, B.S., Platt, J.L. and Kay, N.E. (1985). Monoclonal antibodies to the 140 000 mol. wt glycoprotein on B lymphocyte membranes (CR2 receptor) initiate proliferation of B cells in vitro. *Blood*, **66**, 824–9
13. Melchers, F. and Andersson, J. (1986). Factors controlling the B-cell cycle. *Annu. Rev. Immunol.*, **4**, 13–36
14. Fingeroth, J.D., Weis, J.J., Tedder, T.F., Strominger, J.L., Biro, P.A. and Fearon, D.T. (1984). Epstein-Barr virus receptor of human B-lymphocytes is the C3d receptor CR2. *Proc. Natl. Acad. Sci. USA*, **81**, 4510–3
15. Daha, M.A., Bloem, A.C. and Ballieux, R.E. (1984). Immunoglobulin production by human peripheral lymphocytes induced by anti-C3 receptor antibodies. *J. Immunol.*, **132**, 1197–201
16. Roitt, I. (1986). *Essential Immunology* (4th Edn.). (Oxford: Blackwell Scientific Publishers)
17. Paul, W.E. (ed.) (1984). *Fundamental Immunology.* (New York: Raven Press)
18. Miedema, F. and Melief, C.J.M. (1985). T-cell recognition of human B-cell activation. A reappraisal of the role of interleukin-2. *Immunol. Today*, **6**, 258–9
19. De Franco, A.L., Ashwell, J.D., Schwartz, R.H. and Paul, W.E. (1984). Polyclonal stimulation of resting B lymphocytes by antigen-specific T lymphocytes. *J. Exp. Med.*, **159**, 861–80
20. Stohe, W., Posnett, D.N. and Chiorazzi, N. (1987). Induction of T cell-dependent B-cell differentiation by anti-CD3 monoclonal antibodies. *J. Immunol.*, **138**, 1667–73
21. Killar, L., MacDonald, G., West, J., Woods, A. and Bottomly, K. (1987). Cloned Ia-restricted T cells that do not produce interleukin-4/B cell stimulatory factor 1 (BSF-1) fail to help antigen-specific B cells. *J. Immunol.*, **138**, 1674–9
22. Andersson, J., Schreier, M.H. and Melchers, F. (1980). T cell-dependent B cell stimulation is H-2 restricted and antigen-dependent only at the resting B cell level. *Proc. Natl. Acad. Sci. USA*, **77**, 1612–6
23. Tzehoval, E., De Baetselier, P., Ron, Y., Tartakovsky, B., Feldman, M. and Segal, S. (1983). Splenic B cells function as immunogenic antigen-presenting cells for the induction of effector T cells. *Eur. J. Immunol.*, **13**, 89–94
24. Lanzavecchia, A. (1985). Antigen-specific interaction between T and B cells. *Nature*, **314**, 537–9
25. Krieger, J.I., Grammer, S.F., Grey, H.M. and Chestnut, R.W. (1985). Antigen presentation by splenic B cells: resting B cells are ineffective, whereas activated B cells are defective accessory cells for T-cell responses. *J. Immunol.*, **135**, 2937–45

26. De Rie, M.A., Kabel, P., Sauerwein, R.T., Van Lier, R.A.W., Von dem Borne, A.E.G. Kr., Melief, C.J.M. and Miedema, F. (1987). Anti-HLA class II monoclonal antibodies inhibit polyclonal B-cell differentiation in vitro at the accessory cell level. *Eur. J. Immunol.*, **17**, 881–6

27. Howard, M., Nakanishi, K. and Paul, W.E. (1984). B cell growth and differentiation factors. *Immunol. Rev.*, **78**, 185–210

28. Schimpl, A. (1984). Lymphokines active in B cell proliferation and differentiation. *Springer Semin. Immunopathol.*, **7**, 299–310

29. Hamaoka, T. and Ono, S. (1986). Regulation of B-cell differentiation; interactions of factors and corresponding receptors. *Annu. Rev. Immunol.*, **4**, 167–204

30. Oppenheim, J.J., Kovacs, E.J., Matsushima, K. and Durum, S.K. (1986). There is more than one interleukin-1. *Immunol. Today*, **7**, 45–56

31. Matsushima, K., Akahoshi, T., Yamada, M., Furutami, Y. and Oppenheim, J.J. (1986). Properties of a specific interleukin-1 (IL-1) receptor on human Epstein-Barr virus transformed B lymphocytes: identity of the receptor for IL-1-$\alpha$ and IL-1-$\beta$. *J. Immunol.*, **136**, 4496–500

32. Scala, Y., Kuang, D., Hall, R.E., Muchmore, A.V. and Oppenheim, J.J. (1984). Accessory cell function of human B cells. I. Production of both interleukin 1-like activity and an interleukin 1 inhibitory factor by an EBV-transformed human B cell line. *J. Exp. Med.*, **159**, 1637–52

33. Matsushima, K., Procopio, A., Abe, H., Scala, G., Ortaldo, J.R. and Oppenheim, J.J. (1985). Production of interleukin-1 activity by normal human peripheral blood B lymphocytes. *J. Immunol.*, **135**, 1132–6

34. Miedema, F., Van Oostveen, J.W., Sauerwein, R.W., Terpstra, F.G., Aarden, L.A. and Melief, C.J.M. (1984). Induction of immunoglobulin synthesis by interleukin-2 is T4$^+$8$^-$ cell dependent. A role for IL-2 in the pokeweed mitogen driven system. *Eur. J. Immunol.*, **15**, 107–12

35. Nakagawa, T., Kakagawa, N., Goldstein, H., Volkman, D.J. and Fauci, A.S. (1986). Demonstration that human B cells respond differently to IL-2 and B cell differentiation factor based on their stages of maturation. *J. Immunol.*, **137**, 3175–82

36. Nakagawa, T., Nakagawa, N., Volkman, D.J., Ambrus, J.L. and Fauci, A.S. (1987). The role of interleukin-2 in inducing Ig production in a pokeweed mitogen-stimulated mononuclear cell system. *J. Immunol.*, **138**, 795–801

37. Miedema, F., Van Oostveen, J.W., Terpstra, F.G., Bake, A., Willemze, R., Rauws, E.A.J., Breger, R., V.'t Veer, M., Catovsky, D. and Melief, C.J.M. (1985). Analysis of helper activity on pokeweed mitogen- and interleukin 2-driven immunoglobulin synthesis by neoplastic T4$^+$ cells. *J. Clin. Invest.*, **76**, 2139–43

38. Yokota, T., Otsuka, T., Mosmann, T., Banchereau, J., DeFrance, T., Blanchard, D., De Vries, J., Lee, F. and Arai, K. (1986). Isolation and characterization of a human interleukin cDNA clone, homologous to mouse BSF-1, which expresses B cell and T cell stimulating activities. *Proc. Natl. Acad. Sci. USA*, **83**, 5894–8

39. Noma, Y., Sideras, P., Naito, T., Bergstedt-Lindquist, S., Azuna, C., Severinson, E., Tanabe, T., Kinashi, T., Matsuda, F., Yaoita, Y. and Honjo, T. (1986). Cloning of cDNA encoding the murine IgG1 induction factor by a novel strategy using sp6 promotor. *Nature*, **319**, 640–2

40. Lee, F., Yokota, T., Otsuka, T., Meyerson, P., Villaret, D., Doffman, R., Mosmann, T., Rennick, D., Roehm, N., Smith, C., Zlotnik, A. and Arai, K. (1986). Isolation and characterization of a mouse interleukin cDNA clone that expresses B-cell stimulatory factor 1 activities and T-cell and mast-cell-stimulatory activities. *Proc. Natl. Acad. Sci. USA*, **83**, 2061–5

41. Howard, M., Farrar, J., Hilfiker, M., Johnson, B., Takatsu, K., Hamaoka, T. and Paul, W.E. (1982). Identification of a T cell derived B cell growth factor distinct from interleukin-2. *J. Exp. Med.*, **155**, 914–23

42. Oliver, K., Noelle, R.J., Uhr, J.W., Krammer, P.H. and Vitetta, E.S. (1985). B cell growth factor (B-cell growth factor 1 or B-cell stimulating factor, provision 1) is a differentiation factor for resting B cells and may not induce growth. *Proc. Natl. Acad. Sci. USA*, **82**, 2465–7

43. Roehm, N.W., Liebson, J., Zlotnik, A., Kappler, J., Marrack, P. and Cambier, J.C. (1984). Interleukin-induced increase in Ia expression by normal mouse B cells. *J. Exp. Med.*, **160**, 679–94

44. Noelle, R., Krammer, P.H., Ohara, J., Uhr, J.W. and Vitetta, E.S. (1984). Increased expression of Ia antigens on resting B cells: an additional role for B-cell growth factor. *Proc. Natl. Acad. Sci. USA*, **81**, 6149–53
45. Vitetta, E.S., Ohara, J., Myers, C.D., Layton, J.E., Krammer, P.H. and Paul, W.E. (1985). Serological, biochemical and functional identity of B cell stimulatory factor 1 and B cell differentiation factor for IgG₁. *J. Exp. Med.*, **162**, 1726–31
46. Coffman, R.L., Ohara, J., Bond, M.W., Carty, J., Zlotnik, A. and Paul, W.E. (1986). B cell stimulatory factor 1 enhances the IgE response of lipopolysaccharide-activated B cells. *J. Immunol.*, **136**, 4538–41
47. Rabin, E.M., Mond, J.J., Ohara, J. and Paul, W.E. (1986). Interferon-γ inhibits the action of B cell stimulatory factor BSF-1 on resting B cells. *J. Immunol.*, **137**, 1573–6
48. Rabin, E.M., Mond, J.J., Ohara, J. and Paul, W.E. (1986). B cell stimulatory factor a (BSF-1) prepares resting B cells to enter S phase in response to anti-IgM and lipopolysaccharide. *J. Exp. Med.*, **164**, 517–31
49. Hu-Li, J., Shevach, E.M., Mizuuchi, J., Ohara, J., Mosmann, T. and Paul, W.E. (1987). B cell stimulatory factor 1 (IL-4) is a potent costimulant for normal resting T lymphocytes. *J. Exp. Med.*, **165**, 157–72
50. Fernandez-Botran, R., Sanders, V.M., Oliver, K.G., Chen, Y-W., Krammer, P.H., Uhr, J.W., Vitetta, E.S. (1986). Interleukin 4 mediates autocrine growth of helper T cells after antigenic stimulation. *Proc. Natl. Acad. Sci. USA*, **83**, 9689–93
51. Mosmann, T.R., Bond, M.W., Coffman, R.L., Ohara, J. and Paul, W.E. (1986). T-cell and mast cell lines respond to B-cell stimulatory factor 1. *Proc. Natl. Acad. Sci. USA*, **93**, 5654–8
52. Nakagawa, T., Hirano, T., Nakagawa, N., Yoshizaki, K. and Kishimoto, T. (1985). Effect of recombinant IL-2 and γ-IFN on proliferation and differentiation of human B cells. *J. Immunol.*, **134**, 959–63
53. DeFrance T., Aubry, J.P., Vandervliet, B. and Banchereau, J. (1986). Human interferon-γ acts as a B cell growth factor in the anti-IgM antibody costimulatory assay but has no direct B cell differentiation activity. *J. Immunol.*, **137**, 3861–7
54. Okada, M., Sakaguchi, N., Yoshimura, N., Hara, H., Shimizu, K., Yoshida, N., Yoshizaki, K., Kishimoto, S., Yamamura, Y. and Kishimoto, T. (1983). B cell growth factors and B cell differentiation factor from human T hybridomas. *J. Exp. Med.*, **157**, 583–90
55. Hirano, T., Teranishi, T., Iin, B. and Onoue, K. (1984). Demonstration of a human late-acting B cell differentiation factor acting on *Staphylococcus aureus* Cowan I-stimulated B cells. *J. Immunol.*, **133**, 798–802
56. Butler, J., Falkoff, R.J.M. and Fauci, A.S. (1984). Development of a human T-cell hybridoma secreting separate B-cell growth and differentiation factors. *Proc. Natl. Acad. Sci. USA*, **81**, 2475–8
57. Kikutani, H., Taga, T., Akira, S., Kishi, H., Miki, Y., Saiki, O., Yamamura, Y. and Kishimoto, T. (1985). Effect of B cell differentiation factor (BCDF) on biosynthesis and secretion of immunoglobulin molecules in human B cell lines. *J. Immunol.*, **134**, 990–5
58. Hirano, T., Yasukawa, K., Harada, H., Taga, T., Watanabe Y., Matsuda, T., Kashiwamura, S., Nakajima, K., Koyama, K., Iwawamatsu, A., Tsunasawa, S., Sakiyama, F., Matsui, H., Takahara, Y., Taniguchi, T. and Kishimoto, T. (1986). Complementary DNA for a novel human interleukin (BSF-2) that induces B lymphocytes to produce immunoglobulin. *Nature*, **324**, 73–6

# 11
# Immunopathology of Sjögren's syndrome: a review

B. PAL and I. D. GRIFFITHS

## INTRODUCTION

Sjögren's syndrome may be defined as an autoimmune exocrinopathy with a predilection for multisystem involvement. It is one of the more common chronic inflammatory rheumatic disorders; its prevalence in the population may approach that of rheumatoid arthritis. Although isolated features of the disorder were described by various authors[1,2] from 1882 onwards – it was Gougerot[3] in France who in 1925 first recognized the systemic nature of this illness, with dry eyes being only one of the more obvious manifestations. However, the term Sjögren's syndrome has been given to this disorder in recognition of the work by Henrick Sjögren, a Swedish ophthalmologist, following his monograph on the disorder published in 1933[4]. Mikulicz's disease, described in 1888, is actually the same disease as Sjögren's syndrome[5].

Studies on series of patients since then have established the autoimmune nature of the condition and the protean manifestations associated with it. Several recent large series of patients have been reported by Bloch et al.[6], Shearn[7], Whaley and Buchanan[8] and Fox et al.[9].

Sjögren's syndrome is characterized by at least two of the following three criteria:

(1)  keratoconjunctivitis sicca (KCS/dry eyes);

(2)  xerostomia (dry mouth);

(3)  presence of another connective tissue disease.

Customarily the syndrome has been classified[6] into two categories: primary Sjögren's syndrome or the Sicca syndrome when only the first two criteria are present; and secondary Sjögren's syndrome when either KCS or xerostomia is associated with a definable connective tissue disorder – most commonly rheumatoid arthritis but it may be any of systemic lupus erythematosus, scleroderma, dermatomyositis, primary biliary cirrhosis, chronic active hepatitis and others.

A third category recently recognized is the so-called pseudolymphoma group where florid and widespread lymphocytic infiltration of various tissues occurs associated with lymphadenopathy. It is in this form and in patients with extraglandular involvement such as vasculitis and neuropathy that the risk of non-Hodgkins lymphoma is particularly increased.

## CLINICAL FEATURES

The clinical manifestations of Sjögren's syndrome are protean reflecting the widespread tissue infiltrations with mononuclear cells and immune injury[7-10]. Patients commonly complain of dryness and/or grittiness of eyes and dryness of mouth. There may be angular stomatitis and lingual papillary atrophy[7,8].

Systemic manifestations include low grade fever, weight loss, vasculitis in about 10% of patients and more commonly Raynaud's phenomenon (20%).

Cutaneous manifestations consist of dry and occasionally pruritic skin and impaired sweating. Vitiligo may be seen and there may be purpuric rashes on the lower limbs particularly in patients who have hyperglobulinaemia.

Pulmonary manifestations may be in the form of pleurisy, dry and non-productive cough (bronchitis, sicca) and migratory lung infiltrations. Recurrent infections may lead to bronchiectasis. Pulmonary interstitial fibrosis may occur. Respiratory function test abnormalities may be more common than overt pathology as described above. Common defects include decrease in diffusing capacity and transfer factor defects[8,9].

Gastrointestinal manifestations are common. Apart from xerostomia, impaired taste and severe dental caries may occur. Patients may have difficulty in mastication and dysphagia[7,9]. Abdominal pain may be a feature and pancreatitis is a rare but recognized complication. Chronic atrophic gastritis[9,11,12], malabsorption and diarrhoea may occur. A variety of liver disorders may be seen in patients with Sjögren's syndrome and these include primary biliary cirrhosis, chronic active hepatitis and cryptogenic cirrhosis[7-9].

Cardiac problems may arise due to pericarditis or secondary to pulmonary involvement. Myocarditis is rare[8,9].

Renal features are only occasionally of any clinical significance. However, some renal involvement occurs in up to a quarter of the patients and the pathology has varied from glomerular arteriolitis to glomerulonephritis[7]. The typical pathology, however, is interstitial nephritis[7,9]. Tubular dysfunction may result causing renal tubular acidosis or nephrogenic diabetes insipidus[7,9].

Thyroid disorders may be subclincal more often than overt as shown by the presence of raised thyroid stimulating hormone levels in patients and also the presence of thyroid antibodies[8,9]. In addition to goitre, both hypoactivity and hyperactivity of thyroid functions may occur.

Neuromuscular features classically include trigeminal neuropathy and peripheral neuropathy but other focal cranial nerve deficits and transient neurological deficits such as hemiparesis and transverse myelitis have also

185

been described recently[9,13]. Myalgia is common but overt myositis may also occur.

In the musculoskeletal system the commonest complaint is arthralgias but arthritis may also occur and is typically non-erosive affecting mainly the small joints[8,9,14]. Up to two-thirds of patients with secondary Sjögren's syndrome have an associated rheumatic disorder, commonly rheumatoid arthritis.

## PATHOLOGY: PERIPHERAL BLOOD LYMPHOCYTES

Lymphocyte (B-cell) hyperactivity such as polyclonal hyperglobulinaemia and induction of a variety of autoantibodies occurs in Sjögren's syndrome (SS); there are also alterations in lymphocyte subsets in the peripheral blood. Changes in the ratios of T-helper and suppressor cells have been shown previously in other autoimmune disorders such as systemic lupus erythematosus[15]. Using monoclonal antibodies and the fluorescence activated cell sorter (FACS) the percentage of T-cells was found to be decreased in patients with Sjögren's syndrome compared to controls[16,17]. Some authors have found the number of Leu3/OKT4 cells (helper cells) to be relatively normal while the number of Leu2+/T8 cells (suppressor cells) are significantly diminished in patients with primary Sjögren's syndrome[16] thus giving rise to an increased T4/T8 ratio. Others have found both types of cells decreased proportionately with an unchanged helper/suppressor cell ratio[17]. In the latter study there was a significant decrease in only the suppressor cell subsets in patients with secondary Sjögren's syndrome. There are not only quantitative changes in lymphocyte subsets but also changes in Leu2a expression which suggest abnormal differentiation of the suppressor cell. These alterations may contribute to the immune disturbances characteristic of Sjögren's syndrome.

The reasons for the decreased number of suppressor cells are not clear. Some patients with lupus have lymphocytotoxic antibodies directed against the suppressor cells[18] but such antibodies were not found in patients with Sjögren's syndrome[16].

The natural killer cell (NK) activity of peripheral blood lymphocytes has been reported to be diminished by some authors[19] but these findings have been disputed[20].

The autologous mixed lymphocyte response (AMLR) provides an *in vitro* model for Ia antigen recognition by T-cells. Defective AMLR has been demonstrated previously in other disorders including systemic lupus erythematosus[21]. A high percentage of patients with Sjögren's syndrome also have impaired AMLR[22] and this is apparently associated with an increase in peripheral blood Ia positive T-cells as demonstrated by monoclonal antibody and indirect immunofluorescence techniques[23].

Salivary gland lymphocytes function adequately, as do the peripheral blood cells, in stimulating production of immunoglobulin. In addition they can produce rheumatoid factor which peripheral lymphocytes cannot. Salivary gland lymphocytes, however, have less natural killer cell activity and antibody-dependent cellular cytotoxicity when compared to peripheral blood lymphocytes in this disorder.

## PATHOLOGY: TARGET ORGANS

Tissue infiltration of mononuclear cells occurs in this condition not only in the salivary and lachrymal glands but also in many other organs such as the lungs, kidneys, gastrointestinal tract and others[7-9]. Changes in the salivary and lachrymal glands are the most pronounced and will be discussed here in detail.

At the ordinary microscopic level both minor and major salivary glands show changes from slight lymphocytic infiltrations to florid destructive changes. In the early stages the mononuclear cells infiltrate in a periductal fashion, germinal centres are not usually formed but are occasionally seen in the major glands, where most of the acini show infiltrations. The cells are mainly distributed in the centre of the lobular structure and less often in the periphery[25,25]. The cells may invade the acini and ducts. The latter may enlarge and inspissated substances may accumulate. There is often myoepithelial cell proliferation. Despite these extreme changes the lobular pattern of the glandular structure is retained – a discriminating feature in comparison with changes seen in lymphoma with which diagnostic confusion may arise. Another feature which may differentiate Sjögren's syndrome from lymphoma is the so-called 'benign myoepithelioma' which is characteristically found in the major salivary glands in Sjögren's syndrome. The origin of these lesions is believed to be the proliferating myoepithelial cells of the ducts. This view is further supported by the use of monoclonal antibody staining[26].

Vessels within the lymphocytic infiltrate of the salivary glands in Sjögren's syndrome were found to be identical to those specialized for lymphocyte transport in lymph nodes. These vessels may represent a mechanism for increased lymphocyte traffic into the gland and thereby contribute significantly to the inflammatory process[27].

Using double immunoenzymatic staining techniques, glandular epithelial cells of the salivary glands in patients with Sjögren's syndrome were shown to be HLA-DR positive in contrast to HLA-DR negativity in controls. These HLA-DR positive cells were seen in close proximity to the periphery of dense lymphocytic infiltrates[28].

Electron microscopy reveals further detailed abnormalities such as diminution of secretory granules and mitochondria and the appearance of tubuloreticular structures. The latter were at one time thought to represent viral particles but are now regarded as a non-specific result of tissue insult.

As the severity of the lymphocyte infiltration and other changes in the glands vary and because mononuclear cell aggregates occur in a proportion of normal controls (principally in elderly persons) diagnostic difficulties very often arise. The problem is compounded by the fact that some elderly individuals have a number of autoantibodies including SSA and SSB but lack any histopathological features of Sjögren's syndrome. In general minor labial salivary glands reflect the pathological changes occurring in the major salivary glands as well as non-glandular structures. The ease with which the labial salivary glands can be obtained from a lower lip biopsy is exploited for diagnostic purposes. A number of different arbitrary grading systems have been proposed to indicate mononuclear cell infiltration – some incorporating

187

parenchymal changes[25] while others ignore them for the purposes of grading[24]. There are advantages and disadvantages with all these different systems.

For examination of the lymphocyte subsets in salivary tissues, biopsy specimens are first frozen and tissue sections are then fixed in acetone. Monoclonal antibodies are used as lymphocyte subset markers in a four-step biotin–avidin immunoperoxidase technique[17]: Leu3a or OKT4 mark the T-helper/inducer cells; Leu2a and/or OKT8 mark the T-suppressor/cytotoxic cells; the antibody B532 marks a B-cell subset[16,17]. Other methods that have been used to examine cell types, prior to availability of the monoclonal antibody markers, include the rosetting technique with red blood cells and use of specific serum against immunoglobulin. These methods are less reliable than the more modern technique of using the monoclonal markers.

Using these techniques, a predominance of Leu7 or OKT3 marking T lymphocytes can be found in salivary tissues of which the majority of the cells are helper cell subset marked by Leu3a or OKT4. A small proportion of B-cells may be found but the subset defined by B352 which is absent from peripheral blood is present in salivary tissues[16,17]. A high prevalence of Ia positive or activation antigens marked by OKT10 has been demonstrated in the T-cells in tissues compared to peripheral blood T-cells[16]. These findings show that cellular infiltration at the primary site of tissue injury differs from changes found in the peripheral blood.

The study by Fox et al. showed that salivary gland lymphocytes differed from peripheral blood lymphocytes because they (i) lacked lymphocyte reactive with anti-Leu7 and anti-Leu11 monoclonal antibodies, (ii) lacked NK activity and (iii) lacked the ability to suppress polyclonal B-cell responses in the presence of complement fragment C3a[16].

Monoclonal markers show a similar composition in lymphocytic infiltration in other tissues such as in the stomach where atrophic gastritis may occur[11,12].

As well as the elucidation of the pathology of the cellular infiltration, monoclonal antibodies have a further useful role in practical terms. Non-Hodgkin's lymphomas are usually due to B-cell proliferation. In pseudolymphoma, on the other hand, widespread infiltration of T-cells occurs, the majority of which are Leu2a and/or helper cells. Monoclonal staining is obviously capable of differentiating pseudolymphoma from lymphoma[29,30]. Another use of monoclonal marking is the study of the possible progression of pseudolymphoma to lymphoma by looking for monoclonal light chain patterns. In pseudolymphoma both $\kappa$ and $\lambda$ are expressed whereas in lymphoma only one light chain is present. Screening of serum or urine for the type of light chain could be valuable in the follow-up of Sjögren's syndrome patients in whom risk for malignancy is high[31,32].

It is important to realize that patients with Sjögren's syndrome have a very much increased risk of developing non-Hodgkin's lymphoma[33]. There is also a propensity to develop monoclonal gammopathy[34] and immunoblastic sarcoma[35]. The risk factors in the patients are believed to be persistent lymphoadenopathy, splenomegaly, parotid enlargement, previous radio-therapy or other evidence of aggressive disease such as vasculitis or neuropathy. Other possible indicators of impending malignancy are decreasing levels of serum immunoglobulin especially IgM or autoantibody titres[36].

Treatment with cytotoxic drugs or irradiation may increase the risk[7].

A more recent development is the use of monoclonal antibodies to non-immunoglobulin antigen on B-cells and the complement of C3 receptors which revealed B-cell markers in up to a quarter of lymphoid cells in salivary tissue in patients with primary Sjögren's syndrome.

In the study by Bakshi et al.[17], distinguishing primary and secondary Sjögren's syndrome in patients, certain differences have been noted. For example, a higher proportion of B-cells occurred in tissue in patients having secondary Sjögren's syndrome compared to primary Sjögren's syndrome.

The pathological features detailed above may be seen in addition to the salivary and lachrymal glands in various other tissues and organs such as the bronchi, kidneys and stomach; Sjögren's syndrome is a systemic illness. Lymphocytic infiltrations are also seen in the conjunctivae. Mononuclear cell infiltrations and the resultant immune injury to tissue and local inflammatory reaction lead to tissue damage which in turn causes the various clinical manifestations as described above.

## AUTOANTIBODIES IN SJÖGREN'S SYNDROME

The clinical complexities of Sjögren's syndrome are mirrored by the immunological variabilities. The presence of circulating precipitating autoantibodies directed at cellular antigens was described in 1958[37]. Interest was reawakened by the reports of Alspaugh and Tan in 1975[38] of antibodies to cellular nuclear antigens in Sjögren's syndrome. The antigen source was a human lymphoid cell line (WiL2). Three distinct precipitating antibodies were identified and termed SSA, SSB and SSC. Nomenclature became confused for several years as independent groups identified further precipitating antibodies to either cellular or cytoplasmic antigens from a wide variety of human and mammalian sources in patients with Sjögren's syndrome, these included anti-La[39], anti-Ha[40], anti-Ro[41], and anti-RANA.

Exchange of sera between laboratories subsequently demonstrated that many of these antibody antigen systems were detecting common antibodies, despite the heterogeneity of antigen sources[42]. The presently accepted classification is shown in Table 11.1.

The past eight years have seen a steady increase in the number of autoantibodies detected in connective tissue disorders. Many of these appear to have some diagnostic specificity but are never found uniquely in one clearly defined clinical group and with absolute sensitivity. As Sjögren's

**Table 11.1**  Antibody–antigen reactions in Sjögren's syndrome

| Antibody | Synonyms | Main disease associations | Antigen characteristics |
|---|---|---|---|
| Anti-SSA | Ro | Sjögren's (primary); SLE | ribonucleoprotein (2 bands: 40 kDa and 30 kDa) |
| Anti-SSB | La, Ha | Sjögren's (primary); SLE | nucleoprotein (2 bands: 40 kDa and 29 kDa) |
| Anti-SSC | RANA | RA (with and without Sjögren's) | EBV-related nuclear antigen (EBNA) |

189

syndrome may accompany many of these connective tissue disorders, it is only to be expected that these autoantibodies will be detected in any large series of 'Sjögren's syndrome', where secondary Sjögren's syndrome is included. For completeness the present classification of autoantibodies with their main disease associations is shown in Table 11.2.

However, it appears that anti-SSA (Ro) and anti-SSB (La) remain the most clinically relevant circulating autoantibodies in Sjögren's syndrome and these are discussed more fully.

### Anti-SSA (Ro) antibodies

*Antigen sources and characterization*
The antigen has been extracted from rapidly dividing human cell lines (WiL2 and HEP-2), human spleen, human thymus and calf thymus. It may occur in both the nuclear and cytoplasmic compartments but is predominantly nuclear and gives rise to a speckled immunofluorescent pattern. The antigen appears to be a ribonucleoprotein. Antigenicity is confined to the protein fraction and RNAse digestion does not influence antigenicity. Affinity chromatography using anti-SSA (Ro) sera has been used to further characterize the antigen, Western blotting reveals an antigenic protein band of 60 kDa bound to the non-antigenic 24 kDa RNA component[43].

*Assay methods*
Most assay methods have depended upon showing a precipitation line in either gel diffusion[38] or counter-immunoelectrophoresis (CIE)[44] between the test sera and a crude cellular extract containing SSA (Ro). Inevitably other antigens are present in the cell extract and identification of the antibody antigen line as being anti-SSA (Ro) relies upon showing a line of identity with an adjacent well containing a reference serum with known anti-SSA (Ro) activity.

More recently solid phase ELISA assays have been developed using affinity column purified SSA (Ro) and expressing the antibody activity of the test sera quantitatively in respect to a known standard serum with anti-SSA (Ro) activity[43,45].

**Table 11.2**  Antinuclear antibodies and main disease associations

| Antibody | Primary disease associations |
| --- | --- |
| DNA | Systemic lupus erythematosus (SLE) |
| DNA-histone | SLE, drug-induced LE |
| RNP | Mixed connective tissue disease, overlap syndromes, SLE |
| Sm | SLE |
| SSA (Ro) | Primary Sjögren's |
| SSB (Ha,La) | Primary Sjögren's |
| SSC (RANA) | Rheumatoid arthritis |
| Centromere | Primary biliary cirrhosis |
| PM1 | Myositis |
| Scl70 | Systemic sclerosis |
| Jo1 | Myositis and pulmonary fibrosis |
| SL (Ki) | SLE |

*Clinical significance*
It has become apparent that anti-SSA (Ro) antibodies are not confined to patients with Sjögren's syndrome. Depending upon the sensitivity of the assay system, antibodies have been detected in patients with systemic lupus erythematosus (LE), 'ANA negative' systemic LE, C2-deficient LE, subacute cutaneous LE and neonatal LE[43,46,47]. A clear association between maternal anti-sera (Ro) antibodies and congenital heart block has been demonstrated[48]. The maternal antibody appears to cross the placenta and can only be detected in the neonate during the first three months after birth. One postmortem examination on an infant with congenital heart block revealed anti-SSA (Ro) antibody in atrial tissue by immunofluorescence[49]. The presence of maternal anti-SSA (Ro) was not inevitably associated with any clinical features of a connective tissue disorder in the mother[48].

Systemic LE (SLE) patients with anti-SSA (Ro) antibodies tend to have a lower incidence of significant renal disease and absence of DNA binding[50]. One group however found an association between SSA (Ro) antibodies and membranous glomerulonephritis[51]. Elderly onset SLE is more usually associated with anti-SSA (Ro) antibodies, the prevalence rising from 36% in patients less than 55 years of age at onset, to over 90% in the elderly[52].

In patients with Sjögren's syndrome the prevalence of anti-SSA (Ro) antibodies depends upon disease associations. The prevalence is lowest in patients with secondary Sjögren's syndrome associated with RA and greatest in patients with primary Sjögren's syndrome and an associated vasculitis[53]. The presence of anti-SSA (Ro) is associated with extraglandular features of Sjögren's syndrome including vasculitis, purpura, lymphadenopathy, leucopenia and thrombocytopenia[54]. RA patients with anti-SSA (Ro) antibodies had an increased incidence of adverse reactions to D-penicillamine compared with the antibody negative group[55].

Employing a sensitive solid phase ELISA assay Harley *et al.*[45] detected elevated levels of anti-SSA (Ro) antibody in all subjects with primary Sjögren's syndrome and in 75% of RA Sjögren's patients. The titres of anti-SSA (Ro) were considerably greater in the primary Sjögren's syndrome group. Within the primary Sjögren's group they observed an association of high anti-SSA (Ro) titres with increased serum IgG levels, rheumatoid factor titres and a trend towards association with leukocytoclastic vasculitis. Although anti-SSA (Ro) and anti-SSB (La) titres tended to correlate, no association of anti-SSA (Ro) and other antinuclear antigens, including Sm and RNP occurred.

Low titres of antibodies to SSA (Ro) can be found in normal sera using a sensitive ELISA assay and this binding can be inhibited by prior incubation of the sera with purified SSA (Ro), suggesting that the differences between normal and disease is a quantitative rather than qualitative phenomenon[43].

## Anti-SSB (LA) antibodies

*Antigen sources and characteristics*
The SSB (LA) is a soluble nuclear antigen which can be isolated from a wide variety of sources including rabbit and calf thymus, rat liver, human spleen and human lymphocytes. The antigen is sensitive to trypsin digestion.

Antibodies to this antigen, like anti-SSA, produce a speckled nuclear immunofluorescent pattern. Characterization of the antigen, using column affinity chromatography with linked anti-SSB (La) antibody, has shown two protein bands on Western blotting at 29 kDa and 40 kDa[56].

*Assay methods*
Antibodies were originally detected by precipitating lines in immuno-diffusion[38]. Subsequently counter-immunoelectrophoretic assays were developed[44]. More recently, with the purification of the antigen by affinity chromatography, ELISA assays have been developed[45,56]. Not surprisingly the prevalence of anti-SSB antibodies and their disease associations have changed with the development of more sensitive and quantitative assays.

*Clinical significance*
As with anti-SSA (Ro), the most consistent association of anti-SSB (La) antibodies is with Sjögren's syndrome and primary Sjögren's syndrome in particular[53]. They are also present in SLE and SLE/Sjögren's[47,56]. Evidence for an association with RA/Sjögren's syndrome is conflicting. Venables et al.[56], using an ELISA assay, did not find a striking association whereas Harley et al.[45], using a similar assay, found increased levels of anti-SSB (La) in most RA/Sjögren's patients. Elkon et al.[57], employing a CIE precipitation assay, failed to find antibodies to either SSB (La) or SSA (Ro) in patients with RA/Sjögren's syndrome. Alspaugh et al.[53] using a double diffusion assay detected precipitation lines to SSB (La) in only 8% of RA/Sjögren's compared to 40% of primary Sjögren's.

Most studies have found the prevalence of anti-SSB (La) to be less than SSA (Ro) in both primary Sjögren's syndrome and SLE, and it is very uncommon to detect anti-SSB (La) activity in the absence of anti-SSA (Ro) antibody[58]. However, quantitative assays have shown a strong correlation between SSA (Ro) and SSB (La) antibody levels[45].

The diagnostic significance of anti-SSB (La) was evaluated by Isenberg et al.[59], who identified 15 sera in the laboratory with anti-SSB (La) activity; subsequent clinical evaluation of these patients revealed that eleven had Sjögren's syndrome, which most commonly was either primary or associated with SLE. In only three had the diagnosis been made prior to the re-evaluation.

The presence of anti-SSB (La) antibodies in patients with SLE or SLE/Sjögren's syndrome seems, like anti-SSA (Ra) antibodies, to be associated with a reduced incidence of renal involvement[50,58].

## IMMUNOGENETIC ASSOCIATIONS IN SJÖGREN'S SYNDROME

An association between primary Sjögren's syndrome and the class II MHC antigen, DR3 is well established[60,61]. The prevalence of HLA-DR3 rises from approximately 30% in the normal population to approximately 80% in patients with primary Sjögren's syndrome. Other HLA antigens which are in linkage disequilibrium with HLA-DR3, i.e. A1 and B8, are also increased but the strongest association remains with HLA-DR3[61,62].

The HLA-DR3 association is not found in secondary Sjögren's syndrome, regardless of the connective tissue disorder present[63]. Two groups have found that HLA-MT2, a class II antigen, was increased in both primary and secondary Sjögren's, the prevalence increasing from 40% in the normal population to 90% in Sjögren's syndrome[63,64].

Family studies in Sjögren's syndrome are limited. One study of six kindred in whom the proband had primary Sjögren's syndrome and where other family members had either Sjögren's or an autoimmune disease failed to detect any evidence of haplotype sharing between affected individuals, or an increase in HLA-DR3 in any group other than the probands[65]. No evidence of an association with Gm allotypes could be found. A suggestion of haplotype sharing between affected family members with primary Sjögren's was found in a study of three families, but the haplotype was different in each of the families[64].

In patients with primary Sjögren's syndrome, the prevalence of HLA-DR3 increases still further in those with either anti-SSA (Ro) or anti-SSB (La) antibodies[63,66]. This DR3–anti-SSA/B association does not appear to be confined to primary Sjögren's syndrome. Bell and Maddison[67] found that all their SLE patients with anti-SSA (Ro) possessed HLA-DR3. The prevalence of DR3 in SLE patients without anti-SSA (Ro) was similar to that in the normal population.

The combination of primary Sjögren's–DR3–anti-SSA (Ro)/SSB (La) appears to be associated with increased extraglandular features of the disease[66].

## CONCLUSION

Sjögren's syndrome, a common rheumatic disorder, is an autoimmune exocrinopathy characterized by keratoconjunctivitis sicca and xerostomia with or without an associated connective tissue disorder such as rheumatoid arthritis, systemic lupus erythematosus and others. Nomenclature has been confusing and diagnosis often difficult because of variable expression of clinical disease and laboratory features. The aetiology is unknown but the possible implication of infective agents such as the Epstein–Barr virus is being explored. Increased familial incidence is known and genetic factors may be involved, as suggested by the association with HLA-A1, B8 and DR3; more recently MT2, a class II antigen, has been found to be more strongly associated with Sjögren's syndrome. Various organ systems may be affected by immune-mediated injury resulting in a wide spectrum of clinical manifestations including locomotor, pulmonary, cardiac, gastrointestinal, renal and neuro-logical problems. Systemic manifestations consist of low-grade fever, Raynaud's phenomenon and vasculitis. Risk of lymphomatous complications appears to be greatly increased in this disorder.

Immunological abnormalities are the hallmarks of Sjögren's syndrome. Lymphocyte (B-cell) hyperactivity such as polyclonal hypergammaglobulina-emia and induction of a variety of autoantibodies occur. There are also alterations of tissue and peripheral blood lymphocyte subsets, as revealed by the application of monoclonal markers. In the peripheral blood there is often an increase in the T-helper/suppressor cell ratio. Natural killer cell activity and autologous mixed lymphocyte reaction may be abnormal. The spectrum of autoantibodies includes rheumatoid factors, antinuclear antibodies, gastric parietal cell antibodies, thyroid antimitochondrial and salivary gland antibodies but of more practical importance are the more recently described antibodies to cellular antigens – the SS-A and SS-B antibodies. SS-A antibodies may be found in a low frequency in Sjögren's syndrome with rheumatoid arthritis but more often in association with systemic lupus erythematosus; however, the greatest frequency occurs in primary Sjögren's syndrome with associated vasculitis. SS-B antibodies are most consistently found in primary Sjögren's syndrome and may be of diagnostic value in practice. Like the SS-A antibodies, the SS-B antibodies also appear to be associated with a reduced risk of renal involvement.

## References

1. Leber, H. (1882). Uber die Entstehung der Netzhautablosung. *Klin. Mbl. Augenheilk.*, **20**, 165–6
2. Hadden, W.B. (1888). On 'Dry mouth', or suppression of the salivary and buccal secretions. *Trans. Clin. Soc. London.*, **21**, 176–9
3. Gougerot, A. (1925). Insuffisance progressive et atrophie des glandes salivaries et muqueuses de la bouche, des conjunctives (et parfois des muqueuses, nasale, laryngee, vulvaire). 'Secheresse' de la bouche, des conjunctives etc. *Bull. Soc. Derm. Syph.*, **32**, 376–9
4. Sjögren, H.S. (1933). Zur Kenntnis der Keratoconjunctivitis sicca (Keratitis folliformis bei hypofunction der Tranendrusen). *Acta Ophthalmol., (Copenhagen)*, **2**, 1–151
5. Mikulicz, J.H. (1892). Uber eine eigenartige symmetrische Erkrankung der Tranen und Mundspeichelkdrusen. *Beitz Chir. Fortsch. Geuridmet.*, (Stuttgart: Theodor Billroth) pp. 610–630
6. Bloch, K., Buchanan, W., Wohl, M. et al. (1965). Sjögren's syndrome. Clinical, pathological and serological study of 62 cases. *Medicine (Baltimore)*, **44**, 187–231
7. Shearn, M.A. (1971). Sjögren's Syndrome. In Smith, L.H. (ed.) *Major Problems in Internal Medicine*. Vol. II. (Philadelphia, London, Toronto: W.B. Saunders Co.)
8. Whaley, K. and Buchanan, W.W. (1980). Sjögren's syndrome and associated diseases. In Parker, C.W. (ed.) *Clinical Immunology* Vol. 1, p. 632. (Philadelphia, London, Toronto: W.B. Saunders Co.)
9. Fox, R.I., Howell, F.V., Bone, R.C. and Michelson, P. (1984). Primary Sjögren's syndrome: clinical and immunopathological features. *Semin. Arthr. Rheum.*, **14**, 77–105
10. Moutsopoulus, H.M., Webber, B.L., Vlagopoulos, T.P. et al. (1979). Differences in the clinical manifestations of sicca syndrome in the presence and absence of rheumatoid arthritis. *Am. J. Med.*, **66**, 733–6
11. Maury, C.P.J., Rasanen, V., Teppo, A.M. et al. (1982). Serum pepsinogen II in rheumatic diseases: reduced levels in Sjögren's syndrome. *Arthr. Rheum.*, **25**, 1059–63
12. Kilpi, A., Bergroth, V., Kontinnen, Y.T. et al. (1983). Lymphocyte infiltrations of the gastric mucosa in Sjögren's syndrome: an immunoperoxidase study using monoclonal antibodies in the avidin-biotin-peroxidase method. *Arthr. Rheum.*, **26**, 1196–200
13. Alexander, E.L., Provost, T.T., Stevens, M.B. et al. (1982). Neurologic complications of primary Sjögren's syndrome. *Medicine*, **61**, 247–57
14. Castro-Poltronieri, A. and Alarcon-Segoria, D. (1983). Articular manifestations of primary Sjögren's Syndrome. *J. Rheumatol.*, **10**, 485–8
15. Marimoto, C., Reinherz, E., Skinberg, A., Schur, P. et al. (1980). Alterations in immunoregulatory T cell subsets in active SLE. *J. Clin. Invest.*, **66**, 1171
16. Fox, R.I., Carstens, S.A, Fong, S., Robinson, C.A. et al. (1982). Use of monoclonal antibodies to analyse peripheral blood and salivary gland lymphocyte subsets in Sjögren's Syndrome. *Arthr. Rheum.*, **25**, 419–26

17. Bakshi, A., Mijasaka, N., Kavathas, P., Daniels, T.E. *et al.* (1983). Lymphocyte subsets in Sjögren's syndrome: A quantitative analysis using monoclonal antibodies and the Fluorescence Activated Cell Sorter. *J. Clin. Lab. Immunol.*, **10**, 63–9

18. Marimoto, C., Reinherz, E., Abe, T., Homma, M. and Schlossman, S. (1980). Characteristics of anti-T-cell antibodies in systemic lupus: evidence for reactivity with normal suppressor cells defined by monoclonal antibodies. *Clin. Immunol. Immunopathol.*, **16**, 474

19. Gioto, M., Tanimoto, K., Chihara, T. and Horuchi, Y. (1981). Natural cell-mediated cytotoxicity in Sjögren's syndrome and rheumatoid arthritis. *Arthr. Rheum.*, **24**, 1377–82

20. Miyasaka, N., Seaman, W., Bakshi, A., Sauvezie, B. *et al.* (1983). Natural killing activity in Sjögren's syndrome: an analysis of defective mechanisms. *Arthr. Rheum.*, **26**, 954

21. Kuntz, N.M., Innes, J.B. and Weksler, M.E. (1979). The cellular basis of the impaired autologous mixed lymphocyte reaction in patients with systemic lupus erythematosus. *J. Clin. Invest.*, **63**, 151–6

22. Miyasaka, N., Sauvezie, B., Pierce, D.A., Davids, T.E. and Talal, N. (1980). Decreased autologous mixed lymphocyte reaction in Sjögren's syndrome. *J. Clin. Lab. Invest.*, **66**, 928

23. Sauvezie, B., Miyasaka, N., Gharrem, D., Kielich, C. *et al.* (1982). An increase in peripheral blood Ia-positive T cells in Sjögren's syndrome correlates with a decrease in the autologous mixed lymphocyte response. *Clin. Exp. Immunol.*, **49**, 50–58

24. Greenspan, J.S., Daniels, T.E., Talol, N. and Sylveston, R.A. (1974). The histopathology of Sjögren's syndrome in labial salivary gland biopsies. *Oral Surg.*, **37**, 217–29

25. Tarpley, T.M., Anderson, L.G. and White, E.C. (1974). Minor salivary gland involvement in Sjögren's syndrome. *Oral Surg.*, **37**, 64–74

26. Faguet, G.B., Webb, H.H., Agree, J.F., Ricks, W.B. *et al.* (1978). Immunologically diagnosed malignancy in Sjögren's pseudolymphoma. *Am. J. Med.*, **65**, 424–9

27. Freemont, A.J. and Jones, C.J.P. (1983). Endothelial specialisation of salivary gland vessels for accelerated lymphocyte transfer in Sjögren's syndrome. *J. Rheumatol.*, **10**, 801–4

28. Lindahl, G., Hedfors, E., Klareskog, L. *et al.* (1985). Epithelial HLA-DR expression and T-lymphocyte subsets in salivary glands in Sjögren's syndrome. *Clin. Exp. Immunol.*, **61**, 475–82

29. Fox, R., Adamson, T., Fong, S. *et al.* (1983). Lymphocyte phenotype and functions in pseudolymphoma associated with Sjögren's syndrome. *J. Clin. Invest.*, **72**, 52–62

30. Zulman, J., Jaffe, R. and Talal, N. (1978). Evidence that the lymphoma of Sjögren's syndrome is a monoclonal B-cell neoplasm. *N. Engl. J. Med.*, **229**, 1215–20

31. Walters, M.T., Stevenson, F.K., Herbert, A. *et al.* (1986). Urinary monoclonal free light chains in primary Sjögren's syndrome: an aid to the diagnosis of maligant lymphoma. *Ann. Rheum. Dis.*, **45**, 210–19

32. Moutsopoulos, H.M., Costello, R., Drosos, A.A., Mavridis, A.K. and Papadopoulos, N.M. (1985). Demonstration and identification of monoclonal proteins in the urine of patients with Sjögren's syndrome. *Ann. Rheum. Dis.*, **44**, 109–12

33. Kassan, S., Thomas, T., Mocitsopalous, H. *et al.* (1978). Increased risk of lymphoma in sicca syndrome. *Ann. Intern. Med.*, **89**, 888–92

34. Sugai, S., Konda, S., Shirasaki, Y., Murayama, T. and Nishilaeva, T. (1980). Non-IgM monoclonal gammapathy in patients with Sjögren's syndrome. *Am. J. Med.*, **68**, 861–6

35. Pierce, D.A., Stern, R., Jaffe, R., Subman, J. and Talal, N. (1979). Immunoblastic sarcoma with features of Sjögren's syndrome and systemic lupus erythematosus in a patient with immunoblastic lymphadenopathy. *Arthr. Rheum.*, **22**, 911–16

36. Talal, N. and Bunim, J.J. (1964). The development òf malignant lymphoma in the course of Sjögren's syndrome. *Am. J. Med.*, **36**, 529–40

37. Jones, B.R. (1958). Lacrimal and salivary precipitating antibodies in Sjögren's syndrome. *Lancet*, **ii**, 773–6

38. Alspaugh, M.A. and Tan, E.M. (1975). Antibodies to cellular antigens in Sjögren's syndrome. *J. Clin. Invest.*, **55**, 1067–73

39. Mattioli, M. and Reichlin, M. (1974). Heterogeneity of RNA protein antigens reactive with sera of patients with SLE. *Arthr. Rheum.*, **17**, 421–9

40. Akizuki, M., Powers, R. and Holman, H.R. (1977). A soluble acidic protein of the cell nucleus which reacts with serum from patients with SLE and Sjögren's syndrome. *J. Clin. Invest.*, **59**, 264–72

41. Clark, G.M., Reichlin, M. and Tomasi, T.B. (1968). Characterisation of a soluble cytoplasmic antigen reactive with sera from patients with SLE. *J. Immunol.*, **102**, 117–22
42. Alspaugh, M.A. and Maddison, P.J. (1979). Resolution of the identity of certain antigen antibody systems in SLE and Sjögren's syndrome. An interlaboratory collaboration. *Arthr. Rheum.*, **22**, 796–8
43. Yagamata, H., Harley, J.B. and Reichlin, M. (1984). Molecular properties of the Ro/SSA antigen and enzyme linked immunosorbent assay for quantitation of antibody. *J. Clin. Invest.*, **74**, 625–33
44. Kurata, N. and Tan, E.M. (1976). Identification of antibodies to nuclear acidic antigens by counter immunoelectrophoresis. *Arthr. Rheum.*, **19**, 574–80
45. Harley, J.B., Alexander, E.L., Bias, W.B., Fox, O.F., Provost, T.T., Reichlin, M., Yamagata, H. and Arnett, F.C. (1986). Anti-Ro (SSA) and anti-La (SSB) in patients with Sjögren's syndrome. *Arthr. Rheum.*, **29**, 196–206
46. Maddison, P.J., Provost, T.T. and Reichlin, M. (1981). Serological findings in patients with 'ANA' negative SLE. *Medicine (Baltimore)*, **60**, 87–94
47. Hughes, G.R.V. (1984). Auto-antibodies in lupus and its variants: experience in 1000 patients. *Br. Med. J.*, **289**, 339–42
48. Scott, J.S., Maddison, P.J., Taylor, P.V., Esscher, E., Scott, O. and Skinner, R.P. (1983). Connective tissue disease, antibodies to ribo-nucleoprotein and congenital heart block. *N. Engl. J. Med.*, **309**, 209–12
49. Litsey, S.E., Noonan, J.A., O'Connor, W.N., Cottrill, C.M. and Mitchell, B. (1984). Maternal connective tissue disease and congenital heart block. Demonstration of immunoglobulin in cardiac tissue. *N. Engl. J. Med.*, **312**, 98–9
50. Reichlin, M. (1982). Clinical and immunological significance of antibodies to Ro and La in SLE. *Arthr. Rheum.*, **25**, 767–72
51. Venables, P.J., Yi, T., Woodrow, D.F., Moss, J. and Maini, R.N. (1983). Relationship of precipitating antibodies to soluble cellular antigens and histologically defined renal lesions in SLE. *Ann. Rheum. Dis.*, **42**, 17–22
52. Catoggio, L.J., Skinner, R.P., Smith, G. and Maddison, P.J. (1984). SLE in the elderly: clinical and serological characteristics. *J. Rheumatol.*, **11**, 175–81
53. Alspaugh, M., Buchanan, W.W. and Whaley, K. (1978). Precipitating antibodies to cellular antigens in Sjögren's syndrome, rheumatoid arthritis and other organ and non-organ specific auto-immune diseases. *Ann. Rheum. Dis.*, **37**, 244–46
54. Alexander, E.L., Arnett, F.C., Provost, T.T. and Stevens, M.B. (1983). Sjögren's syndrome: association of anti-Ro (SSA) antibodies with vasculitis; haematological abnormalities and serologic hyper-reactivity. *Ann. Intern. Med.*, **98**, 155–9
55. Moutsoponlus, H.M., Skoponli, F.N., Sarras, A.K., Tsamponlas, C., Mavridis, A.K., Constantoponlos, S.H. and Maddison, P.J. (1985). Anti-Ro (SSA) positive RA: a clinicosero-logical group of patients with high incidence of D-penicillamine side effects. *Ann. Rheum. Dis.*, **44**, 215–19
56. Venables, P.J., Charles, P., Buchanan, R.C., Yi, T., Mumford, P.A., Schreiber, L., Room, G.R. and Maini, R.N. (1983). Quantification and detection of isotypes of anti-SSB antibodies by ELISA and Farr assay using affinity purified antigens. *Arthr. Rheum.*, **26**, 146–55
57. Elkon, K.Z., Gharavi, A.E., Hughes, G.R.U. and Montsoupoulos, H.M. (1984). Auto-antibodies in the sicca syndrome (primary Sjögren's syndrome). *Ann. Rheum. Dis.*, **43**, 243–5
58. Editorial (1984). Antinuclear antibodies. *Lancet*, **ii**, 611–13
59. Isenberg, D.A., Hammond, L., Fisher, C., Griffiths, M., Stewart, J. and Bottazzo, G.F. (1982). Predictive value of SSB precipitating antibodies in Sjögren's syndrome. *Br. Med. J.*, **284**, 1738–40
60. Moutsopoulos, H.M., Mann, D.L., Johnson, A.H. and Chused, T.M. (1979). Genetic differences between primary and secondary sicca syndrome. *N. Engl. J. Med.*, **301**, 761–3
61. Fye, K.H., Teraksi, P.I., Michalski, J.P., Daniels, T.E., Opelz, G. and Talal, N. (1978). Relationship of HLA DRw3 and HLA B8 to Sjögren's syndrome. *Arthr. Rheum.*, **21**, 337–42
62. Whittingham, S., Mackay, I.R. and Tait, B.D. (1983). Auto-antibodies to small ribonucleo-proteins. A strong association between anti-SSB (LA), HLA B8, and Sjögren's syndrome. *Aust. NZ. J. Med.*, **13**, 565–70
63. Wilson, R.W., Provost, T.T., Bias, W.B., Alexander, E.L., Edlow, D.W., Hochberg, M.C., Stevens, M.B. and Arnett, F.C. (1984). Sjögren's syndrome; influence of multiple HLA-D region alloantigens on clinical and serological expression. *Arthr. Rheum.*, **27**, 1245–53

64. Mann, D.L. and Moutsopoulos, H.M. (1983). HLA-DR alloantigens in different subsets of patients with Sjögren's syndrome and in family members. *Ann. Rheum. Dis.*, **42**, 533–6
65. Reveille, J.D., Wilson, J.D., Provost, T.T., Bias, W.B. and Arnett, F.C. (1984). Primary Sjögren's syndrome and other auto-immune diseases in families. *Ann. Intern. Med.*, **101**, 748–56
66. Vitali, C., Tavoni, A., Rizzo, G., Neri, R., D'Ascanio, A., Cristofani, P. and Bombardier, S. (1986). HLA antigens in Italian patients with primary Sjögren's syndrome. *Ann. Rheum. Dis.*, **45**, 412–16
67. Bell, D.A. and Maddison, P.J. (1980). Serological subsets in SLE. *Arthr. Rheum.*, **23**, 1268–73

# 12
# Systemic lupus erythematosus

D. ALARCÓN-SEGOVIA

## INTRODUCTION

Systemic lupus erythematosus (SLE) is an autoimmune disease occurring preferentially in young women. There are complex interactions between genetic, environmental and hormonal factors that participate in its aetiopathogenesis. In turn, these result in an immune dysregulation in which T-cells, the products of mononuclear cells (lymphokines and monokines), and the resulting abnormal cell functions all participate to cause activation and premature differentiation of B-cells into autoantibody-producing cells. Autoantibodies can have deleterious effects that modulate the clinical expressions of the disease either by direct interaction with self antigens or by forming immune complexes that can deposit themselves in various locations. Lastly, autoantibodies may also appear that, by reacting with immunoregulatory cells, may influence their function and accentuate the immune dysregulation.

These levels of the pathophysiology of SLE are depicted in Table 12.1. They illustrate the interactions of most of the immunopathogenic mechanisms dealt with in previous chapters of this book.

**Table 12.1**  Pathophysiology of systemic lupus erythematosus

| Level 1: Aetiopathogenesis | | |
|---|---|---|
| Genetic | Environmental | Hormonal factors |
| Level 2: Pathogenesis | | |
| Cells | Functions | Mediators |
| Level 3: Disease mechanisms | | |
| Immune complex deposition | Direct antibody effect | Immunoregulatory antibodies |

## AETIOPATHOGENESIS

Genetic, environmental and hormonal factors all seem to participate in the development of the immune dysregulation causing SLE. Their role in its aetiopathogenesis has been likened to a troika, the carriage pulled by three horses[1].

### Genetic factors

The participation of genetic factors is suggested by the familial aggregation of SLE cases and by the occurrence of SLE in identical twins[2]. Discordance for SLE, however, does exist and familial aggregation could also occur through environmental factors[2]. Studies of autoantibodies in relatives from patients with SLE have shown a higher prevalence in consanguineous relatives from SLE patients than in normal unrelated subjects[3]. The presence of autoantibodies in non-consanguineous relatives sharing the same household with SLE is more frequent than in normal subjects, although it is less than that occurring in consanguineous ones[3,4]. This finding suggests that environmental factors are at play. More striking would be the finding of decreased suppressor cell function in relatives from patients with SLE[5].

The disease is particularly frequent in some ethnic groups even when sharing similar environments. In New York City, for instance, SLE was found to be more frequent in Blacks than in Puerto Ricans and in the latter more than Whites[6]. SLE seems to be particularly common in Mexico[1]. This observation appears to be at odds with findings related SLE to the haplotype HLA-A1, B8, Dr3 which is uncommon in Mexico. Studies of Mexican Mestizo families with multiple SLE members have suggested that another HLA haplotype, which is common in Mexico, relates to development of SLE in this ethnic group. This haplotype, the HLA-A9, B35, Dr4, has been found in Mexican Indians as part of an extended haplotype that includes the SC31 complotype and the GL02 allele of the erythrocyte enzyme glyoxalase[7]. As such, it is common in Mexico and may explain the high frequency of SLE in that country[7]. A relationship between SLE and Gm groups of immunoglobulins has also been proposed but more striking has been the relationship between SLE (seemingly not drug-induced, *vide infra*) and the slow acetylator phenotype[8,9]. This relationship could be pointing to an interaction of genetic and environmental factors where the genetically determined activity of hepatic acetyl transferase could modulate the effect of environmental agents that are catabolized by this mechanism[8].

Patients with SLE have also been found to have decreased erythrocytic receptors for C3b[10] as well as decreased clearance of immune complexes by the spleen[11]. Both abnormalities can be genetically determined but could conceivably be acquired. Sequential studies have suggested that this could be the case in SLE[11].

## Environmental factors

That environmental factors can also operate in the aetiopathogenesis of SLE is suggested by the aforementioned finding of autoantibodies in non-consanguineous relatives from SLE patients who share their household[3]. Also suggestive are the findings of antilymphocytic[12], anti-DNA[13] and anti-idiotypic for anti-DNA[14] antibodies in physicians and laboratory workers who handle blood samples from SLE patients.

A disease akin to SLE has been described as being elicited by various drugs. Some of these drugs are particularly prone to cause antinuclear antibodies (ANA) in a large proportion of patients who ingest them for long periods of time and a fully fledged clinical picture of SLE in a smaller proportion of individuals[15]. Table 12.2 lists the drugs with these properties that have been recognized. Other drugs are less regularly associated with the causation of ANA and/or SLE and their triggering mechanism may be an allergic reaction to the drug rather than resulting from a pharmacological property of the drug[15]. These drugs are listed in Table 12.3.

An important recent observation is that of the development of an SLE-like

**Table 12.2** Drug-related lupus syndrome: drugs commonly associated with causation of SLE and/or antinuclear antibodies

|  |
|---|
| Hydralazine |
| Procainamide |
| Isoniazid |
| D-penicillamine |
| Chlorpromazine |
| Anticonvulsants |
|    diphenylhydantoin |
|    mephenytoin |
|    trimethadione |
|    primidone |
|    ethosuximide |
|    carbamazepine |
| Methyldopa |
| ? Practolol |
| ? Cimetidine |

**Table 12.3** Drug-related lupus syndrome: other drugs that have occasionally been described to cause SLE

| | |
|---|---|
| Aminosalicylic acid | Oxyphenisatin |
| Chlorthalidone | Penicillin |
| Griseofulvin | Phenylbutazone |
| Guanoxan | Propylthiouracil |
| Hydrochlorothiazide | Quinidine |
| Isoquinazepon | Reserpine |
| Levodopa | Streptomycin |
| Lithium carbonate | Sulphonamides |
| Methysergide | Tetracycline |
| Methylthiouracil | Tolazamide |
| Nalidixic acid | |
| Oral contraceptives | |

illness in monkeys fed alfalfa sprouts or the non-protein amino acid L-canavanine that they contain[16]. Onset or exacerbation of SLE in humans consuming alfalfa tablets have both been described[17] and, in a recent investigation, it has been found that L-canavanine may cause an abrogation of suppressor cell function that results in the *in vitro* production of anti-DNA antibodies even by normal B-cells[18]. This nutritional triggering mechanism for immune dysregulation could be operative in more SLE patients than are currently recognized.

## Hormonal factors

SLE occurs in females in a proportion of 10 to 1. In addition, it might be more common in patients with Klinefelter's syndrome who are males with an XXY phenotype and primary testicular failure than in normal XY males[19].

Patients with SLE have been found to have abnormal oestrogen as well as androgen metabolism. Thus, both males and females with SLE have been found to have increased C-16 hydroxylation of oestrone with resulting increased levels of 16α-hydroxyoestrone and oestriol which are more oestrogenic metabolites[20]. In females, but not in males, with SLE there is a concomitant decrease in the C-2 hydroxylation that results in lower levels of 2-hydroxyoestrone and 2-methoxyoestrone with little or no peripheral oestrogenic activity. Therefore patients with SLE would tend to have higher oestrogenic activity than non-SLE subjects of the same sex. Females with SLE have also been found to have a distinct abnormality of androgen metabolism that causes increased oxidation at C-17. Testosterone metabolites oxidized at C-17 are both less potent androgens and liable to become oestrogens[21]. This abnormality was not found in males. It would seem, therefore, that although some abnormalities occur in both male and female SLE patients, females with SLE have more pronounced changes that may lead to increased oestrogen/androgen activity ratios.

These observations could be meaningful from the standpoint of immunoregulation. Thus, oestrogens may have stimulatory effects on the immune system whereas testosterone tends to have an inhibitory effect[22–24]. In accordance with this, oestrogen administration may cause exacerbation of SLE in female patients[25]. Patients with Klinefelter's syndrome and SLE have been found to have both an increase in C-16 hydroxylated active oestriol and a decrease in 2-hydroxyoestrone thus resembling the oestrogen metabolism of female SLE patients more than that of male SLE patients.

The course of SLE can be modified by pregnancy[26]. Onset of the disease may occur during pregnancy or, more frequently, in the postpartum. Immunoregulation can be influenced by pregnancy or by hormones related to it such as chorionic gonadotrophin or prolactin[27,28]. Hyperprolactinaemia may be more frequent in SLE than in non-SLE females.

## PATHOGENESIS (IMMUNE DYSREGULATION)

Immune dysregulation can occur by a decrease or increase in the absolute number of cells that exert a function, by a dysfunction proper of cells without numerical change or by increase or decrease in the production of, or the response to, soluble factors that mediate their functions or serve as links of communication between cells.

The immunoregulatory T-cell pathways serve in man, as they do in the mouse, as a mechanism for obtaining an adequate, both quantitatively as well as qualitatively, production of antibodies. A dysregulation causing increased stimulation of B-cells could result in increased amounts of antibodies (hypergammaglobulinaemia) as well as production of autoantibodies[29]. It is normal for there to be a potential for the production of autoantibodies but this is suppressed by the normal net balance of immune regulation.

## Cells

Patients with SLE characteristically have decreased total lymphocytes in their peripheral blood when their disease is active[30]. T-cells with receptors for the Fc portion of immunoglobulin G are also decreased in SLE as are T-cells that form autologous rosettes (Tar cells)[31,32]. T-cells identified by monoclonal antibodies T4 or T8 have been found to be diminished in the peripheral blood of patients with active SLE when considered as a group[33,34]. Individual patients may have diminution of T4 (helper/inducer) cells, of T8 (cytotoxic/suppressor) cells or of both[35].

Cells that can cause killing of tumoral or virus modified cells without prior stimulation are also numerically diminished in SLE which is, in part, responsible for a decrease in natural killer (NK) cells function[36].

B-cells do not seem to be diminished in patients with SLE but there are several indications of their being in an activated state in the peripheral blood of SLE patients. This does not happen in normal subjects[37,38].

## Functions

T-cells from patients with SLE have been found to respond poorly to activation with mitogens such as concanavalin A or phytohaemagglutinin. This early finding, that correlated well with the presence of cutaneous anergy in patients with SLE gave insight into the presence of an immune dysregulation of T-cells in this disease.

The function of suppression by T lymphocytes of other T lymphocytes or B lymphocytes has been found to be diminished in SLE[39-44]. The non-specific suppression of T-cells on B-cells could be activated by concanavalin A or appear spontaneously in culture after several days[44]. Each seems to be a distinct function[45], and they are diminished, albeit heterogeneously, in SLE[44].

Tar cells have many of the characteristics of post-thymic precursor T-cells that have been described in the mouse as peculiar to the Lyt 1,2,3 cell[46,47]. By co-culturing Tar cells with T-cells with receptors for the Fc portion of IgM (Tμ cells) which are mainly helper cells, as well as B-cells, all in the presence of pokeweed mitogen, it has been determined that these cells cause feedback inhibition[47], a function also ascribed in the mouse to the Lyt 1,2,3 cell. This function is also decreased in SLE[32].

Helper cell function has not yet been adequately studied in SLE. In an ongoing study with allogenic combinations of T- and B-cells we have found some patients who seem to have a predominance of excess helper function (F. Guadarrama, L. Llorente and D. Alarcón-Segovia, unpublished observations).

The role of each function in the resulting net regulation is difficult to assess. Contrasuppression, a function exerted by a subpopulation of T8 cells that abrogates the suppressive action of T-cells on helper cells seems to be increased in SLE (A. Palacios, J. Alcocer-Varela and D. Alarcón-Segovia, unpublished observations).

Normal human T lymphocytes proliferate when co-cultured *in vitro* with inactivated autologous non-T mononuclear cells[48]. This phenomenon is known as the autologous mixed lymphocyte reaction (AMLR) and has been found to have both immunological memory and specificity[49]. The maximum reaction which occurs on the seventh day of co-culture has been found to be depressed in SLE patients. When the day to day kinetics of the response have been studied, it has been observed that in some SLE patients the low seventh day response may be preceded by a peak response on day 5[50].

NK cell function is found to be diminished in SLE when studied in assay of $^{51}$Cr release by K562 target cells. It also responds poorly to interleukin-2[36]. At the single cell level this seems to be due to an intrinsic defect in the lytic capacity of NK cells[36]. Patients with SLE have been found to have decreased response to IL-2[51] a function primarily, but not exclusively, performed by T8 cells. Also diminished in SLE is the response to the monocyte product IL-1[52].

## Mediators

Mononuclear cells produce, particularly on activation, diverse non-immuno-globulin factors that act on other leukocytes and have therefore been termed interleukins or growth or differentiation factors. Thus, communication within the immune system, as well as between the immune and other systems may take place through these mediators as well as by direct cell–cell interaction. The monocyte factor interleukin-1, acts primarily on the T4 cell, particularly that which forms autologous rosettes[53]. This monokine, however has multiple effects on diverse targets including fibroblasts and endothelial cells suggesting it to be a pluripotential mediator. The production of IL-1 by monocytes from patients with SLE has been found defective[52]. This might indicate, by involving a cell different from T- and B-cell, that the immunological aberration of SLE is either multicentric or originates in a stem cell precursor of all three mononuclear cells[52].

Interleukin-2 is produced by T lymphocytes, particularly those that form autologous rosettes[53], which are the same cells that respond best to IL-1. The cells that respond best to IL-2, are the T8 cells that do not form autologous rosettes[53].

T-cells from patients with SLE produce IL-2 less efficiently than those of normal subjects[51,54]. This defect is more pronounced in cells from patients with active disease than in those of patients with inactive disease. In turn, there are observations indicating that an OKT8 cell whose population seems to be expanded in SLE has the potential to suppress the production of IL-2 in SLE patients. Its removal causes increased production of IL-2 by SLE cells and its re-addition causes it to fall[55]. Whether this cell could be the contrasuppressor cell which seems also to be increased in SLE has not been determined.

Interleukin-3 is another T-cell-derived lymphokine that acts preferentially on B-cell precursors[56]. T-cells from autoimmune MRL/Mp/lpr mice produce IL-3 spontaneously[57]. In an ongoing study we have found that T-cells from SLE patients produce spontaneously an IL-3-like activity detectable in murine bone-marrow cells as well as in an IL-3-dependent cell clone[58]. Production of this activity upon phytohaemagglutinin (PHA) stimulation is similar to that of normal subjects whereas its release in AMLR is decreased, particularly in patients with active disease. All of this suggests an *in vivo* preactivation of T-cells that produce this IL-3-like activity in patients with active SLE.

Another lymphokine, preliminarily termed B-cell growth factor, is also produced more readily by T-cells from patients with active disease than by those in remission[59]. Production by T-cells of a factor capable of inducing differentiation of B-cells to immunoglobulin-secreting cells (B-cell differentiation factor) is also increased in SLE patients, particularly those with active disease[59].

The immunoregulatory abnormalities found in SLE in the number of cells, the function of cells (independent of their number since these are corrected in the respective assays), and in the production of interleukins and similar mediators all tend to favour an increased activation and differentiation of B-cells. Indeed, it is peculiar that those functions that either suppress or favour abrogation of this activation are all decreased, whereas those that either counteract this suppression or induce B-cell activation or differentiation are augmented. As a result, there is excess production of autoantibodies which themselves have pathogenetic implications and seem to actually be more directly implicated in disease manifestations. This takes us to the third level, that leading more directly to disease expression on the one hand but also, to the capabilities, on the other, of accentuating, or perhaps even initiating, disease manifestations.

## MECHANISM OF THE DISEASE

Autoantibodies that are formed as a result of a positive net regulation that leads to increased activation and differentiation of B-cells may be deleterious and cause disease by several mechanisms:

(1)  They can participate in the formation of immune complexes leading to this particular form of immune-mediated damage;

(2)  They can have a direct effect by interacting with self antigens and causing cytotoxicity, often with the mediation of, or amplification by, complement;

(3)  They may interact, in various ways, with cells of the immune system and accentuate or modulate their dysregulation.

Autoantibodies found in SLE range from antibodies reactive with nuclear components including nucleic acids, histones, non-histone acidic proteins and centromere proteins, to antigens from other organelles[60]. There are also autoantibodies that react with the surface of such cells as lymphocytes, other leukocytes, erythrocytes, platelets, neurons, or with antigenic molecules present in various cell populations such as Ia antigens. Other autoantibodies react with immunoglobulins, whether at their constant regions (rheumatoid factors) or at their variable regions (anti-idiotypic antibodies).

## Immune complex deposition

The role of immune complex deposition in disease pathogenesis has been unravelled since the classical experiments on the induction of serum sickness. Circulating immune complexes are present in SLE and have some correlation with disease activity[61,62]. Through elution, immunofluorescence and electron microscopic studies they have been found to be deposited in glomeruli, small vessels, and choroid plexi[63]. The main components of the immune complexes found in SLE are antinuclear antibodies, particularly anti-double-stranded DNA, and their respective antigens[62]. Complement components, capable of inducing damage, have also been found[63]. Immune complexes may also saturate Fc receptors in the spleen and other reticuloendothelial cell-bearing organs causing their dysfunction; this may also have a genetic basis as explained in the above discussion of aetiopathogenesis[11].

Clinical manifestations resulting from immune complex deposition include glomerulonephritis, small and perhaps medium-sized vessel vasculitis and some of the neuropsychiatric manifestations[63]. They could also have a role in the causation of the salivary gland damage which is so frequent, both clinically and subclinically, in SLE[64] or play a role in pulmonary manifestations such as the dreadful pulmonary haemorrhage[65]. The varied manifestations they may cause depend on their immunochemical characteristics, their ability to fix complement, their association with rheumatoid factors, their modulation by anti-idiotypic antibodies, and the presence of receptors for the Fc portion of the immunoglobulins or for complement (C3b)[63].

## Direct antibody effect

Autoantibodies in SLE may react with antigens that either adhere to the cell membrane or are part of it. There, complement components that bind to the hinge region of the antibody, including the membrane attack complex, may cause inflammation, cell lysis or both. Binding of DNA to the basal membrane of glomeruli may cause damage that has been postulated to be as important as, if not more important than circulating immune complexes trapped there[62].

Antibodies to neurons, which often share cross-reactivity with antilymphocytic antibodies, may be responsible for some of the neuropsychiatric manifestations of SLE. The best example, however, of the direct antibody effect is that causing red cell, platelet or leukocytic cytolysis. Haemolytic anaemia, thrombocytopenic purpura, and leukopenia may all result from this

205

type of effect. Lymphopenia, which is almost uniformly present in SLE, may be a primary phenomenon manifesting the immune dysregulation or be a secondary event leading to it.

## Immunoregulatory autoantibodies

Antibodies may influence immune regulation in various ways. There are antilymphocytic antibodies that may react with various lymphocyte subpopulations including antibodies to Ia$^+$ cells[66]. Presence of antibodies to T4$^+$ or T8$^+$ seem to correlate inversely with the number of the respective T-cells in the peripheral blood of patients with SLE[67]. Antibodies that do not fix complement may, by adhering to lymphocytes, cause them to be lysed by killer cells by the damage mechanism known as antibody-mediated cellular cytotoxicity[68]. Anti-lymphocytic antibodies may also penetrate into lymphocytes where they cause them damage[69].

The penetration of antinuclear antibodies into cells bearing Fc receptors and mediated by them is an interesting phenomenon that may contribute to immune dysregulation[70]. It has been found to permit the entrance of anti-RNA or anti-DNA antibodies all the way to the nucleus where the antigen resides. It occurs probably by means of receptor-mediated endocytosis through clathrin-coated vesicles[71]. The transport of antibodies across cells via this mechanism and involving Fc receptors has been described, and the presence of coated vesicles has been determined in lymphocytes[72,73]. Penetration of antinuclear antibodies into cells has been found to cause protracted cell death as well as abrogation of suppressor cell function[74]. Circulating T-cells from SLE patients have been found to have a peculiar cytofluorographic pattern when stained with Acridine Orange[38]. This pattern, showing activation with increased RNA content but no concomitant increase in DNA content can be reproduced in normal activated T-cells with receptors for the Fc portion of IgG incubated in anti-DNA antibodies[38].

This novel mechanism of immune-mediated damage may contribute to immune dysregulation. Because T cells bearing Fc receptors for IgG are mainly suppressor lymphocytes, their loss through antibody penetration mainly causes abrogation of suppressor cell function[74]. Immune regulation may also be influenced by the presence of rheumatoid factor which occurs in a quarter of SLE patients.

Anti-idiotypic antibodies to DNA may contribute to modulation of the disease by various mechanisms. These could include interaction with anti-DNA antibodies preventing their formation of immune complexes with DNA, or interacting with it at the skin's membrane or in the glomerulus or preventing their penetration into cells.

## CONCLUSIONS

Systemic lupus erythematosus is indeed a complex disease; genetic, environmental and hormonal factors all contribute, like the horses of a troika, to the development of immune dysregulation. In SLE, cells, functions and their mediators participate, again as a troika, in causing activation of B-cells with production of autoantibodies. These, in turn, can cause damage (another troika) either through formation of immune complexes, directly by causing cell cytolysis, or by interacting with cells of the immune system to accentuate the dysregulation. The overlapping of all three of these levels of pathophysiology is quite marked in SLE but for analytical purposes they should be separately considered – each level embracing its troika of factors or mechanisms all of which are pulling towards disease.

## Acknowledgements

Work from our laboratory that is mentioned in this chapter was supported by grants from the Consejo Nacional de Ciencia y Technologia, the Fondo para Estudios e Investigaciones Ricardo J. Zevada, the Fundación Mary Street Jenkins and the Programa Universitario para Investigación Clinica from the Universidad Nacional Autónoma, all from Mexico.

## References

1. Alarcón-Segovia, D. (1984). The pathogenesis of immune dysregulation in systemic lupus erythematosus. A troika. *J. Rheumatol.*, **11**, 588–90
2. Kaplan, D. (1984). The onset of disease in twins and siblings with systemic lupus erythematosus. *J. Rheumatol.*, **11**, 648–52
3. De Horatius, R.J., Pillarisetty, R., Messner, R.P. and Talal, N. (1975). Antinucleic acid antibodies in systemic lupus erythematosus patients and their families. Incidence and correlation with lymphocytotoxic antibodies. *J. Clin. Invest.*, **56**, 1149–54
4. De Horatius, R.J., Alarcón-Segovia, D., Messner, R.P. and Fishbein, E. (1981). Lymphocytotoxic antibodies in Mexican patients with systemic lupus erythematosus and their families. Relationship of disease activity in the probands to antibody cytotoxicity in their relatives. *Rev. Invest. Clin. (Mex.)*, **33**, 161–64
5. Miller, K.B. and Schwartz, R.S. (1979). Familial abnormalities of suppressor cell function in systemic lupus erythematosus. *N. Engl. J. Med.*, **301**, 803–9
6. Siegel, M., Lee, S.L. and Peress, N.S. (1967). The epidemiology of drug-induced systemic lupus erythematosus. *Arthr. Rheum.*, **10**, 407–15
7. Granados, J., Frajman, M., Terán, L. and Alarcón-Segovia, D. (1983). Haplotipos implicados en la predisposición genética al lupus eritematoso generalizado (LEG) en familias Mexicanas. In *XI Congreso Mexicano de Reumatologia*. p. 11. (Mérida, Yucatán, México: Sociedad Mexicana de Reumatología)
8. Reidenberg, M.M., Levy, M., Drayer, D.E., Zylber-Katz, E. and Robbins, W.C. (1980). Acetylator phenotype in idiopathic systemic lupus erythematosus. *Arthr. Rheum.*, **23**, 569–73
9. Fishbein, E. and Alarcón-Segovia, D. (1979). Slow acetylation phenotype in systemic lupus erythematosus. *Arthr. Rheum.*, **22**, 95–6
10. Nojima, Y., Terai, C., Minota, S., Takana K., Myakawa, Y. and Tokaku, F. (1985). Low capacity of erythrocytes to bind immune complexes via C3b receptor in patients with systemic lupus erythematosus: correlation with pathological proteinuria. *Clin. Immunol. Immunopathol.*, **34**, 109–117
11. Frank, M.M., Hamburger, M.I., Lawley, T.J., Kimberly, R.P. and Plotz, P.H. (1979). Defective reticuloendothelial system Fc-receptor function in systemic lupus erythematosus. *N. Engl. J. Med.*, **300**, 518–23
12. De Horatius, R.J., Rubin, R., Messner, R.P. and Carr, R.I. (1979). Lymphocytotoxic antibodies in laboratory personnel exposed to SLE sera. *Lancet*, **ii**, 1141–42

13. Tan, E.M. (1982). Autoantibodies to nuclear antigens (AN): their immunobiology and medicine. *Adv. Immunol.*, **33**, 167–240
14. Abdou, N.I., Wall, H., Lindsley, H.B., Halsey, J.F. and Susuki, T. (1981). Network theory of autoimmunity. *In vitro* suppression of serum anti-DNA antibody binding to DNA by anti-idiotypic antibody in systemic lupus erythematosus. *J. Clin. Invest.*, **67**, 1297–1304
15. Alarcón-Segovia, D. and Kraus, A. (1984). Drug-related lupus syndromes. In Lemberger, L. and Reidenberg, M.M. (eds.) *Proceeding of the Second World Conference on Clinical Pharmacology and Therapeutics.* pp. 187–206
16. Malinow, M.R., Bardana, E.J., Pirofsky, B. and Craig, S. (1982). Systemic lupus erythematosus-like syndrome in monkeys fed alfalfa sprouts: role of a nonprotein aminoacid. *Science*, **216**, 415–17
17. Roberts, J.L. and Hayashi, J.A. (1983). Exacerbation of SLE associated with alfalfa ingestion (Letter). *N. Engl. J. Med.*, **308**, 1361
18. Alcocer-Varela, J., Iglesias, A., Llorente, L. and Alarcón-Segovia, D. (1985). Effects of L-canavanine on T cells may explain the induction of systemic lupus erythematosus by alfalfa. *Arthr. Rheum.*, **28**, 52–57
19. Alarcón-Segovia, D. and Sauza, J. (1984). Systemic lupus erythematosus and Klinefelter's syndrome. In Bandmann, H-J. and Breit, R. (eds.) *Klinefelter's Syndrome.* (Berlin: Springer Verlag)
20. Lahita, R.G., Bradlow, H.L., Kunkel, H.G. and Fishman, J. (1981). Increased 16α-hydroxylation of oestradiol in systemic lupus erythematosus. *J. Clin. Endocrinol. Metab.*, **53**, 174–8
21. Lahita, R.G., Bradlow, H.L. and Kunkel, H.G. (1983). Testosterone oxidation in systemic lupus erythematosus. *Arthr. Rheum.*, **26**, (Suppl.), 570 (Abstract)
22. Talal, N. (1981). Sex steroid hormones and systemic lupus erythematosus. *Arthr. Rheum.*, **24**, 1054–56
23. Raveche, E.S., Tijio, J.H., Boegel, W. and Steinber, A.D. (1979). Studies on the effects of sex hormones on autosomal and X-linked genetic control of induced and spontaneous antibody production. *Arthr. Rheum.*, **22**, 1177–87
24. Chávez de la Lama, O., Llorente, L. and Alarcón-Segovia, D. (1983). Efecto de las hormonas androgénicas sobre las funciones linfocitarias. In *Congreso Mexicano de Reumatología.* p. 16. (Mérida, Yucatán, México: Sociedad Mexicana de Reumatología)
25. Jungers, P., Dougados, M., Pelissier, C., Kuttenn, F., Tron, F., Lasavre, P. and Bach, J.F. (1981). Influence of oral contraceptive therapy on the activity of systemic lupus erythematosus. *Arthr. Rheum.*, **25**, 618–23
26. Gutiérrez, G., Jiménez, J. and Mintz, G. (1981). Results of a prospective multidisciplinary approach to pregnancy in systemic lupus erythematosus (SLE). *Arthr. Rheum.*, **24** (Suppl.) S107
27. Frajman, M., Díaz-Jouanen, E., Alcocer-Varela, J., Fishbein, E., Guevara, M. and Alarcón-Segovia, D. (1983). Effect of pregnancy on functions of circulating T cells from patients with systemic lupus erythematosus: correction of T cell suppression and autologous mixed lymphocyte responses. *Clin. Immunol. Immunopathol.*, **29**, 94–102
28. Vidaller, A., Llorente, L., Larrea, F., Méndez J.P., Alcocer-Varela, J. and Alarcón-Segovia, D. (1986). T-cell dysregulation in patients with hyperprolactinemia. Effect of bromocriptine treatment. *Clin. Immunol. Immunopathol.*, **38**, 337–43
29. Alarcón-Segovia, D., Alcocer-Varela, J. and Díaz-Jouanen, E. (1985). The connective tissue diseases as disorders of immune regulation. *Clin. Rheum. Dis.*, **11**, 451–69
30. Rivero, S.J., Díaz-Jouanen, E. and Alarcón-Segovia, D. (1978). Lymphopenia in systemic lupus erythematosus. Clinical, diagnostic and prognostic significance. *Arthr. Rheum.*, **21**, 295–302
31. Alarcón-Segovia, D. and Ruiz-Argüelles, A. (1978). Decreased circulating thymus-derived cell with receptors for the Fc portion of immunoglobulin G in systemic lupus erythematosus. *J. Clin. Invest.*, **62**, 1390–94
32. Palacios, R., Alarcón-Segovia, D., Llorente, L., Ruíz-Argüelles, A. and Díaz-Jouanen, E. (1981). Human post-thymic precursor cells in health and disease. II their loss and dysfunction in systemic lupus erythematosus and their partial correction with serum thymic factor. *J. Clin. Lab. Immunol.*, **5**, 71–80
33. Bekke, A.C., Kirkland, P.A., Kitridou, R.C. *et al.* (1983). T lymphocyte subsets in systemic lupus erythematosus. *Arthr. Rheum.*, **26**, 745–50

34. Morimoto, C., Reinherz, E.L., Schlossman, S.F. *et al.* (1982). Alterations in immunoregulatory T cell subsets in active systemic lupus erythematosus. *J. Clin. Invest.*, **66**, 1171–74
35. Melendro, E.I., Saldate, C., Rivero, S.J. and Alarcón-Segovia, D. (1983). T-cell subpopulations in the peripheral blood of patients with connective tissue diseases as determined by flow cytometry using monoclonal antibodies. *Clin. Immunol. Immunopathol.*, **27**, 340–47
36. Gónzalez-Amaro, R., Alcocer-Varela, J. and Alarcón-Segovia, D. (1985). Caracterización de la función citotóxica natural (NK) en enfermedades del tejido conjunctivo. In *Abstracts XIII Congreso Mexicano de Reumatología*. p. 40. (Guanajuato, México: Sociedad Mexicana de Reumatología)
37. Ginsburg, W.W., Finkelman, F.D. and Lipsky P.E. (1979). Circulating and pokeweed mitogen-induced immunoglobulin-secreting cell in systemic lupus erythematosus. *Clin. Exp. Immunol.*, **35**, 76–88
38. Alarcón-Segovia, D., Llorente, L., Fishbein, E. and Díaz-Jouanen, E. (1982). Abnormalities in the content of nucleic acids of peripheral blood mononuclear cells from patients with systemic lupus erythematosus. Relationship to DNA antibodies. *Arthr. Rheum.*, **23**, 304–17
39. Abdou, N.I., Sagawa, A., Pascual, E., Herbert, J. and Sadeghee, S. (1976). Suppressor T cell abnormality in idiopathic systemic lupus erythematosus. *Clin. Immunol. Immunopathol.*, **6**, 192–99
40. Bresnihan, B. and Jasin, H.G. (1977). Suppressor function of peripheral blood mononuclear cells in normal individuals and patients with systemic lupus erythematosus. *J. Clin. Invest.*, **59**, 106–16
41. Horowitz, S., Borcherding, W., Moorthy, A.V. *et al.* (1977). Induction of suppressor T cells in systemic lupus erythematosus by thymosin and cultured thymic epithelium. *Science*, **197**, 999–1001
42. Sakane T., Steinberg, A.D. and Green, I. (1978). Studies of immune functions of patients with systemic lupus erythematosus. I. Dysfunction of suppressor T-cell activity related to impaired generation of, rather than response to suppressor cells. *Arthr. Rheum.*, **21**, 657–64
43. Kaufman, D. B. and Bostwick, E. (1979). Defective suppressor T-cell activity in systemic lupus erythematosus. *Clin. Immunol. Immunopathol.*, **13**, 9–18
44. Ruíz-Argüelles, A., Alarcón-Segovia, D., Llorente, L. and Del Giudice-Knipping, J.A. (1980). Heterogeneity of the spontaneously expanded and mitogen-induced generation of suppressor cell function of T cells on B cells in systemic lupus erythematosus. *Arthr. Rheum.*, **23**, 1004–9
45. Galanaud, P., Grevor, M.C., Delfraissy, J.F. *et al.* (1979). Regulation of the primary *in vitro* antibody response in human peripheral blood lymphocytes: different effects of mitogen-induced and spontaneous suppressor cells. *Clin. Exp. Immunol.*, **38**, 106–16
46. Palacios, R., Alarcón-Segovia, D., Llorente, L., Ruíz-Argüelles, A. and Díaz-Jouanen, E. (1981). Human post-thymic precursor cells in health and disease. I. Characterization of the autologous rosette-forming T cell as post-thymic precursors. *Immunology*, **42**, 127–35
47. Heijnen, C.J., Pot, K.H., Kafer, L. *et al.* (1982). Functional analysis of the defective T cell regulation of the antigen specific PFC response in SLE patients: differentiation of suppressor effector cells. *Clin. Exp. Immunol.*, **47**, 359–67
48. Opetz, G., Kuchi, M., Takasugi, M. and Terasaki, P.I. (1975). Autologous stimulation of human lymphocyte subpopulation. *J. Exp. Med.*, **142**, 1327–33
49. Weksler, M.E. and Kosak, R. (1977). Lymphocyte transformation induced by autologous cells. V. Generation of immunologic memory and specificity during the autologous mixed lymphocyte reaction. *J. Exp. Med.*, **146**, 1833–38
50. Laffón, A., Alcocer-Varela, J. and Alarcón-Segovia, D. (1983). Differences in the kinetics of the autologous mixed lymphocyte reaction between the various connective tissue diseases. *Rheumatol. Int.*, **3**, 117–28
51. Alcocer-Varela, J. and Alarcón-Segovia, D. (1982). Decreased production of and response to interleukin-2 by cultured lymphocytes from patients with systemic lupus erythematosus. *J. Clin. Invest.*, **69**, 1388–92
52. Alcocer-Varela, J., Laffón, A. and Alarcón-Segovia, D. (1984). Defective monocyte production of, and T lymphocyte response to, interleukin-1 in the peripheral blood of patients with systemic lupus erythematosus. *Clin. Exp. Immunol.*, **55**, 125–32
53. Fishbein, E., Alcocer-Varela, J. and Alarcón-Segovia, D. (1983). Cellular bases of the production of and response to interleukin-2 in man: role of autologous rosette-forming T-cell subsets defined with monoclonal antibodies. *Immunology*, **50**, 233–7

54. Linker-Israeli, M., Bakke, A.C., Kitridou, R.C. *et al.* (1983). Defective production of interleukin-1 and interleukin-2 in patients with systemic lupus erythematosus (SLE). *J. Immunol.*, **130**, 2651−55
55. Linker-Israeli, M., Bakke, A.C., Quismorio, F.P. and Horwitz, D.A. (1985). Correction of interleukin-2 production in patients with systemic lupus erythematosus by removal of spontaneously activated suppressor cell. *J. Clin. Invest.*, **75**, 762−68
56. Palacios, R., Henso, G., Steinmetz, M. and McKearn, J.P. (1984). Interleukin-3 supports growth of mouse pre-B-cell clones *in vitro*. *Nature*, **309**, 126−31
57. Palacios, R. (1984). Spontaneous production of interleukin-3 by T lymphocytes from autoimmune MRL-MP-1pr/pr mice. *Eur. J. Immunol.*, **14**, 599−605
58. Palacios, M.E., Alcocer-Varela, J. and Alarcón-Segovia, D. (1987). Spontaneous production of interleukin-3-like activity by T lymphocytes from patients with systemic lupus erythematosus. (Submitted for publication)
59. Martínez-Cordero, E., Alcocer-Varela, J. and Alarcón-Segovia, D. (1986). Stimulating and differentiation factors for human B lymphocytes in systemic lupus erythematosus. *Clin. Exp. Immunol.*, **65**, 598−604
60. Alarcón-Segovia, D. (1983). Antibodies to nuclear and other intracellular antigens in the connective tissue diseases. *Clin. Rheum. Dis.*, **9**, 161−75
61. Abrass, C.K., Nies, K.M., Lovie, J.S., Border, W.A. and Glassock, R.J. (1980). Correlation and predictive accuracy of circulating immune complexes with disease activity in systemic lupus erythematosus. *Arthr. Rheum.*, **23**, 273−82
62. Izui, S., Lambert, P.H. and Mischer (1976). *In vitro* demonstration of a particular affinity for glomerular basement membrane and collagen for DNA. *J. Exp. Med.*, **144**, 428−43
63. Inman, R.D. (1982). Immune complexes in SLE. *Clin. Rheum. Dis.*, **8**, 49−62
64. Alarcón-Segovia, D., Ibáñez de Kasep, G., Velázquez-Forero, F., Hernández-Ortíz, J. and González-Jiménez, Y. (1974). Sjögren's syndrome in systemic lupus erythematosus. Clinical and subclinical manifestations. *Ann. Intern. Med.*, **81**, 577−83
65. Abud-Mendoza, C., Díaz-Jouanen, E. and Alarcón-Segovia, D. (1985). Fatal pulmonary haemorrhage in systemic lupus erythematosus. Occurrence without hemoptysis. *J. Rheumatol.*, **12**, 558−66
66. Okudaira, K., Searles, R.P., Ceuppens, J.L., Goodwin, J.S. and Williams, R.C. Jr. (1982). Anti-Ia reactivity in sera from patients with systemic lupus erythematosus. *J. Clin. Invest.*, **69**, 17−24
67. Morimoto, C., Reinherz, E.L., Distaso, J.A., Steinberg, A.D. and Schlossman, S.F. (1984). Relationship between systemic lupus erythematosus T cell subsets, anti-T-cell antibodies, and T cell functions. *J. Clin. Invest.*, **73**, 689−700
68. Kumagai, S., Steinberg, A.D. and Green, I. (1981). Antibodies to T cells in patients with systemic lupus erythematosus can induce antibody-dependent cell-mediated cytotoxicity against human T cells. *J. Clin. Invest.*, **67**, 605−614
69. Okudaira, K., Searles, R.P., Tanimoto, K., Horuchi, Y. and Williams, R.C. (1982). T lymphocyte interaction with immunoglobulin G antibody in systemic lupus erythematosus. *J. Clin. Invest.*, **69**, 1026−38
70. Alarcón-Segovia, D. and Ruíz-Argüelles, A. (1980). Antibody penetration into living cells: mechanisms and consequences. In Larralde, C., Willms, K., Ortíz-Ortíz, L. and Sela, M. (eds.) *Molecules, Cells and Parasites in Immunology.* pp. 53−64. (New York: Academic Press)
71. Goldstein, J.L., Anderson, R.G.W. and Brown, M.S. (1979). Coated pits, coated vesicles and receptor-mediated endocytosis. *Nature*, **279**, 679−85
72. Rodewald, R. (1980). Immunoglobulin transmission in mammalian young and the involvement of coated vesicles. In Ockleford, C.D. and Whyte, A. (eds.) *Coated Vesicles.* p. 69−98. (Cambridge: Cambridge University Press)
73. Nevorotin, A.J. (1980). Coated vesicles in different cell types: some functional implications. In Ockleford, C.D. and Whyte, A. (eds.) *Coated Vesicles.* p. 25−53. (Cambridge: Cambridge University Press)
74. Alarcón-Segovia, D., Ruíz-Argüelles, A. and Llorente, L. (1979). Antibody penetration into living cells II. Anti-ribonucleoprotein IgG penetrates into T cells causing their deletion and the abrogation of suppressor function. *J. Immunol.*, **122**, 1855−62

# 13
# Immunopathogenetic mechanisms of arthritis and modes of action of anti-rheumatic therapies

A. C. ALLISON

## INTRODUCTION

The aetiology of rheumatoid arthritis (RA) remains unknown. There is no evidence for bacterial involvement, which is the case in rheumatic fever, Lyme arthritis and Reiter's disease. Although acute viral infections such as rubella can produce arthritis, there is no evidence that rubella or any other virus is specifically associated with RA. While responses of lymphocytes from RA patients to Epstein-Barr virus have provided interesting information[1], no causal relationship has been established. The pattern of disease, and responses to immunosuppressive drugs, leave little doubt that immune reactions to an exogenous agent or agents, or to host components, are involved. In other words, the pathogenesis of RA is an immunologically driven, chronic inflammatory reaction. There are certainly autoimmune manifestations in RA, notably production of antiglobulins or rheumatoid factors; but the aetiology of autoimmunity is itself obscure and likely to be due to complex interactions of host genetic and environmental factors[2,3]. Whether rheumatoid factors play a causal role in RA is an unresolved question, which will be discussed below.

Despite our lack of understanding of the aetiology of RA, a great deal of information has accumulated about the immunopathogenesis of the disease, including interactions of lymphocytes, macrophages and various cell types derived from connective tissue, as well as the production of several mediators. Nevertheless many points remain uncertain, for example the relative importance of immunopathological reactions involving primarily T lymphocytes as opposed to those dependent on B lymphocytes, and the relative importance of lipid-derived mediators such as prostaglandins and leukotrienes on the one hand and peptide mediators, such as activated complement components, on the other. In recent years the potential role of interleukin-1s (IL-1s) in the pathogenesis of RA has emerged, so that endogenous mediators and drugs regulating the formation of IL-1 become relevant to understanding the disease process and how it can be controlled.

Effects of therapies, including different classes of drugs (immunosuppressives, glucocorticoids, inhibitors of prostaglandin synthesis and long-acting, disease-remitting drugs), as well as procedures that more or less selectively alter the migration pattern of or deplete lymphocytes (thoracic duct drainage and total lymphoid irradiation), represent useful methods for analysing the pathogenesis of RA. Indeed pathogenesis and therapy are so intimately related that they cannot adequately be discussed apart. In this chapter novel information will be provided about the mode of action of glucocorticoids, long-acting anti-rheumatic drugs and effects of total lymphoid irradiation (TLI). This information will be used as a guide through the complex pattern of interactions, involving many cell types and mediators, which contribute to the immunopathogenesis of RA. Following a brief review of antigen presentation, the principal cell types participating in immune responses in RA synovia will be considered, then the mediators will be listed and finally the effects of drugs and other therapies will be discussed.

## CELL TYPES PARTICIPATING IN PATHOGENESIS OF ARTHRITIS

### Interactions of cell types and mediators in immune responses (Figure 13.1)

On the T-cell arm of the immune response, antigen (Ag) associated with type II major histocompatibility complex (MHC) glycoproteins on the surface of interdigitating cells is presented to receptors on the surface of helper T cells ($T_H$), which then, in the presence of IL-1, secrete IL-2 (see Figure 13.1). Ag is presented in the same way to precursors of effector T cells ($T_{EP}$). In the presence of Ag and IL-2 the latter proliferate and produce mediators, including IL-4 and IFN-$\beta_2$. A population of specific memory T lymphocytes with distinctive surface markers[4], is also developed.

On the B cell arm of the immune response, antigen in the form of an immune complex and C3b (AgC) is localized on the surface of follicular dendritic cells. There it interacts with surface membrane Ig receptors on precursor B lymphocytes ($B_p$). In the presence of Ag, IL-1 and IL-4, B-cells proliferate. A differentiation factor from T lymphocytes (IFN-$\beta_2$) induces the cells to differentiate into Ig-secreting effector cells ($B_E$). A specific memory population ($B_M$) is also generated.

### Polymorphonuclear leukocytes

Polymorphonuclear leukocytes (PMN) are found in RA synovial fluid, sometimes in large numbers. Presumably the PMN are responding to chemotaxis by mediators such as $LTB_4$ and C5a, which are present in synovial fluid[5,6]. It has been suggested that lytic enzymes released from PMN may degrade cartilage in RA[7]. However, systematic histopathological studies of

212

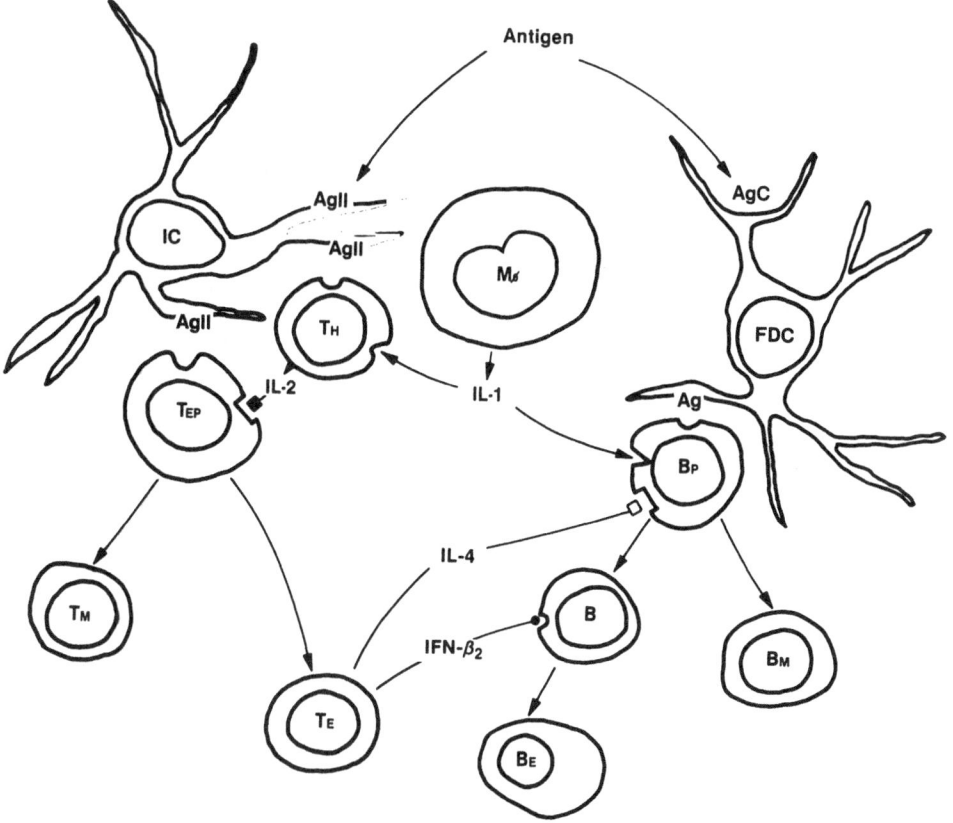

**Figure 13.1** Diagram of cell and mediator interactions in humoral and cell-mediated responses to antigens (see text)

RA tissues by Fassbender and colleagues[8], as well as others, have shown that cartilage and bone erosion occur from the edges, adjacent to areas of proliferating pannus, in which there are few, if any, PMN. This contrasts with septic arthritis in which there is degradation of cartilage adjacent to the joint space. PMN can be regarded as a manifestation of an acute inflammatory response superimposed at intervals on the chronic inflammation of RA.

## Cells of the monocyte–macrophage lineage

Better candidates for a central role in pathogenesis of RA are monocytes and macrophages which are present in pannus. Monocytes and macrophages are major producers of IL-1, which is likely to be an important mediator of

213

inflammation, and of cartilage and bone erosion. The suggestion will be made below that one of the modes of action of long-acting anti-rheumatic drugs is to inhibit the proliferation of monocyte precursors and to accelerate their differentiation. It is therefore necessary to consider these processes in more detail.

Monocytes arise in the bone marrow from common precursors which are induced by colony-stimulating factors (CSFs) to proliferate and to differentiate into cells of the granulocyte or monocyte lineage. Three human CSFs have been cloned, sequenced and expressed by recombinant DNA technology. G-CSF is a glycoprotein of relative molecular mass 20 000 ($M_r = 20\,K$) which induces the proliferation of precursors and their differentiation into granulocytes[9]. M-CSF (formerly known as CSF-1) is a heavily glycosylated 45 K glycoprotein which induces proliferation of the same precursors and their differentiation into monocytes[10]. GM-CSF is a 22 K glycoprotein that induces proliferation of the common precursors and their differentiation into both granulocytes and monocytes[11]. The receptor for M-CSF is the product of the c-fms proto-oncogene[12], a 165 K transmembrane protein with tyrosine kinase activity.

Binding of a glycoprotein growth factor to a receptor is followed by transduction of the signal for proliferation within the cell. Often lipid mediators are involved, for example increased turnover of phosphatidyl inositol, liberation of diacylglycerol and activation of protein kinase C[13,14]. We have analysed the role of products of arachidonate metabolism as regulators of proliferation and differentiation in the human pluripotential precursor cell line HL-60 and in the promonocytic cell line U-937[15]. We found that inhibitors of phospholipase A, inhibitors of the 5-lipoxygenase pathway of arachidonate metabolism, combined 5-lipoxygenase and cyclo-oxygenase inhibitors, and antagonists of leukotriene $D_4$ inhibit the proliferation of these cells and induce their differentiation into cells with markers of monocytes and macrophages: increased Fc$\gamma$ and C3b receptor expression and increased lysozyme and lysosomal enzyme production (Figures 13.2 and 13.3). Agents inhibiting the cyclo-oxygenase but not the lipoxygenase pathway of arachidonate metabolism have no such effect. We postulate that while M-CSF and GM-CSF are exogenous glycopeptide growth factors for monocytic precursors, the intrinsic lipid-derived factors by which signals for growth are transduced are the sulphidopeptide leukotrienes LTC$_4$ and LTD$_4$[15].

Monocytes are recruited into the rheumatoid synovium, presumably because endothelial cells in that site are activated by IL-1 and other mediators to become more adhesive for circulating leukocytes (see below). Cells with markers typical of monocytes and monocyte-derived macrophages are present in rheumatoid synovium[16,17]. These cells express class II MHC glycoproteins, Fc$\gamma$ receptors, monocyte lineage differentiation antigens, are phagocytic and have non-specific esterase.

### Dendritic cells (interdigitating cells and follicular dendritic cells)

In synovial tissue there are several cell types with dendritic (branching) shapes. Some of these are probably of mesenchymal origin (see below), while others

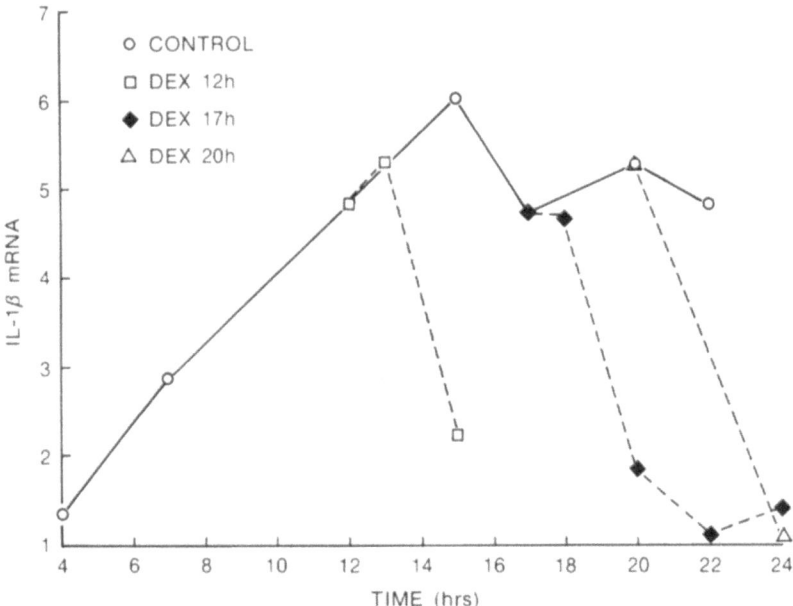

**Figure 13.2** Production of IL-1β messenger RNA in a human promonocytic cell line (U-937) primed with phorbol myristate acetate and induced with lipopolysaccharide. At the times indicated, dexamethasone (10 μmol L⁻¹) was added. After 1 h, levels of IL-1β mRNA rapidly fall. (Data of Lee *et al.*, reference 78)

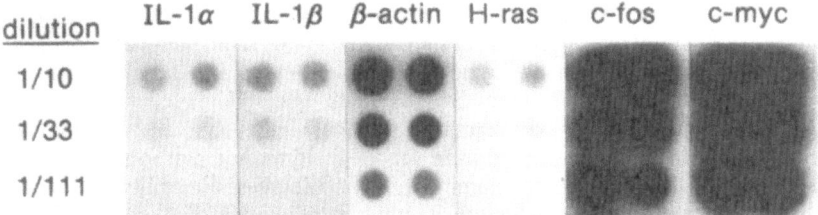

**Figure 13.3** Messenger RNA extracted from RA synovial tissue hybridized with probes for IL-1α, IL-1β, and the proto-oncogenes, *H-ras*, *c-fos* and *c-myc*. Substantial amounts of mRNAs for *c-fos* and *c-myc* are present, and both IL-1α and IL-1β genes are expressed (S.W. Lee and A.C. Allinson)

are probably of the same lineages as the principal antigen-presenting cells in lymphoid tissues, namely follicular dendritic cells (FDC) and interdigitating cells (IDC). The relationships and markers of these cell types are too complex to discuss here in detail. Briefly, IDC originate from the bone marrow and migrate through tissues and then lymphatics to the T-dependent areas of lymph nodes, where they extend their processes among T lymphocytes[18]. During their brief sojourn in the skin they are known as Langerhans cells. These cells constitutively express class II MHC glycoproteins[19], and we have found them constitutively to produce IL-1s, unlike monocytes, in which both processes require activation. Hence IDC are well adapted to their function of

215

presenting antigens to T lymphocytes. In RA synovia immunohistological examination shows large, dendritic cells with strong HLA-DR expression to be associated with Leu 3a[+]T4[+] lymphocytes[20]. Staining with OKT6 confirms the suspicion that these cells are of the IDC lineage.

There is also evidence that localization of antigens to FDC, in the form of complement-activating immune complexes, efficiently stimulates the generation of B lymphocyte memory[21,22], which presumably requires proliferation of clones of B lymphocytes with high-affinity surface membrane immunoglobulin (SMIg) receptors for that antigen. Self-associating IgG rheumatoid factors, which activate complement[23], are likely to be localized in this way. The properties of FDC, reviewed by Tew[22], coincide with those in follicles in RA synovia, as well as some cells in diffuse infiltrates.

## B lymphocytes

The presence in RA synovia of B lymphocytes and their terminally differentiated forms, plasma cells, has long been recognized[24]. In some synovia the B lymphocytes are grouped into typical follicles, but in the majority B lymphocytes are diffusely distributed[25]. There is both morphological and immunochemical evidence that B lymphocytes are activated in rheumatoid synovia, and also in the peripheral blood and extra-articular tissues of patients with active RA. Some B lymphocytes in RA synovia stain with monoclonal antibody B532, a marker of activation[25]; this is true both within follicles and in diffuse infiltrates. RA synovial tissue in culture incorporates labelled amino acids into Ig at rates comparable to those of stimulated lymphoid tissues[26]. Both IgG and IgM rheumatoid factors are among the Igs synthesized by cultured RA synovia[27]. IgG synthesis by RA synovia *in vivo* has also been demonstrated[28]. Hence in RA synovia B lymphocytes are fully activated to produce their characteristic secretory products, Igs.

In the circulating blood of many patients with RA, B lymphocytes, but not T lymphocytes, incorporate labelled thymidine without additional stimulation[29]. Of 28 patients examined, 13 had increased numbers of *in vivo* active immunoglobulin-producing B lymphocytes detected by a reverse plaque-forming cell assay[30]. Most of these had extra-articular manifestations of disease (nodules and vasculitis). About one half of the remaining patients had increased numbers of Ig-secreting B lymphocytes in synovial fluid. These studies imply that in RA patients whose disease is primarily articular, Ig synthesis is restricted to the synovial compartment, while in those with extra-articular features Ig-producing B cells are present also in the circulation.

The presence of a polyclonal B-cell activator associated with $\alpha_2$-macroglobulin in the serum of patients with RA has also been reported[31]; whether this is related to the known effect of proteinases in activating B lymphocytes remains to be established.

## Leu-1[+] B lymphocytes

IgM rheumatoid factor is secreted by a subset of B lymphocytes that express at low density in mice the pan-T-cell glycoprotein Ly-1 and in humans the pan-T-cell homologous glycoprotein Leu-1 (CD5)[32,33]. Leu-1[+] B cells in humans can be identified and purified by double labelling for B1 and Leu-1, followed by fluorescence-activated cell sorting. The Leu-1$^+$ B cells can then be activated to secrete Igs by Epstein-Barr virus[32] or *Staphylococcus aureus*[33]. These studies provide evidence that Leu-1 B cells are the principal source of IgM-anti-Fc$\gamma$ (rheumatoid factor) as well as IgM and IgG antibodies against single-stranded DNA and IgM autoantibodies with specificity for insulin and thyroglobulin[32]. Thus major products of this subset of lymphocytes are IgM autoantibodies. However, in persons immunized with tetanus toxoid, Leu-1$^+$ B cells also produce IgM antibodies against the antigen, whereas IgG anti-toxoid is produced exclusively by Leu-1$^-$ B cells[32].

Leu-1$^+$ B cells in humans and Ly-1$^+$ B cells in mice appear to be a distinct lineage of B lymphocytes with a limited repertoire of $V_H$ genes in the unmutated (germline) configuration. This subset of B cells is abundant in the embryo and newborn, including umbilical cord blood. In normal adults the number of Leu-1$^+$ B cells in peripheral blood is low (about 3%), but it is increased in patients with rheumatoid arthritis (about 20%)[34]. The proportion of Leu-1$^+$ B cells is higher in lymph nodes and tonsils than in peripheral blood. In autoimmune NZB and Me$^v$ mice, the proportion of Ly-1$^+$ B cells is higher than in other strains, especially in old animals with high levels of IgM autoantibodies. Thus increased proliferation of this subset of B lymphocytes may be a common feature in the pathogenesis of autoimmune diseases. It will be interesting to know whether antibodies against double-stranded DNA, which are thought to be pathogenic in systemic lupus erythematosus, are produced by Leu-1$^+$ B cells. Since production of rheumatoid factors is not affected by total lymphoid irradiation, it may be thymus independent. Ascertaining whether immune responses of Leu-1$^+$ B cells are thymus independent, as well as what stimuli and mediators are required for their proliferation and differentiation, are goals of future research.

## T lymphocytes

There is widespread misunderstanding about subsets of T lymphocytes, their distinguishing characteristics, how they are activated and markers of activation. Current information will be reviewed briefly as necessary background to discussion of the findings in RA. Cloning of T lymphocytes in the presence of antigen and IL-2, and the molecular biological definition of receptors for antigen on subsets of T lymphocytes, have clarified many problems associated with helper and cytotoxic subsets of T lymphocytes. However, while there is strong evidence that suppressor T lymphocytes exist, and probably play an important role in preventing autoimmunity[2], it has only recently been possible to clone these cells and their properties are still poorly defined.

In the mouse there are two types of helper T lymphocyte clones, designated $T_H1$ and $T_H2$[35]. The $T_H2$ subset produces IL-3 and IL-4 but does not produce IL-2 or IFN-$\gamma$ whereas the $T_H1$ subset produces IL-2, IFN-$\gamma$, IL-3 and GM-CSF. Unfortunately there are still no surface markers for these subsets and whether there are human equivalents is not yet known.

Three sequential events are required to propel primary resting T lympho-cytes through the cell cycle[36]. First, antigenic or mitogenic stimulation induces a $G_0$–$G_1$ transition, which is associated with the synthesis of the IL-2 receptor and its expression on the cell surface. IL-1 may be required for this process. In a second phase, without additional mitogenic or antigenic stimulation clones of helper T lymphocytes express the IL-2 receptor and $\beta$-chain T-cell receptor. However, further antigenic or mitogenic stimulation is required for transcription of the IL-2, IL-3, GM-CSF and IFN-$\gamma$ genes[37]. In a third phase of activation, interaction of IL-2 with its receptor propels the cell through $G_1$ and into S phase, a change that is associated with the expression of transferrin receptors on the cell surface[36]. Control of the second and third phases seems to be independently affected not only by antigenic stimulation but also by humoral factors: glucocorticoids, for example, do not inhibit expression of the IL-2 receptor and $\beta$-chain T-cell receptor whereas they do inhibit production of IL-2, IL-3, GM-CSF and IFN-$\gamma$[37]. Prostaglandin $E_2$ does not inhibit expression of the IL-2 receptor but does inhibit IL-2 production and expression of transferrin receptors[38].

When the monoclonal antibodies OKT4 and OKT8 were introduced it was thought that they were markers for helper T cells and suppressor/cytotoxic T cells respectively. However, it is now clear that suppressor cells can be found in the $T4^+$ subset and cytotoxic cells in the $T8^+$ subset. In fact, T4 (CD4) appears to define genetic restriction of interactions with cells bearing class II MHC structures and T8 (CD8) restriction of interactions with cells bearing class I MHC structures, rather than specific functions[39]. Likewise the inclusion of suppressor/cytotoxic cells in the Leu-2a subset and helper/inducer cells in the Leu-3a subset, as defined by other monoclonal antibodies, is an over-interpretation. These antibodies are certainly useful for defining changes in ratio of subsets in some diseases, notably AIDS, in which human immunodeficiency virus enters T lymphocytes following attachment to the CD4 molecule[40] and the subset of lymphocytes expressing the receptor is depleted. However, conclusions about the functional consequences of changes in subsets defined by surface markers must be made with caution.

Analyses of cells isolated from RA synovia[41], as well as immunohistological examination of the synovial tissues[20,25], have shown the presence of more T lymphocytes than B lymphocytes. Moreover, nearly one half of the T lymphocytes express HLA-DR, a marker of activation[42]; this is a much higher proportion than in peripheral blood. However, T lymphocytes in RA synovia do not express transferrin receptors[25], as expressed in fully activated cycling T cells. The distribution of T lymphocyte subsets varies in different synovia and even in different parts of the same synovial sample. In nodular infiltrates containing relatively large numbers of B lymphocytes and plasma cells, the ratio of Leu $3^+4^+$ to Leu $3^+8^+$ T lymphocytes is high (6 to 14/1), whereas in diffuse infiltrates the Leu $4^+/8^+$ ratios are more like those in peripheral blood (2 to 4/1)[20].

Some authors have suggested that in the peripheral blood of patients with active RA the proportion of CD4/CD8 cells is abnormally high, and returns towards to normal with successful treatment[43]. However, others have found the CD4/CD8 ratios in peripheral blood to be within normal limits, so this ratio does not appear to be a generally useful guide to disease activity and efficacy of therapy[44].

### Endothelial cells, fibroblasts and cells of mesenchymal origin

Just as synovial dendritic cells are heterogeneous, synovial 'fibroblasts' represent a variety of cell types of mesenchymal origin which may well contribute to the pathogenesis of RA. Markers of these cell types, their subsets and states of differentiation are still limited.

In rheumatoid synovia endothelial cells are often quite prominent and they may be stimulated to proliferate by growth factors which are locally produced. The receptor for epidermal growth factor can be demonstrated by staining with monoclonal antibody 455 on endothelial cells in rheumatoid synovia[25]; such staining is rare in sections of synovial tissue obtained from osteoarthritic joints or joints of persons with traumatic injury.

Fassbender and his colleagues[8,24], who have extensive experience of the histological and electron microscopic appearances of operation specimens of synovia from patients with RA, have paid particular attention to the tissue in closest contact with eroded cartilage. They conclude that erosion is associated with the presence of immature-looking mesenchyme-like cells with large nuclei. These cells encroach on the articular cartilage from the area of junction with the synovium, often following the presence of a fibrinous inflammatory exudate. Such infiltrations of immature cells are short lived, and they are replaced by cells of fibroblastic appearance, laying down the collagen that is characteristic of mature pannus overlying eroded cartilage. The fibroblasts may be differentiated forms of the immature cells in the erosive lesions. However, erosive immature cells can reappear during the intermittent course of the disease after periods of quiescence and acute inflammation. Because the presence of immature cells is transient, they are seen in only about 5% of synovial tissues sampled.

A report from the United States[25] has provided evidence that in about one-third of RA specimens examined, synovial and subsynovial and perivascular tissues show markers of activation and proliferation even though there are few infiltrating lymphocytes. Many cells bear HLA-DR and HLA-DS glycoproteins, as well as transferrin receptors demonstrated with monoclonal antibody L22[25].

Adherent fibroblasts freshly isolated from RA synovium respond to stimulation with IL-1 by production of large amounts of collagenase and $PGE_2$ (see below); following several subcultures these responses decrease, possibly because one subset of fibroblast-type cells overgrows others present in the synovium. As a generalization it can be stated that the role of connective tissue cells in the pathogenesis of RA is poorly understood, although it may be important, especially in a subgroup of cases.

## MEDIATORS PARTICIPATING IN PATHOGENESIS OF ARTHRITIS

### Interleukin-1

Evidence has accumulated that IL-1 may be a central mediator in the pathogenesis of RA. For this reason IL-1 is described in more detail than other mediators and information is given about assays for the two known varieties of IL-1 and the corresponding messenger RNAs (mRNAs). These assays provide a secure foundation for analyses of the role of IL-1 in RA and other inflammatory arthritides as well as for studies of the effects of drugs, such as glucocorticoids, and procedures, such as total lymphoid irradiation, which will be described in the section on therapies.

*Structure*
Cloning investigations[45-47] have demonstrated that there are two human IL-1 genes (IL-1$\alpha$ and IL-1$\beta$) producing in several cell types primary translation products with 271 and 269 amino acids, having $M_r$ 30 606 and 30 749 (31K) for IL-1$\alpha$ and IL-1$\beta$, respectively. The primary gene product of IL-1$\alpha$ is biologically active whereas that of IL-1$\beta$ is not; both are cleaved to biologically active forms of 17.5 K. The 17.5 K IL-1$\beta$ molecule is also known as the pI7 form, whereas the 17.5 K IL-1$\alpha$ molecule is also termed the pI5 form. Human IL-1$\beta$ has only 26% amino acid homology with human IL-1$\alpha$, although the homology of the nucleic acids is greater (45%), suggesting that the two genes arose by duplication of a common precursor in the distant past. Nevertheless IL-1$\alpha$ and IL-1$\beta$ bind to the same receptor on several cell types[48]. It is not surprising that IL-1$\alpha$ and IL-1$\beta$ share many biological activities in which they are usually about equipotent.

*Immunoassay*
IL-1 has usually been measured by bioassays, especially the murine thymocyte co-mitogenic (lymphocyte-activating factor or LAF) assay. However, the assay is ambiguous because IL-1$\alpha$ and IL-1$\beta$ are both active, and factors other than IL-1 (e.g. IL-2) can have thymocyte co-stimulatory activity. Moreover other mediators such as $PGE_2$ (which are often present in synovial fluid or supernatants of synovial cell cultures) can inhibit the response, and are not easily eliminated by dialysis. For these reasons we and others have developed DNA probes for measurement of mRNAs for IL-1$\alpha$ and IL-1$\beta$, as well as immunoassays for the proteins. Our assay for IL-1$\beta$ is a sandwich ELISA using two monoclonal antibodies against distinct epitopes with co-operative binding[49]. It can detect IL-1$\beta$ in concentrations down to 15 pg ml$^{-1}$ in serum, other biological fluids, culture media, and released from cells by Triton X-100 lysis. This is close to the sensitivity of most bioassays. We have also developed a slightly less sensitive immunoassay for IL-1$\alpha$.

*Control of IL-1 formation*
Human peripheral blood monocytes or U-937 cells in culture are used to study the control of IL-1 formation. In both cell types levels of IL-1$\alpha$ and IL-1$\beta$ mRNAs are barely detectable. When monocytes are stimulated with lipopolysaccharide (LPS), substantial amounts of IL-1$\beta$ mRNA and lesser amounts of IL-1$\alpha$ mRNA are found (ratio about 15 to 1). Hence the control is at the level of transcription of the IL-1$\alpha$ and IL-1$\beta$ genes. U-937 cells respond maximally to LPS only when they are primed with phorbol-12-myristate-13-acetate (PMA: see Figure 13.2). Beginning about 2 h after stimulation, increased levels of IL-1$\beta$ are detectable in the cells by immunoassay. In human peripheral blood monocytes stimulated with LPS, a substantial

amount of IL-1$\beta$ is formed. The IL-1 is readily demonstrable by immuno-fluorescence in the cytoplasm of the cell[50]. Western blots show that intracellular IL-1$\beta$ is predominantly the 31 K form, whereas the secreted form is 17.5 K[50]. In fact, the mechanism of secretion of IL-1 is not understood since the molecule lacks the typical leader sequence found in most secreted proteins; possibly cleavage of the 31 K to the 17.5 K form is linked with secretion.

*Production of IL-1 by RA synovia*
Several groups of investigators found IL-1 by bioassays in synovial fluid[51,52]. We have consistently observed IL-1$\beta$ mRNA and some IL-1$\alpha$ mRNA in RA synovial tissue (Figure 13.3), as well as IL-1$\beta$ in supernatants of RA synovial cell cultures (Figure 13.4). IL-1$\beta$ is released first, then PGE$_2$. The delayed release of PGE$_2$ is presumably due in part to escape from control of drugs used by the patient and in part to IL-1-induced production of PGE$_2$ by synovial cells in culture. The amounts of IL-1 produced (several nanograms

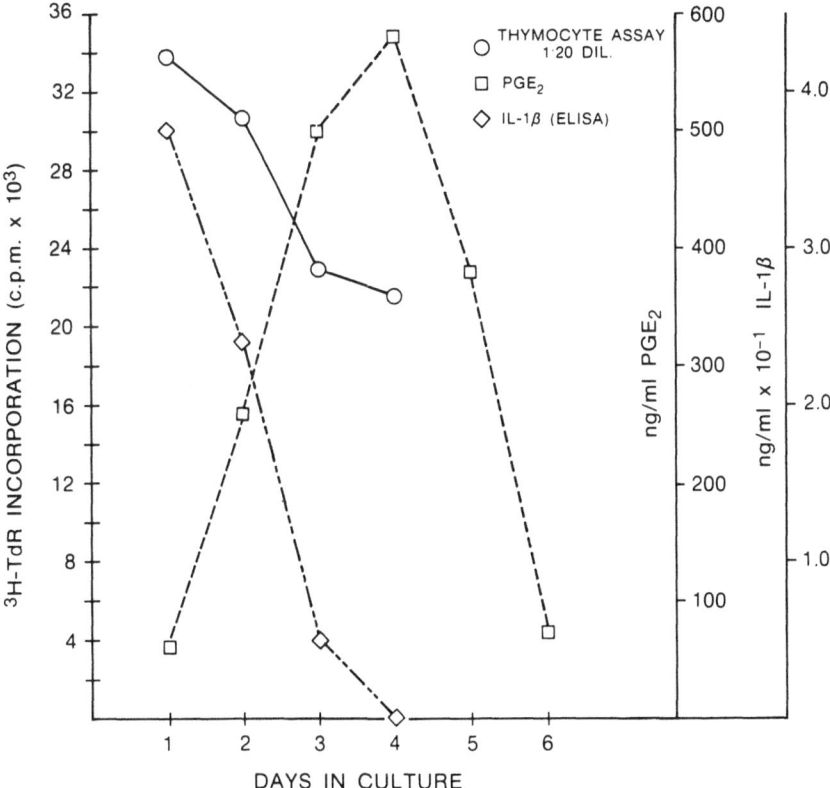

**Figure 13.4** Release from cultured RA synovial tissue of IL-1$\beta$ measured by immunoassay, of lymphocyte-activating activity and of PGE$_2$. (Observations of E.M. Eugui, M. Masada, J. Kenney, B. DeLustro and A.C. Allison)

221

per ml of culture fluid) are sufficent to induce cartilage proteoglycan degradation and bone erosion. We have also found that total lymphoid irradiation (a treatment decreasing the signs and symptoms of RA) reduces production of IL-1 by RA synovial cultures[53] (see below). Mechanisms inducing IL-1 formation that might be operative in RA synovia, and effects of IL-1 that might contribute to the pathogenesis of different types of arthritis are therefore of interest.

*Inducers of IL-1 formation*
Four classes of inducers of IL-1 formation by monocytes and macrophages have been described. One class includes inorganic crystals such as silica[54] and monosodium urate[55]; the former may be relevant to the pathogenesis of silicotic fibrosis and the latter to the pathogenesis of gout. Hydroxyapatite crystals are less potent inducers of IL-1 formation by human monocytes than are monosodium urate crystals, and calcium pyrophosphate dihydrate does not stimulate IL-1 release[55]. IL-1 acting on endothelial cells could increase attachment of PMN (see below), facilitating their recruitment to the joint in crystal-mediated arthritis.

The second class of IL-1 inducers includes bacterial products such as lipopolysaccharide[54], the muramyl dipeptide components of bacterial cell walls[56] and whole bacteria, including the spirochaete of Lyme disease[57]. This may be relevant to the pathogenesis of Reiter's disease and Lyme disease, respectively. We have recently injected recombinant human IL-1$\alpha$ and IL-1$\beta$ into rhesus monkeys, and a major side effect is the development of anterior uveitis. From our previous experience with muramyl peptides in rabbits[58], accumulation of leukocytes in the uveal tract and prostaglandin formation contribute to the pathogenesis of anterior uveitis. IL-1 produces both of these effects, as discussed below, so IL-1 could be a major mediator of the arthritis and anterior uveitis that are components of Reiter's disease. Whether products of the Gram negative bacteria associated with this disease induce IL-1 formation by acting directly on monocytes or through an immunological mechanism is unknown. Bacteria in dental plaque induce chronic inflammatory periodontal disease, in which we again find formation of substantial amounts of IL-1$\beta$.

The third class of inducers of IL-1 formation comprises immune complexes[59], including self-associating IgG rheumatoid factors[60]. Obviously this could play a role in the pathogenesis of RA, as discussed below. The fourth class of inducers includes T lymphocyte products. Evidence has been presented that T lymphocytes and macrophages can interact by a genetically-restricted mechanism requiring cell contact to produce lymphocyte-activating factor (LAF)[61]. Macrophages stimulated with media containing GM-CSF, a product of activated T lymphocytes (among other cells), also produce LAF[62]. These experiments should be repeated with cloned GM-CSF and immunoassays for IL-1, but it seems likely that some products of activated T lymphocytes induce IL-1 formation in cells of the monocyte-macrophage lineage. IFN-$\gamma$ does not itself induce production of IL-1 by human monocytes, but it enhances and maintains the capacity of the cells to respond to LPS by IL-1 formation[63].

*Effects on endothelial cells*

Effects of IL-1 that could be relevant to the pathogenesis of arthritis will now be considered. IL-1 acts on endothelial cells in culture to increase adhesion of PMN, monocytes and lymphocytes[64,65]. This could be a stage in the recruitment of cells from the circulation into the joints, thereby initiating or perpetuating an inflammatory reaction.

*Induction of prostaglandin formation*

IL-1 acts on synovial fibroblast-type cells to induce the production and release of $PGE_2$[66] and on endothelial cells to induce production of prostacyclin[67]. In view of the likely contribution of prostaglandin formation to pain and other manifestations of RA, and the beneficial effects of cyclo-oxygenase inhibitors in the disease, this effect could be important in the pathogenesis of pain and other manifestations of inflammation.

*Induction of metalloproteinase secretion by chondrocytes*

IL-1 also induces the production of substantial amounts of $PGE_2$ by chondrocytes. However, the most interesting effect of IL-1 on chondrocytes is the induction of a neutral metalloproteinase that can degrade cartilage proteoglycan[68,69]. This is the outcome of a series of investigations beginning with the observation of Fell and Jubb[70] that co-culture of porcine synovial connective tissue and cartilage led to proteoglycan degradation. The factor produced by synovial tissue responsible for this effect was eventually purified and termed catabolin, which is the porcine homologue of IL-1[71]. Human monocyte-derived IL-1 and recombinant human IL-1$\alpha$ and IL-1$\beta$ are potent inducers of metalloproteinase secretion by isolated rabbit chondrocytes[68]. Since tumour necrosis factor (TNF-$\alpha$) shares some properties of IL-1, it is interesting that recombinant human TNF-$\alpha$ did not induce prostaglandin or neutral metalloproteinase release by chondrocytes, although it decreased production of plasminogen activator. In chondrocytes activated by IL-1 indomethacin does not influence metalloproteinase secretion or proteoglycan degradation, suggesting that prostaglandins do not mediate this effect[68,69].

*Induction of procollagenase secretion*

The metalloproteinase just described also cleaves procollagenase to active collagenase that can degrade collagen in cartilage, bone and loose connective tissue. IL-1 induces the release of procollagenase by synovial fibroblast-type cells[66] and by chondrocytes[72]. Thus IL-1 induces the synthesis and release of both types of enzymes required for breakdown of connective tissue matrix and fibres. This could explain cartilage erosion in sites of highest concentrations of IL-1 adjacent to proliferating pannus in RA and alongside the joint space in septic arthritis.

223

*Bone demineralization*

Following studies with IL-1-containing supernatants[72], it has been shown that recombinant human IL-1$\alpha$ and IL-1$\beta$ are able to induce the release of calcium from organ cultures of calvaria and long bones[73]. In this assay IL-1$\beta$ is active in concentrations less than $10^{-11}$ mol L$^{-1}$, somewhat more active than IL-1$\alpha$; IL-1$\beta$ is the most potent known inducer of demineralization, about one thousand times as active as parathyroid hormone. Recombinant tumour necrosis factor (TNF-$\alpha$) also induces demineralization although it is less potent than IL-1; the two have synergistic effects, as does TNF-$\beta$ (lymphotoxin) and PGE$_2$ with IL-1[73]. By inducing demineralization of bone and degrading intercellular matrix and collagen fibres, IL-1 could contribute to joint erosion in RA and loss of alveolar bone in chronic inflammatory periodontal disease. IL-1-induced loss of calcium from bone cultures is inhibited by drugs blocking cyclo-oxygenase.

*Spontaneous IL-1 production by mononuclear phagocytes of RA patients*

Shore and colleagues[74] reported that cultured peripheral blood monocytes from RA patients who had a recent (less than 6 months) onset of their disease or exacerbation of existing RA, showed spontaneous IL-1 secretion. Adherent peripheral blood cells from patients with equally active RA but with historically stable disease did not. These observations suggest that production of IL-1 by circulating monocytes activated only by adherence may be temporally linked to an early event in the onset, or exacerbation, of RA. IL-1 production by peripheral blood monocytes and synovial monocyte-derived cells of RA patients activated only by adherence has also been reported by Danis and colleagues[75].

*Effects of IL-1 on haemopoiesis*

Recent studies have shown IL-1 to have major effects on haemopoiesis. IL-1 acts on stromal cells in the bone marrow to induce the production of G-CSF and GM-CSF[76]. IL-1 acts synergistically with these factors in stimulating the proliferation of granulocyte–monocyte precursors; IL-1 is, in fact, identical to a factor previously termed haemopoietin-1.

In addition, we have found that IL-1$\alpha$ and IL-1$\beta$ (but not TNF-$\alpha$) antagonize effects of erythropoietin on late erythroid precursors[77]. We suggest that IL-1 production may be a factor in the pathogenesis of hypoplastic anaemia in RA and systemic lupus erythematosus. IL-1 may exert this effect indirectly by inducing the formation of an intermediate cytokine.

*IL-1 production is influenced by the state of differentiation of cells of the monocyte–macrophage lineage*

Our studies with the human promonocytic cell line U-937, show that these cells do not respond to lipopolysaccharide by producing IL-1 unless they are primed by phorbol myristate acetate[78]. PMA induces competence for IL-1 production as well as expression of typical markers of differentiation (Fc$\gamma$ and C3b receptors and increased lysozyme and lysosomal enzymes). Induction of differentiation by other agents, including auranofin and 5-lipoxygenase inhibitors, shows expression of the same markers but the fully differentiated

cells do not express increased competence for IL-1 production. If these findings can be extrapolated to normal differentiation of cells of this series, precursors up to the level of promonocytes in the bone marrow would have not yet acquired competence to produce IL-1. In view of the effects of IL-1 on haemopoiesis, production of IL-1 in the bone marrow would normally be under tight control. Circulating monocytes show maximal production of IL-1, and presumably this is also true of cells recently recruited into RA synovia. Fully differentiated cells that have resided in tissues for some time lose their competence to produce IL-1 when appropriately stimulated. Consistent with this interpretation are findings that cultured monocytes rapidly lose capacity to produce IL-1[63,79] and that pulmonary alveolar macrophages, which are known to have a haematogenous origin, produce much less IL-1 than monocytes when the two cell types are stimulated under comparable conditions[79]. Macrophage-type cells from RA synovia activated by LPS also produce less IL-1 than do peripheral blood monocytes from the same individuals[75].

## Interleukin-2

In view of the presence in RA synovia of many T cells, quite a high proportion expressing markers of activation (class II MHC glycoproteins), production of IL-2 might have been expected. However, the situation regarding IL-2 production by RA synovial and peripheral blood T cells is confusing. Despite some claims to the contrary, most investigators have been unable to detect IL-2 in RA synovia or synovial fluid[80,81]. Moreover, production of IL-2 by synovial lymphocytes stimulated by mitogens or by antibody against CD3, as well as proliferative responses to added IL-2, may be deficient[82–84]. These effects have been attributed by Miossec et al.[83] to the presence in RA synovial fluid of a macromolecular inhibitor of IL-2, which blocks responses of mitogen-stimulated human peripheral blood T cells and mouse thymocytes to IL-2. The production of IL-2 by peripheral blood T cells activated with mitogens or Epstein-Barr virus is often decreased, especially in patients with active disease[84]. This is attributed to a monocyte-derived inhibitor of IL-2 and IFN-$\gamma$. However, production of IL-2 by peripheral blood cells of patients with active RA, as assessed by a limiting dilution method (which would reduce effects of inhibitors), is actually reported to be increased[85].

## Interferon-$\gamma$

In view of evidence that T lymphocytes are activated in RA synovia, production of IFN-$\gamma$ might have been expected. Since IFN-$\gamma$ increases expression of class II MHC glycoproteins in macrophages and other cell types, it would be a possible mediator of this effect in RA synovia, in which a relatively high proportion of mononuclear and dendritic cells express HLA-DR and HLA-DS. Interest in this possibility was intensified by a report of spontaneous production of an acid-labile IFN in systemic lupus erythematosus (SLE); however, examination of serum IFN in SLE showed it to be acid-labile

IFN-$\alpha$, not IFN-$\gamma$[86]. We have been unable to demonstrate IFN-$\gamma$ in RA synovial culture supernatants, which contain abundant IL-1 and PGE$_2$. According to Husby and Williams[81], IFN-$\gamma$ is not readily detectable in RA synovial tissue by fluorescence microscopy and Malaise and Franchimont[87] reported that only a few of the RA synovial samples studied with an enzyme-linked immunoabsorbent assay showed detectable levels of IFN-$\gamma$. Using what has now become the standard radioimmunoassay for IFN-$\gamma$, J. Vilcek (personal communication) has not detected this mediator in RA synovial fluids.

There is also evidence for defective production of IFN-$\gamma$ when peripheral blood mononuclear cells from patients with active RA are stimulated with PHA or by autologous Epstein-Barr virus-transformed B lymphocytes, despite normal proliferative responses[88]. Depressed IFN-$\gamma$ production following autologous stimulation appears to be due to the release by stimulated adherent mononuclear cells of PGE$_2$; production of IFN-$\gamma$ by lymphocytes of patients with active RA is unusually sensitive to inhibition by E-type prostaglandins[88].

## Interleukin-4 (B-cell stimulatory factor BSF-1)

The existence of distinct T lymphocyte-derived helper factors that increase B lymphocyte proliferation and differentiation into antibody-secreting cells has long been recognized. IL-4 is a 20 K protein produced by some activated T lymphocytes[89]. It acts on resting B cells to increase their expression of MHC class II molecules, is a co-factor for entry into S-phase of mouse cells stimulated with antibodies against surface membrane Ig, and increases the production of IgG$_1$ and IgE by mouse B cells stimulated with lipopolysaccharide. Cloning and expression of murine and human IL-4 genes established that IL-4 is not only a co-activator of B cells: it can also stimulate some T cell lines and mast cell lines. Whether IL-4 is produced in RA synovia is not yet established. Since some products of activated T lymphocytes, such as IL-2 and IFN-$\gamma$, are not produced in RA synovial tissue, the question remains open.

## B-cell differentiation factor BSF-2 (interferon-$\beta_2$)

The human B-cell differentiation factor otherwise known as BSF-2 (B-cell stimulating factor 2) has been characterized in activated T lymphocytes as well as in human T-cell lines that secrete this factor constitutively[90,91]. Human BSF-2 has the following effects:

(i)    Increasing synthesis of secretory type heavy chains of Igs as well as their messenger RNAs;

(ii)   Inducing IgM and IgG secretion in *Staphylococcus aureus* Cowan-I-activated normal human B lymphocytes; and

(iii)  Inducing IgG or IgM secretion in Epstein-Barr virus-transformed B cell lines in the absence of an effect on proliferation.

When BSF-2 was purified to homogeneity, cloned, expressed and sequenced, it transpired that BSF-2 is identical with interferon-$\beta_2$, a protein that had been independently studied for other reasons[91].

IFN-$\beta_2$ is distinct from other interferons in several respects. Its constitutive expression in human diploid fibroblasts is increased by other cytokines, including IL-1$\alpha$ and IL-1$\beta$, TNF-$\alpha$ and platelet-derived growth factor. IFN-$\beta_2$ is also expressed in monocytes and increases the expression of cell surface histocompatibility antigens in some cell types. Mature IFN-$\beta_2$ is a 21 K glycoprotein with 184 amino acid residues derived from a precursor of 212 amino acids. The carboxy terminal of IFN-$\beta_2$ has some sequence homology with IFN-$\beta_1$ and the amino terminal with GM-CSF[91].

Disorders in the regulation of IFN-$\beta_2$ production may play a role in the pathogenesis of autoimmunity, for example, in MRL/*lpr* and Motheaten mice[90]. T lymphocytes of MRL/*lpr* mice constitutively produce B-cell differentiation factor, and B-cells of Motheaten mice spontaneously produce a B-cell maturation factor, both presumably IFN-$\beta_2$. Cardiac myxomas are rare tumours associated with hypergammaglobulinaemia, autoantibodies and connective tissue disorders. These disappear following surgical removal of the tumour, suggesting that tumour products are involved in the autoimmune manifestations of the patients. Cardiac myxomas produce large amounts of IFN-$\beta_2$, and a particular carcinoma of the cervix from a patient with autoantibodies also produced IFN-$\beta_2$. These associations suggest that production of IFN-$\beta_2$ may be involved in the induction of certain autoimmune diseases[90].

It has long been known that RA synovial fluid contains a factor or factors inducing Ig secretion in B lymphocytes activated by pokeweed mitogen[29]. We have found this activity in supernatants of RA synovial cultures. Studies are in progress to ascertain whether the activity is attributable to IFN-$\beta_2$.

## THERAPY OF RHEUMATOID ARTHRITIS

For therapy of RA four classes of drugs (immunosuppressives, glucocorticoids, cyclo-oxygenase inhibitors and long-acting antirheumatic agents) and two immunosuppressive procedures (thoracic duct drainage and total lymphoid irradiation) have been used. Since novel interpretations of the modes of action of glucocorticoids and long-acting agents are presented here, they will be discussed in more detail than the other therapies. Some basic information about experimental animal models of inflammation and arthritis is included because unambiguous differences in the mode of action of classes of drugs (e.g. immunosuppressives and long-acting agents) are revealed.

### Immunosuppressive drugs

These suppress antibody formation and cell-mediated immunity in conventional tests, as well as adjuvant arthritis in rats and type II collagen arthritis in mice. They are not anti-inflammatory in models such as carrageenan-induced oedema and they are not directly analgesic. Several immunosuppressive drugs have been used with varying degrees of success in RA, including cyclophosphamide, azathioprine, methotrexate and cyclosporin. The relative efficacies of high and low doses of immunosuppressive drugs and their side effects, which are often serious, have been widely discussed.

Cyclosporin has recently been shown to be efficacious in RA patients. This has been taken as evidence in support of a T-cell-mediated pathogenesis of RA. However, cyclosporin inhibits not only cytotoxic T lymphocytes but also T-cell-dependent antibody formation as well as the formation of some supposedly T-independent antibodies[92]. Moreover, cyclosporin can affect the function of antigen-presenting cells[93].

## Glucocorticoids

Unlike polypeptide hormones, which usually interact with cell surface receptors, steroids enter cells by passive diffusion through the plasma membrane and within the cell bind high-affinity protein receptor molecules which have specificity for different classes of steroids[94]. The binding of the steroid leads to activation of the receptor–steroid complex, which is thought to involve a conformational change in the protein. The steroid-bound receptor molecules in the nucleus bind to enhancer regions of many genes and act as specific transcriptional regulators to induce or repress the transcription of certain target genes[94].

Although glucocorticoids are among the most potent and widely used anti-inflammatory agents, their mode of action is poorly understood. The most popular theory has been that glucocorticoids induce the formation of a group of proteins, collectively termed lipocortins, that inhibit phospholipase $A_2$ activity, thereby decreasing the production of pro-inflammatory prostaglandins and 5-lipoxygenase products[95,96]. A human lipocortin of $M_r$ 40 K has been cloned and expressed[97]. However, proteins of the lipocortin family (also known as calpactins), which are membrane-associated cytoskeletal proteins serving as substrates for tyrosine kinase phosphorylation[98], are present in rather high concentrations in many cell types. They are glucocorticoid inducible to a very limited degree, if at all, and they are not phospholipase inhibitors but phospholipid-binding proteins[99]. Although there may be other proteins with properties more closely matching those originally postulated for lipocortin, alternative or supplementary mechanisms by which glucocorticoids might exert anti-inflammatory effects deserve consideration.

One such mechanism is inhibiting the formation of varieties of IL-1, which are mediators of inflammation and tissue degradation (see above). Glucocorticoids have been reported to inhibit the release of IL-1 by mouse peritoneal macrophages stimulated with lipopolysaccharide (LPS)[100]. Because inhibition of IL-1 formation by glucocorticoids has interesting implications for immunopharmacology, we have analyzed the phenomenon at the molecular level in the human promonocytic cell line U-937 and in cultured human peripheral blood monocytes[78]. Dexamethasone and other glucocorticoids were found in therapeutic concentrations to inhibit selectively the transcription of IL-1$\alpha$ and IL-1$\beta$ genes and to induce the degradation of IL-1$\beta$ messenger RNA (mRNA, Figure 13.4). The formation and stability of other mRNAs, for $\beta$-actin and the proto-oncogene c-fos, were unaffected by dexamethasone.

The effect of glucocorticoids on mRNA stability is unusual, although some other examples of regulation dependent on mRNA stability are known. Glucocorticoids also inhibit expression on cells of the monocyte macrophage lineage of class II MHC glycoproteins which are required for antigen presentation[100].

Our molecular biological studies support the generalization that IL-1 and glucocorticoids have antagonistic effects, the former pro-inflammatory and the latter anti-inflammatory. Glucocorticoids not only suppress the transcription of IL-1 genes; they reinforce these effects by degrading IL-1 mRNA already formed, thereby rapidly inhibiting IL-1 formation, and by antagonizing the effects of IL-1 on target cells. An example of the latter is the induction by IL-1 of collagenase in synovial cells[66] and suppression of collagenase gene transcription in these cells by dexamethasone[101]. IL-1$\alpha$ and IL-1$\beta$ stimulate the activity of plasminogen activator in synovial cells[102], whereas glucocorticoids suppress transcription of the gene encoding this enzyme[103]. IL-1 increases formation of PGE$_2$ in several cell types[66] and PGI$_2$ in endothelial cells[67], whereas glucocorticoids inhibit the production of PGE$_2$ in several cell types[104] and PGI$_2$ in endothelial cells[105]. The antagonism can also be effected in the opposite direction: IL-1 decreases the induction by glucocorticoids of phosphoenolpyruvate carboxykinase in liver cells[106] and alkaline phosphatase in endothelial cells[107].

Inhibition of MHC II expression and IL-1 formation in antigen-presenting and accessory cells contribute to the immunosuppressive effects of glucocorticoids. However, the expression of specific genes in helper T lymphocytes is also inhibited. Biological studies show that some T lymphocyte helper effects on antibody formation are sensitive to glucocorticoids[108]. Effects of these drugs on mRNA production by two types of murine helper T lymphocytes (T$_H$1 and T$_H$2) have been analysed by Culpepper and Lee[37]. Some mRNAs (for the IL-2 receptor, $\beta$-chain T-cell receptor and Thy-1) are constitutively expressed in these cells, and levels of their mRNAs are unaffected by glucocorticoids. Transcription of other genes (IL-2, IL-3, GM-CSF and IFN-$\gamma$) requires stimulation with mitogen or antigen, and mRNA levels are markedly decreased by glucocorticoids. Expression of the preproencephalin gene also requires antigenic or mitogenic stimulation, but glucocorticoids do not decrease the level of the mRNA formed[37]. Proliferation of, and antibody formation by, B lymphocytes in the presence of appropriate growth and differentiation factors are relatively resistant to glucocorticoids[109].

In addition to their effects on monocytes and T lymphocytes, glucocorticoids have many effects on other cell types, which produce undesirable side effects. Examples are inhibition of transcription of the type I procollagen gene[110], which explains skin thinning, and induction of liver enzymes regulating carbohydrate metabolism[106], which is a problem in diabetics. Effects on calcium metabolism of bone are well known but not yet explained at the molecular level.

## Long-acting antirheumatic drugs

The use of gold salts to treat patients with RA, on the assumption that the disease is due to infection, was initiated in 1922[111]. The results of a multi-centre controlled trial, published in 1961, established that gold salts are efficacious in RA, but that efficacy appears only after several months of treatment[112]. Gold salts became the prototype of a class of long-acting antirheumatic drugs, which now include D-penicillamine, chloroquine and hydroxychloroquine, sulphasalazine, laevamisole and dapsone. To the traditional gold salts (gold thiomalate, gold chloride and gold thioglucose) an orally active gold compound, auranofin, has been added.

The mechanism by which long-acting antirheumatic drugs exert their effects has been a mystery. Lipsky provided evidence that gold compounds can under some conditions inhibit mitogen-induced lymphocyte proliferation[113], and that D-penicillamine and copper inhibit helper T cell function[114]. However, the time course of efficacy of these compounds is different from that of immunosuppressive agents, and long-acting drugs have no activity in animal models such as adjuvant arthritis in the rat and monoarticular and type II collagen arthritis in the mouse which are preventible by immunosuppressive drugs[115,116].

Gold salts are bound to and taken up predominantly by monocytes and monocyte-derived macrophages[117]. The number of neutrophils and macrophages in inflammatory responses to implants in rats and mice was found to be reduced by gold salts, which was attributed to decreased proliferation of precursors in the bone marrow[118]. Consistent with this suggestion, gold salts and D-penicillamine have been found to inhibit the formation of granulocyte–macrophage colonies from mouse and human bone marrow[119,120]. The concentration required for inhibition, $10^{-7}$ to $10^{-8}$ mol L$^{-1}$ in the case of human precursors, is in the therapeutic range.

The fact that long-acting antirheumatic drugs exert their effects only after dosage for 3 or 4 months led us to explore further effects on monocyte precursors and differentiation. The timing would be consistent with a mode of action based on cell kinetics. Enzyme inhibitors would be expected to be effective within a few hours, and the rapidity with which cyclo-oxygenase inhibitors exert analgesic effects shows this to be true. Immunosuppressive drugs would be expected to take rather longer to be effective, because ongoing immunopathological events involve complex interactions of lymphocytes and effector cells which are not subject to such rapid regulation. Nevertheless, effects of drugs such as methotrexate and cyclosporin in RA are demonstrable in 1 or 2 months. The time course of long-acting drugs suggests that they may be exerting effects on a population of cells participating in the pathogenesis of RA but turning over rather slowly. Since these drugs are clearly not immunosuppressives, it is unlikely that lymphocytes (or at least major subsets of lymphocytes) are their principal target.

The main cell type co-operating with lymphocytes in the pathogenesis of chronic inflammation is of the monocyte–macrophage lineage. We therefore explored the possibility that long-acting antirheumatic drugs might inhibit the proliferation of monocyte precursors and accelerate their differentiation into mature monocyte-derived macrophages with decreased capacity to produce IL-1 and other inflammatory mediators. As reviewed in the section on IL-1, precursors cells do not produce IL-1; early differentiated cells, corresponding to peripheral blood monocytes, show the maximal response, and terminally differentiated cells such as alveolar macrophages produce very little IL-1 when stimulated. A drug inhibiting the multiplication of monocyte precursors in the bone marrow and accelerating their differentiation might therefore over a period of months reduce the number of cells in rheumatoid synovia producing IL-1 and other mediators of inflammation. This explanation for the efficacy of long-acting antirheumatic drugs is shown diagrammatically in Figure 13.5.

For the initial experiments we used auranofin. As shown in Figures 13.6 and 13.7, auranofin is indeed a potent inhibitor of the proliferation of the U-937 human promonocytic cell line and inducer of differentiation, as manifested by several markers[121].

## Total lymphoid irradiation

A procedure for irradiating the spleen and lymph nodes, but sparing as far as possible the bone marrow, was developed at Stanford University for treatment of Hodgkin's disease. Total lymphoid irradiation (TLI) was found to benefit patients with intractable rheumatoid arthritis. The efficacy of the procedure in the majority of patients, but not all, has been shown in a double-blind, randomized trial at Stanford as well as in other centres.

Recently our group has collaborated with that of S. Strober at Stanford to study in detail immune functions of, and mediator production by, peripheral blood and synovial cells of 11 severe RA patients before treatment and 4 months following TLI[53]. After TLI the most notable change in peripheral blood was a decrease in the number of Leu-3$^+$ T lymphocytes and their capacity to function as helpers for antibody formation in culture. In all patients

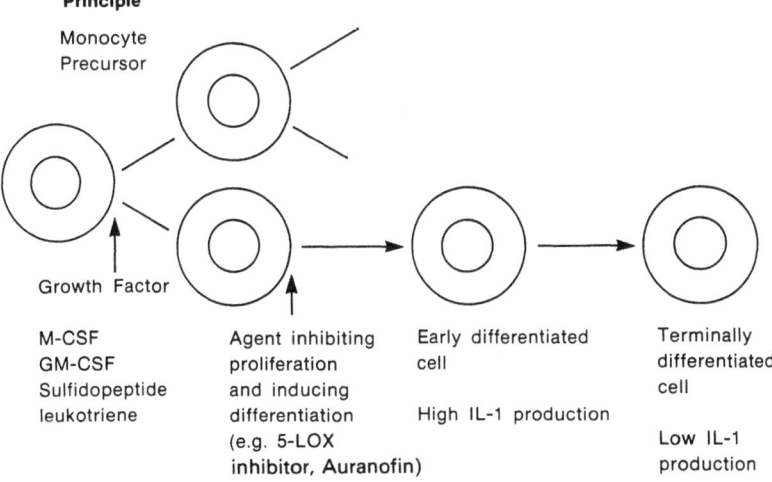

**Figure 13.5**  Diagram of our hypothesis of the mode of action of long-acting antirheumatic drugs. These agents inhibit proliferation and accelerate differentiation of cells of the monocyte–macrophage lineage. Eventually they will deplete the pools of precursors and early differentiated cells, thereby decreasing IL-1 production

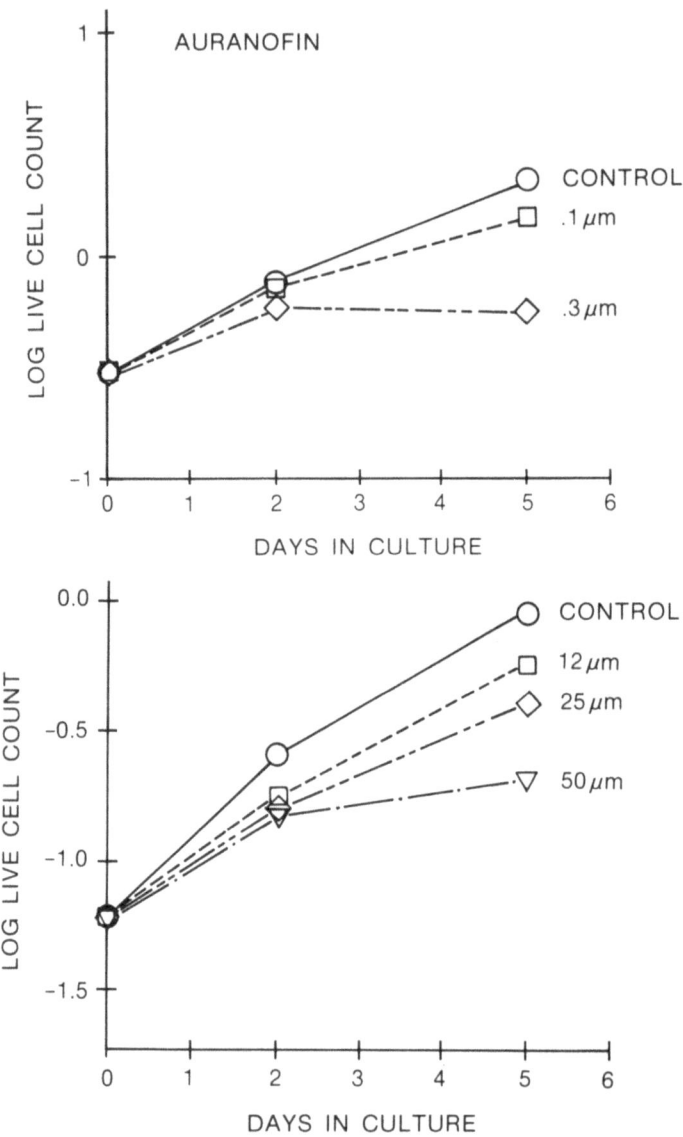

**Figure 13.6** Inhibition by (a) auranofin (above) and (b) a selective 5-lipoxygenase inhibitor, AA 861 (below) of the proliferation of U-937 cells (Data of R. Waters and A.C. Allinson)

who showed clinical improvement, production of IL-1 by RA synovial tissues was decreased (Figure 13.8). In contrast the levels of IgM, IgA and IgG rheumatoid factors, and of C3 in the blood and synovial fluid, did not change significantly. The capacity of peripheral blood mononuclear cells to produce IL-1 following stimulation with LPS was not reduced following TLI, and the number of cells of the monocyte–macrophage lineage (staining with Leu-M3)

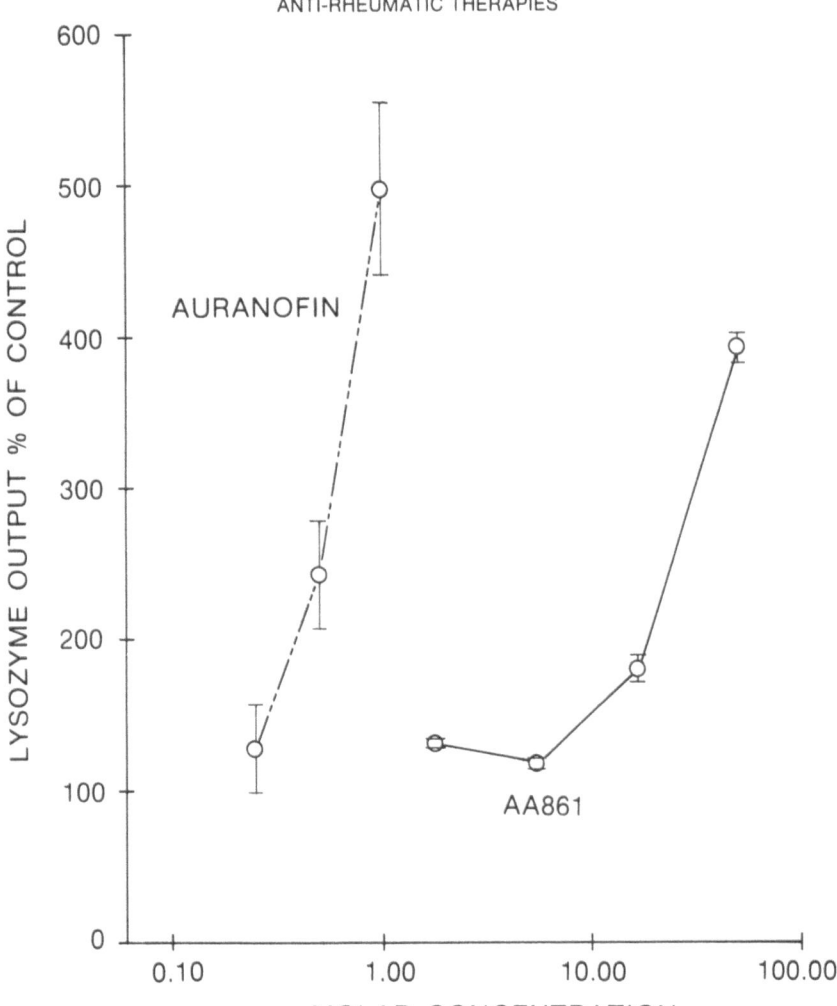

**Figure 13.7** Increased lysozyme output by U-937 cells exposed to auranofin and to a selective 5-lipoxygenase inhibitor AA 861 (Data of R. Waters and A.C. Allinson)

in the synovium showed no detectable change.

These observations are consistent with the interpretation that production of IL-1 by RA synovial tissue contributes to the signs and symptoms of the disease. They also suggest that a radiosensitive cell type migrating from lymphoid tissues to the synovium contributes to IL-1 production. Since the concentrations of rheumatoid factors, including IgG rheumatoid factor, are unchanged following TLI, it seems unlikely that they are driving the immunopathology of RA. The formation of rheumatoid factors may not require T cell help, which is sensitive to TLI. Possibly this is because rheumatoid factors are made by Leu-1[+] B lymphocytes (see page 216).

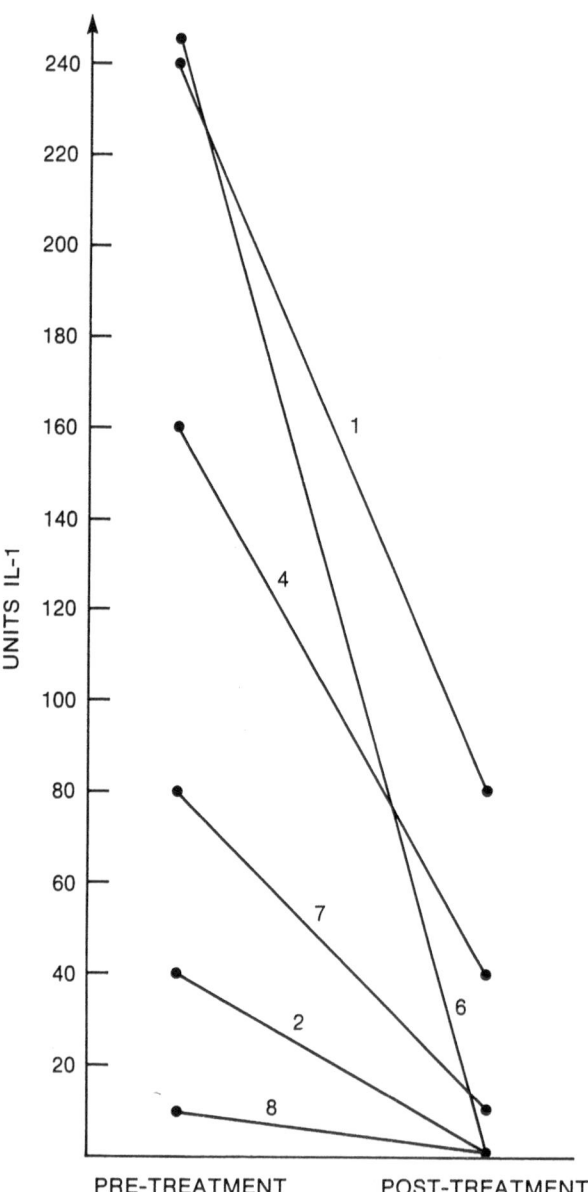

**Figure 13.8** Production of IL-1 by synovial tissue of patients with rheumatoid arthritis before and following treatment with total lymphoid irradiation. The numbers refer to individual patients. Patient number 8 showed no clinical improvement. (Data from reference 53)

## Thoracic duct drainage

Several groups of investigators have reported that thoracic duct drainage (TDD) after a remarkably short interval of a few days can improve symptoms and signs in patients with severe RA[122]. The beneficial effects of TDD have usually been attributed to immunosuppression. However, Ueo et al.[123] found that following TDD the number of mononuclear cells in RA synovia was decreased. They suggest that TDD accelerates the migration of lymphocytes from peripheral tissues to the circulating blood. The same authors point out that thoracic duct lymphocytes contain about 40% B cells, so TDD does not selectively deplete T cells as was formerly thought.

## GENERAL DISCUSSION

With so many cell types and mediators interacting in the pathogenesis of RA (Figure 13.9), no dogmatic conclusions can be given. The discussion of several points that follows is intended as a guide to current thinking and a statement of unresolved questions.

## The role of IL-1

The role of IL-1 as a central mediator of inflammation and joint erosion in RA is conceptually appealing. Among unresolved questions are which cell types in RA synovia produce IL-1 and how they are activated. The most obvious candidates as high producers of IL-1$\beta$ are monocyte-derived macrophages, but immature connective tissue cells associated with areas of cartilage and bone erosion may also be major producers of IL-1$\alpha$, especially in certain phases of the disease. What induces IL-1 production? Self-aggregating IgG can induce IL-1 formation, and C3b, which can activate monocytes to produce prostaglandins, may also induce IL-1 formation. Products of activated T lymphocytes might also be inducers, but since the formation of other T lymphocyte products (IL-2 and IFN-$\gamma$) is suppressed in RA synovia this possibility remains uncertain.

IL-1 formation is naturally regulated by glucocorticoids and inducers of differentiation. These regulatory effects are used in therapy with glucocorticoid analogues and long-acting antirheumatic drugs. Total lymphoid irradiation also decreases IL-1 formation by RA synovia.

## B lymphocytes

B lymphocytes in RA synovia are activated to produce Igs, including rheumatoid factors, at a high rate. In patients with systemic manifestations of disease (nodules and vasculitis) this is also true in extra-articular sites. What is activating the B lymphocytes? Conceivably they are being stimulated by an exogenous antigen not yet defined. They are certainly being stimulated by some autoantigens, notably Ig. An interesting possibility is that some types of rheumatoid factor can cross-link surface membrane Ig on B

235

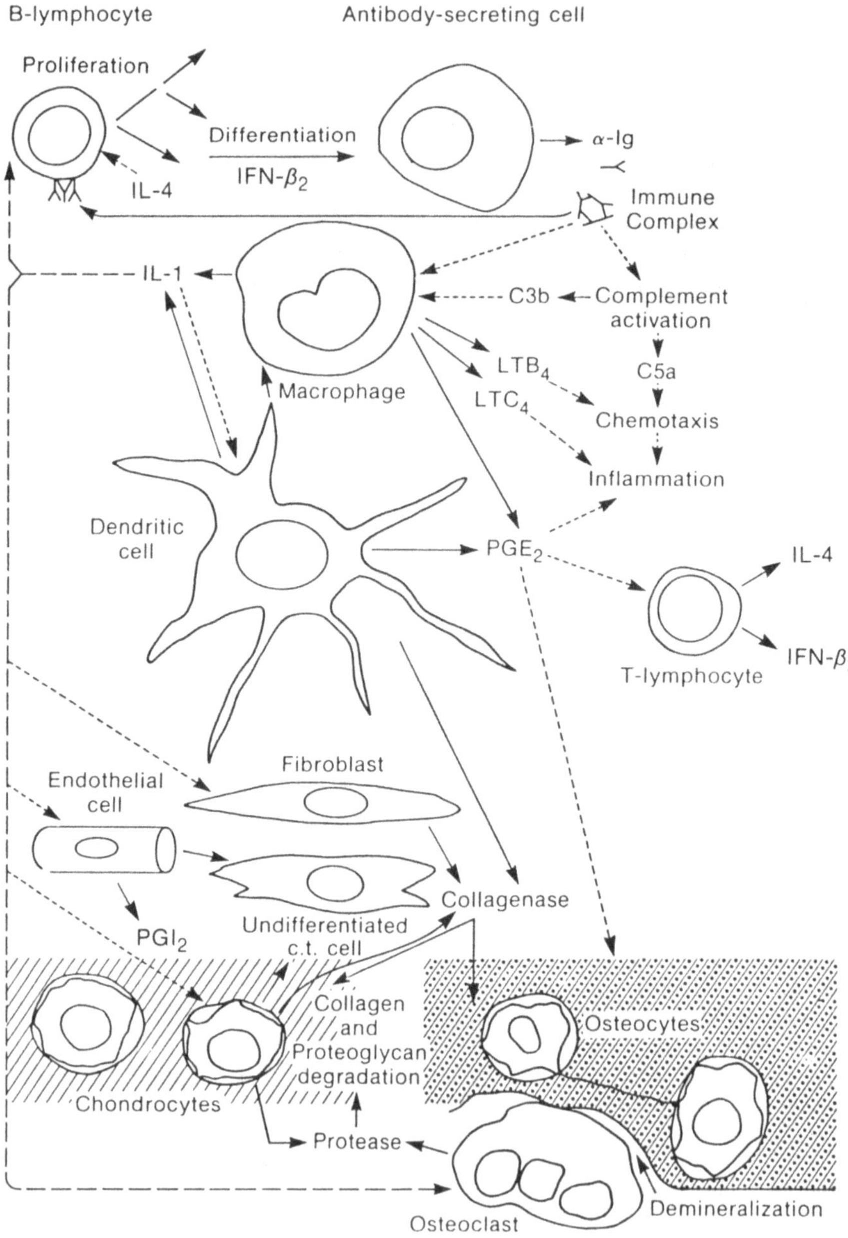

**Figure 13.9** Diagram of interactions of cells and mediators in the pathogenesis of rheumatoid arthritis

lymphocytes and provide one signal for activation, as anti-Ig and Staphylo-coccus protein A can do. Second signals for B lymphocyte proliferation and differentiation might include IL-4 and IFN-$\beta_2$. It would be interesting to know whether these are produced in RA synovia and, if so, by what cell types. The increased production of IFN-$\beta_2$ observed in mice and humans with autoimmune diseases focuses attention on this mediator of B cell growth and differentiation.

Another novel point to emerge during the last few years is the role of the Leu-1$^+$ subset of B lymphocytes in the production of rheumatoid factors and other autoantibodies. More information about how this subset is activated, whether their responses are T-independent, and their capacity to produce mediators other than Igs is required.

## T lymphocytes

The paradox that has recently become apparent is that while there are many T lymphocytes in RA synovia, and about half of them show signs of activation such as expression of MHC II glycoproteins, they are not producing some characteristic mediators of activated T cells, IL-2 and IFN-$\gamma$. This does not appear to be due to the recruitment into the synovium of a subset of T lymphocytes unable to produce these mediators. We have found that lymphocytes recovered from RA synovium activated by mitogens produce abundant IL-2. Although PGE$_2$ is a likely inhibitor of T cell mediator production, there are probably other inhibitors as well. When we cultured RA synovium with indomethacin, their capacity to produce IL-2 was sometimes restored but usually was not. Other inhibitors not yet fully characterized[83,84] may be involved. Inhibitors may also suppress in varying degrees responses of RA peripheral blood cells to mitogens and following Epstein-Barr virus infection[82,84]. However, dilution experiments (which reduce suppression) show that there is no intrinsic deficiency in the capacity of peripheral blood lymphocytes of RA patients to produce IL-2[85].

The suggestion that defective IL-2 production in RA may explain the disorder of immunoregulation in this disease[82] is at present speculative. IL-2 is actually required for suppressor T cell activation[124]. The same is true of suggestions that abnormal ratios of CD4/CD8 T lymphocytes reflect a deficit of suppressor T lymphocytes in RA peripheral blood[43] or synovial tissue[17]. As stated above, CD4 and CD8 appear to define MHC I and MHC II restriction of interactions rather than helper or suppressor phenotypes[39], and full characterization of human suppressor phenotypes and products has not yet been achieved. The complexity of the situation is illustrated by observations that in one model of suppression (responses to Candida and diphtheria toxoid) a subset of CD4$^+$ cells induces CD8$^+$ cells to express a suppressor phenotype[125].

Despite the lack of production of IL-2 and IFN-$\gamma$ in RA synovia, T lymphocytes may be producing other mediators such as GM-CSF, IL-4 and IFN-$\beta_2$; further studies on these points are required.

## Rheumatoid factors

The presence of antiglobulins or rheumatoid factors of various classes in the peripheral blood and synovial fluid of patients with RA has long been recognized. Most attention has been given to IgM, which in the presence of aggregated IgG on a surface, can activate complement by the classical pathway[6]. IgG rheumatoid factors can self-associate to form stable complexes which can also activate complement and induce the production of IL-1 by monocytes[60]. The presence of such complexes in the peripheral blood is associated with decreased serum complement levels. However, levels of IgM, IgG and IgA rheumatoid factors are not decreased in the sera or synovial fluids of severe RA patients showing a good clinical response to total lymphoid irradiation, suggesting that mediators other than rheumatoid factors play a major role in pathogenesis[53].

## Complement

Evidence has accumulated that the classical pathway of complement can be activated in RA synovia and synovial fluid, and sometimes in the peripheral blood of RA patients[6]. The activation of complement is at least partly due to the interaction of IgM rheumatoid factor with aggregated IgG. Self-aggregating IgG–anti-IgG can also activate complement[23]. IgG immune complexes able to activate complement have been extracted from RA synovia; these may partly be composed of self-aggregating IgG.

Among the effects of complement cleavage products, which have been detected in synovial fluid, is chemotaxis of leukocytes, which is mainly due to C5a.

## The state of activation of cells in RA synovia

Evidence has been presented that B lymphocytes in RA synovia are fully activated whereas T lymphocytes show some signs of activation but not others. Cells of the monocyte–macrophage lineage, and perhaps some other cell types, are producing IL-1. Proliferating synovial tissue can invade cartilage, and Harris[126] has suggested that it may be considered 'aggressive, and, in a sense, malignant'. Fassbender[8] also likens the immature connective tissue cells invading cartilage to mesenchymal tumours.

We have found in RA synovia remarkably high levels of expression of the proto-oncogenes c-fos and c-myc (Figure 13.3). These proto-oncogenes are observed in activated promonocytic cell lines[127] and also in activated lymphocytes and fibroblasts[36]. The expression of c-fos and c-myc in rheumatoid synovia is an indication of ongoing activation. Whether this is due to the production of activating factors by an immunopathological reaction, to a virus infection or to a process with some features of malignant transformation is not clear. Since at least some types of malignancy are attributed to unregulated oncogene expression, the distinction between malignancy and non-malignant activation of tissues such as rheumatoid synovia may be semantic rather than real. More important would be establishing the presence of a causative agent such as a virus, and definition of whether the immunopathological reaction is driven by T or B lymphocytes, a question that is still open.

# References

1. Hasler, F., Bluestein, H.G., Zwaifler, N.J. and Epstein, L.B. (1983). Analysis of the defects responsible for the impaired regulation of EBV-induced B-cell proliferation by rheumatoid arthritis lymphocytes. II. Role of monocytes and the increased sensitivity of rheumatoid arthritis lymphocytes to prostaglandin E. *J. Immunol.*, **131**, 768–72
2. Allison, A.C. (1977). Autoimmune diseases: Concepts of pathogenesis and control. In Talal, N. (ed.) *Autoimmunity: Genetic, Virologic, and Clinical Aspects.* pp. 92–139. (New York, London: Academic Press)
3. Schwartz, R.S. and Rose, N.R. (eds.) (1986). Autoimmunity: experimental and clinical aspects. *Ann. N.Y. Acad. Sci.*, **475**, 1–427
4. Budd, R.C., Cerottini, J.-C., Horvath, C., Bron, C., Pedrazzini, T., Howe, R.C. and MacDonald, H.R. (1987). Distinction of virgin and memory T lymphocytes. *J. Immunol.*, **138**, 3120–9
5. Klickstein, L.B., Shapleigh, C. and Goetzl, E.J. (1980). Lipoxygenation of arachidonic acid as a source of polymorphonuclear chemotactic factors in synovial fluid and tissue in rheumatoid arthritis and spondyloarthritis. *J. Clin. Invest.*, **66**, 1166–70
6. Zwaifler, N.J. (1973). The immunopathology of joint inflammation in rheumatoid arthritis. *Adv. Immunol.*, **16**, 265–336
7. Mohr, W., Menninger, H. and Putzier, R. (1979). Morphologische Hinweise für die Beteiligung an der rheumatischen Knorpel-destruktion. *Bull. Schweiz. Akad. Med. Wiss.*, **35**, 443–51
8. Fassbender, H.G. and Simmling-Annefeld, M. (1983). The potential aggressiveness of synovial tissue in rheumatoid arthritis. *J. Pathol.*, **139**, 399–406
9. Souza, L.M., Boone, T.C., Gabrilone, J., Lai, P.H., Zsebo, K.M., Murdock, D.C., Chazin, V.R., Bruszewski, J., Lu, H., Chen, K.K., Barendt, J., Platzer, E., Moore, M.A.S., Mertelsmann, R. and Welta, K. (1986). Recombinant human granulocyte colony-stimulating factor: effects on normal and leukemic myeloid cells. *Science*, **232**, 61–5
10. Kawasaki, E.S., Ladner, M.B., Wang, A.M., Van Arsdell, J., Warren, M.K., Coyne, M.Y., Schweickart, V.L., Lee, M.-T., Wilson, K.J., Boosman, A., Stanley, E.R., Ralph, P. and Mark, D.F. (1985). Molecular cloning of a complementary DNA encoding human macrophage-specific colony-stimulating factor (CSF-1). *Science*, **230**, 291–4
11. Cantrell, M.A., Anderson, D., Cerretti, D.P., Price, V., McKereghan, K., Tushinski, R.J., Mochizuki, D.Y., Larsen, A., Grabstein, K., Gillis, S. and Cosman, D. (1985). Cloning, sequence and expression of a human granulocyte/macrophage colony-stimulating factor. *Proc. Natl. Acad. Sci. USA*, **82**, 6250–4
12 Sherr, C.J., Rettenmeier, C.W., Socca, R., Roussel, M.F., Look, A.T. and Stanley, E.R. (1985). The *c-fms* proto-oncogene product is related to the receptor for mononuclear phagocyte growth factor, CSF-1. *Cell*, **41**, 665–76
13. Nishizuka, Y. (1986). Perspectives on the role of protein kinase C in stimulus-response coupling. *J. Natl. Cancer Inst.*, **763**, 363–70
14. Berridge, M.J. and Irvine, R.F. (1984). Inositol triphosphate, a novel second messenger in cellular signal transduction. *Nature*, **312**, 315–21
15. Waters, R. and Allison, A.C. (1987). Differentiation of promonocytic and promyelocytic human cell lines induced by 5-lipoxygenase inhibitors and leukotriene $D_4$ antagonists. (Submitted)
16. Burmester, G.R., Dimitriu-Bona, A., Waters, S.J. and Winchester, R.J. (1983). Identification of three major synovial lining cell populations by monoclonal antibodies directed to Ia antigens and antigens associated with monocytes/macrophages and fibroblasts. *Scand. J. Immunol.*, **17**, 69–82

17. Duke, O., Panayi, G.S., Janossy, G. and Poulter, L.W. (1982). Immuno-histological analysis of the lymphocytic infiltrates of rheumatoid synovial membrane using monoclonal antibodies. *Ann. Rheum. Dis.*, **41**, 192–3

18. Hoefsmit, E.C.M., Balfour, B.M., Kamperdijk, E.W.A. et al. (1979). Cells containing Birbeck granules in the lymph and the lymph nodes. In Muller-Bucholz, W. and Moller-Hermelinck, H.K. (eds.) *Function and Structure of the Immune System. Adv. Exp. Med. Biol.*, **114**, 389–98

19. Peeler, J.S. and Niederkorn, J.Y. (1986). Antigen presentation by Langerhans cells *in vivo*: donor-derived Ia+ Langerhans cells are required for induction of delayed hypersensitivity but not for cytotoxic T lymphocyte responses to alloantigens. *J. Immunol.*, **136**, 4362–71

20. Meijer, C.J.L.M., de Graaf-Reitsma, C.B. Lafeber, G.J.M. and Cats, A. (1982). *In situ* localization of lymphocyte subsets in synovial membranes of patients with rheumatoid arthritis with monoclonal antibodies. *J. Rheumatol.*, **9**, 359–65

21. Klaus, G.G., Humphrey, J.H., Kunkl, A. and Dongworth, D.W. (1980). The follicular dendritic cell: its role in antigen presentation in the generation of immunological memory. *Immunol. Rev.*, **53**, 3–28

22. Tew, J.G., Phipps, R.P. and Mandel, T.E. (1980). The maintenance and regulation of the humoral immune response: persisting antigen and the role of follicular antigen-binding dendritic cells as accessory cells. *Immunol. Rev.*, **53**, 175–201

23. Mannick, M. and Nardella, F.A. (1983). Self-associating IgG-rheumatoid factors. In Shiokawa, Y., Abe, T. and Yamauchi, Y. (eds. ) *New Horizons in Rheumatoid Arthritis.* pp. 124–31. (Amsterdam: Excerpta Medica)

24. Fassbender, H. (1980). *Pathology of Rheumatoid Disease.* pp. 2–143. (Heidelberg: Springer)

25. Young, C.L., Adamson, T.C. III, Vaughan, J.H. and Fox, R.I. (1984). Immunohistologic characterization of synovial membrane lymphocytes in rheumatoid arthritis. *Arthr. Rheum.*, **27**, 32–9

26. Smiley, J.D., Sachs, C. and Ziff, M. (1968). *In vitro* synthesis of immunoglobulin by rheumatoid synovial membrane. *J. Clin. Invest.*, **47**, 624–32

27. Wernick, R.M., Lipsky, P.E., Marban-Arcos, E., Maliakkol, J.J., Edelbaum, D. and Ziff, M. (1985). IgG and IgM rheumatoid factor synthesis in rheumatoid synovial membrane cell cultures. *Arthr. Rheum.*, **28**, 742–51

28. Sliwinski, A.J. and Zvaifler, N.J. (1970). *In vivo* synthesis of IgG by the rheumatoid synovial membrane. *J. Lab. Clin. Med.*, **76**, 304–10

29. Al-Balaghi, S., Strom, H. and Möller, E. (1984). B-cell differentiation factor in synovial fluid of patients with rheumatoid arthritis. *Immunol. Rev.*, **78**, 7–23

30. Bell, D.A. and Pinto, J. (1984). Distribution of activated B lymphocytes in the circulation and synovial fluid in rheumatoid arthritis. *Clin. Immunol. Immunopathol.*, **31**, 272–81

31. Teodorescu, M., Chang, J.L. and Skosey, J.L. (1981). Polyclonal B-cell activator associated with alpha-2-macroglobulin in the serum of patients with rheumatoid arthritis. *Int. Arch. Allergy Appl. Immunol.*, **66**, 1–12

32. Casali, P., Burastero, S.E., Nakamura, M., Inghirami, G. and Notkins, A.L. (1987). Human lymphocytes making rheumatoid factor and antibody to ssDNA belong to Leu-1+ B-cell subset. *Science*, **236**, 77–81

33. Hardy, R.R., Hayakawa, K., Shimizu, M., Yamasaki, K. and Kishimoto, T. (1987). Rheumatoid factor secretion from human Leu-1+ B-cells. *Science*, **236**, 81–3

34. Plater-Zyberk, C., Maini, R.N., Lam, K., Kennedy, T.D. and Janossy, G. (1985). A rheumatoid arthritis B cell subset expresses a phenotype similar to that in chronic lymphocytic leukemia. *Arthr. Rheum.*, **28**, 971–6

35. Mossman, T.R., Cherwinski, H., Bard, M.W., Giedlin, M.A. and Coffman (1986). Two types of murine helper T-cell clone. I. Definition according to profiles of lymphokine activities and secreted proteins. *J. Immunol.*, **136**, 2348–57

36. Cleveland, J.L., Rapp, U.R. and Farrar, W.L. (1987). Role of *c-myc* and other genes in interleukin-2 regulated CT6 lymphocytes and their malignant variants. *J. Immunol.*, **138**, 3495–504

37. Culpepper, J. and Lee, F. (1987). Glucocorticoid regulation of lymphokine production by murine T lymphocytes. In Webb, D.R. and Goeddel, D.V. (eds.) *Molecular Cloning and Analysis of Lymphokines.* pp. 275–89. (Orlando: Academic Press)

38. Chouaib, S., Welte K., Mortelsman, R. and Dupont, B. (1985). Prostaglandin $E_2$ acts at two distinct pathways of T lymphocyte activation: inhibition of interleukin 2 production and down-regulation of transferrin receptor expression. *J. Immunol.*, **135**, 1172–9

39. Germain, R.N. and Malissen, B. (1986). Analysis of the expression and function of class II major histocompatibility complex-encoded molecules by DNA-mediated gene transfer. *Annu. Rev. Immunol.*, **4**, 281–315
40. McDougal, J.S., Mawle, A., Cort, S.P., Nicholson, J.K.A., Cross, G.D., Scheppler-Campbell, J.A., Hicks, D. and Sligh, J. (1985). Cellular tropism of the human retrovirus HTLV/III/LAV I. Role of T-cell activation and expression of the T4 antigen. *J. Immunol.*, **135**, 3151–62
41. Burmester, G., Irani, Y.D., Kunkel, H., Winchester, R. (1981). Ia⁺ T-cells in synovial fluid and tissues of patients with rheumatoid arthritis. *Arthr. Rheum.*, **24**, 1370–6
42. Reinherz, E.L., Kung, P.C. Pesando, J.M., Ritz, J., Goldstein, R. and Schlossman, S.F. (1979). Ia determinants on human T-cell subsets defined by monoclonal antibody. Activation stimuli required for expression. *J. Exp. Med.*, **150**, 1472–82
43. Veys, E.M., Hermanns, P., Goldstein, G., Kung, P., Schindler, J. and van Wauve, J. (1981). Determination of T lymphocyte subpopulations by monoclonal antibodies in rheumatoid arthritis. Influence of immunomodulating agents. *Int. J. Immunopharmacol.*, **3**, 313–9
44. Forre, O., Thoen, J., Lea, T., Dobloug, J.H., Mellbye, O.J., Natvig, J.B., Pahle, J. and Solheim, B.G. (1982). *In situ* characterization of mononuclear cells in rheumatoid tissues, using monoclonal antibodies: no reduction of T8-positive cells or augmentation in T4-positive cells. *Scand. J. Immunol.*, **16**, 315–9
45. Auron, P.E., Webb, A.C., Rosenwasser, J.J., Mucci, S.F., Rich, A., Wolff, S.M. and Dinarello, C.A. (1984). Nucleotide sequence of human monocyte interleukin-1 precursor cDNA. *Proc. Natl. Acad. Sci. USA*, **81**, 7907–11
46. March, C.J., Mosley, B., Larsen, A., Cerretti, D.P., Braedt, G., Price, V., Gillis, S., Henney, C.S., Kronheim, S.R., Grabstein, K., Conlon, P.J., Hopp, T.P. and Cosman, D. (1985). Cloning, sequence, and expression of two distinct human interleukin-1(IL-1) cDNAs. *Nature*, **315**, 641–7
47. Gubler, V., Chua, A.O., Stern, A.S., Hellmann, C.P., Vitek, M.P., Dechiara, T.M., Benjamin, W.R., Collier, K.J., Dukovitch, M., Familletti, P.C., Fielder-Nagy, C., Jensen, J., Kaffka, K., Kibian, P.L., Stremlo, D., Wittreich, B.H., Woehle, D., Mizel, S.B. and Lomedico, P.T. (1986). Recombinant human interleukin 1α: purification and biological characterization. *J. Immunol.*, **136**, 2492–7
48. Dower, S.K., Kronheim, S.R., March, C.J., Conlon, P.J., Hoff, T.P., Gillis, S. and Urdal, D. (1985). Detection and characterization of high affinity plasma membrane receptors for interleukin 1. *J. Exp. Med.*, **162**, 501–15
49. Kenney, J.S., Masada, M.P., Eugui, E.M., De Lustro, B., Mulkins, M.A. and Allison, A.C. (1987). Monoclonal antibodies to human recombinant interleukin 1β: quantitation of IL-1β and inhibition of biological activity. *J. Immunol.*, **138**, 4236–242
50. Bayne, E.K., Rupp, E.A., Limjuco, G., Chin, J. and Schmidt, J.A. (1986). Immunocyto-chemical detection of interleukin 1 within stimulated human monocytes. *J. Exp. Med.*, **163**, 1267–80
51. Fontana, A., Hengartner, H., Weber, E., Fehr, K., Grob, P.K. and Cohen, G. (1982). Interleukin-1 activity in the synovial fluid of patients with rheumatoid arthritis. *Rheumatol. Int.*, **2**, 49–53
52. Wood, D.D., Ihrie, E.J., Dinarello, C.A. and Cohen, P.L. (1983). Isolation of an interleukin-1-like factor from human joint effusions. *Arthr. Rheum.*, **26**, 975–83
53. Gaston, J.S.H., Strober, S., Solovera, J.J., Gaudow, D., Lane, N., Schurman, D., Hoppe, R.T., Chen, R.C., Eugui, E.M., Vaughan, J.H. and Allison, A.C. (1987). Dissection of the mechanisms of immune injury in rheumatoid arthritis using total lymphoid irradiation. *Arthr. Rheum.* (In press)
54. Gery, I. and Lepe-Zuniga, J.L. (1984). Interleukin 1: uniqueness of its production and spectrum of activities. *Lymphokines*, **9**, 109–25
55. Di Giovine, F.S., Malawista, S.E., Nuki, G. and Duff, G.W. (1987). Interleukin 1 (IL-1) as a mediator of crystal arthritis. Stimulation of T-cell and synovial fibroblast mitogenesis by urate crystal-induced IL-1. *J. Immunol.*, **138**, 3213–8
56. Oppenheim, J.J., Togawa, A., Chedid, L. and Naizel, S. (1980). Components of mycobacteria and muramyl dipeptide with adjuvant activity induce lymphocyte-activating factor. *Cell. Immunol.*, **50**, 71–81
57. Habicht, G.S., Beck, G., Benach, J.L., Coleman, J.L. and Leichtling, K.D. (1985). Lyme disease spirochetes induce human and murine interleukin 1 production. *J. Immunol.*, **134**, 3147–54

241

58. Waters, R.V., Terrell, T. and Jones, G.H. (1986). Uveitis induction in the rabbit by muramyl dipeptides. *Infect. Immun.*, **51**, 816–25
59. Chou, Y.K., Sherwood, T. and Virella, G. (1985). Erythrocyte bound immune complexes trigger the release of interleukin-1 from human monocytes. *Cell. Immunol.*, **91**, 308–14
60. Nardella, F.A., Dayer, J.-M., Roelke, M., Krane, S.M. and Mannik, M. (1983). Self-associating IgG rheumatoid factors stimulate monocytes to release prostaglandins and mononuclear cell factor that stimulates collagenase and prostaglandin production by synovial cells. *Rheumatol. Int.*, **3**, 183–6
61. Farr, A.G., Kiely, J.-M. and Unanue, E.A. (1979). Macrophage-T-cell interactions involving *Listeria monocytogenes:* role of the H2 gene-complex. *J. Immunol.*, **122**, 2395–404
62. Moore, R.N., Oppenheim, J.J., Farrar, J.J., Carter, C.S. Jr., Waheed, A. and Shadduck, R.K. (1980). Production of LAF (IL-1) by macrophages activated with colony-stimulating factors. *J. Immunol.*, **125**, 1302–5
63. Arenzana-Seisdedos, F., Virelizier, J.-L. and Fiers, W. (1985). Interferons as macrophage-activating factors. III. Preferential effects of interferon-γ on the interleukin 1 secretory potential of fresh or aged human monocytes. *J. Immunol.*, **134**, 2444–8
64. Bevilacqua, M.P., Pober, J.S., Wheeler, M.E., Cotran, R.S. and Gimbrone, M.A. Jr. (1985). Interleukin 1 acts on cultured human vascular endothelium to increase the adhesion of polymorphonuclear leukocytes, monocytes and related leukocyte cell lines. *J. Clin. Invest.*, **76**, 2003–11
65. Cavender, D.E., Haskard, D.O., Joseph, B. and Ziff, M. (1986). Interleukin 1 increases the binding of human B and T lymphocytes to endothelial cell monolayers. *J. Immunol.*, **136**, 203–7
66. Dayer, J.-M. and Demczuk, S. (1984). Cytokines and other mediators in rheumatoid arthritis. *Springer Semin. Immunopathol.*, **7**, 387–413
67. Rossi, V., Brevario, F., Ghezzi, P., Dejana, E. and Mantovani, A. (1985). Prostacyclin synthesis induced in vascular cells by interleukin-1. *Science*, **229**, 174–6
68. Schnyder, J., Payne, T. and Dinarello, C.A. (1987). Human monocyte or recombinant interleukin 1's are specific for the secretion of a metalloproteinase from chondrocytes. *J. Immunol.*, **138**, 496–503
69. Smith, R.L., Allison, A.C. and Schurman, D.J. (1987). Inhibition of interleukin-1 (IL-1) induced articular cartilage degradation by actinomycin D and cycloheximide. *J. Orthopaed. Res.* (In press)
70. Fell, H.B. and Jubb, R.W. (1977). The effect of synovial tissue on the breakdown of articular cartilage in culture. *Arthr. Rheum.*, **20**, 1359–71
71. Saklatvala, J., Sarsfield, S.J. and Townsend, Y. (1985). Pig interleukin 1. Purification of two immunologically different leukocyte proteins that cause cartilage resorption, lymphocyte activation and fever. *J. Exp. Med.*, **162**, 1208–20
72. Gowen, M., Wood, D.D., Ihrie, E.J., McGuire, M.K.B. and Russell, R.G.G. (1983). An interleukin-1-like factor stimulates bone resorption *in vitro*. *Nature*, **306**, 378–80
73. Stashenko, P., Dewhirst, F.E., Peros, W.J., Kent, R. and Ago, J.M. (1987). Synergistic interactions between interleukin-1, tumour necrosis factor, and lymphotoxin in bone resorption. *J. Immunol.*, **138**, 1464–8
74. Shore, A., Jaglal, S. and Keystone, E.C. (1986). Enhanced interleukin-1 generation by monocytes is temporally linked to an early event in the onset or exacerbation of rheumatoid arthritis. *Clin. Exp. Immunol.*, **65**, 293–302
75. Danis, V.A., March, L.M., Nelson, D.S. and Brooks, P.M. (1987). Interleukin-1 secretion by peripheral blood monocytes and synovial macrophages from patients with rheumatoid arthritis. *J. Rheumatol.*, **14**, 33–9
76. Pennick, D., Yang, G., Gemmell, L. and Lee, F. (1987). Control of hemopoiesis by a bone marrow stromal cell clone: lipopolysaccharide- and interleukin-1-inducible production of colony-stimulating factors. *Blood*, **69**, 682–91
77. Schooley, J.C., Kullgren, B. and Allison, A.C. (1987). Inhibition of interleukin 1 of the action of erythropoietin on erythroid precursors and its possible role in the pathogenesis of hypoplastic anaemias. *Br. J. Haematol.*, **67**
78. Lee, S.W., Tsou, A.-P., Chan, H., Thomas, J., Petrie, K., Eugui, E.M. and Allison, A.C. (1987). Glucocorticoids selectively inhibit the transcription of interleukin-1 genes and decrease the stability of IL-1β mRNA. *Proc. Natl. Acad. Sci. USA* (In press)

79. Wevers, M.D., Rennard, S.I., Hance, A.J., Bitteman, P.B. and Crystal, R.G. (1984). Normal human macrophages obtained by bronchoalveolar lavage have a limited capacity to release interleukin-1. *J. Clin. Invest.*, **74**, 2208–18

80. Egeland, T. and Lund, H. (1987). Immunoregulating lymphokines in rheumatoid joints. I. Search for interleukin-2 in synovial fluid. *Scand. J. Immunol.*, **25**, 101–6

81. Husby, G. and Williams, R.C. Jr. (1985). Immunohistochemical studies of interleukin-2 and γ-interferon in rheumatoid arthritis. *Arthr. Rheum.*, **28**, 174–81

82. Combe, B., Pope, R.M., Fischbach, M., Darnell, B., Baron, S. and Talal, N. (1985). Interleukin-2 in rheumatoid arthritis: production and response to interleukin-2 in rheumatoid synovial fluid, synovial tissue and peripheral blood. *Clin. Exp. Immunol.*, **59**, 520–8

83. Miossec, P., Kisiwado, T. and Ziff, M. (1987). Inhibitor of interleukin-2 in rheumatoid synovial fluid. *Arthr. Rheum.*, **30**, 121–9

84. Lotz, M., Tsoucas, C.D., Fong, S., Dinarello, C.A., Carson, D.A. and Vaughan, J.H. (1986). Release of lymphokines after infection with Epstein-Barr virus *in vitro*. II. A monocyte-dependent inhibitor of interleukin-2 and interferon-gamma in rheumatoid arthritis. *J. Immunol.*, **136**, 3643–8

85. McKenna, R.M., Ofosu-Apprah, W. and Warrington, R.J. (1986). Interleukin 2 production and responsiveness in active and inactive rheumatoid arthritis. *J. Rheumatol.*, **13**, 28–32

86. Preble, O.T., Black, R.J., Friedman, R.M., Klippel, J.H. and Vilcek, J. (1982). Systemic lupus erythematosus: presence in human serum of an unusual acid-labile leukocyte interferon. *Science*, **216**, 329–41

87. Malaise, M.G. and Franchimont, P. (1987). Defective *in vitro* γ-interferon production in rheumatoid arthritis. *Arthr. Rheum.*, **30**, 230–331

88. Hasler, F., Bluestein, H.G., Zwaifler, N.J. and Epstein, L.B. (1983). Analysis of the defects responsible for the impaired regulation of EBV-induced B-cell proliferation by rheumatoid arthritis lymphocytes. II. Role of monocytes and the increased sensitivity of rheumatoid arthritis lymphocytes to prostaglandin E. *J. Immunol.*, **131**, 768–72

89. Paul, W.E. and Ohara, J. (1987). B-cell stimulatory factor-1/interleukin 4. *Annu. Rev. Immunol.*, **5**, 429–59

90. Hirano, T., Taga, T., Yasukawa, K., Nakajima, K., Nakano, N., Takatsuki, T., Shimizu, M., Murashima, A., Tsunasokawa, S., Sakiyama, F. and Kishimoto, T. (1987). Human B-cell differentiation factor defined by an anti-peptide antibody and its role in autoantibody production. *Proc. Natl. Acad. Sci. USA*, **84**, 228–31

91. Sehgal P.B., May, L.T., Tamm, I. and Vilček, J. (1987). Human $\beta_2$-interferon and B-cell differentiation factor BSF-2 are identical. *Science*, **235**, 731–2

92. Klaus, G.C.B. and Havrylowicz, C.M. (1984). Activation and proliferation signals in mouse B cells. II. Evidence for activation ($G_0$ to $G_1$) signals differing in sensitivity to cyclosporine. *Eur. J. Immunol.*, **14**, 250–4

93. Varey, A.-M., Champion, B.R. and Cooke, A. (1986). Cyclosporine affects the function of antigen-presenting cells. *Immunology*, **57**, 111–4

94. Yamamoto, K.R. (1985). Steroid receptor regulated transcription of specific genes and gene networks. *Annu. Rev. Genet.*, **19**, 209–15

95. Flower, R.J. and Blackwell, G.J. (1979). Anti-inflammatory steroids induce synthesis of a phospholipase-$A_2$ inhibitor which prevents prostaglandin generation. *Nature*, **278**, 456–9

96. Hirata, F., Schiffman, E., Venkatsubramanian, K., Solomon, D. and Axelrod, J. (1980). A phospholipase $A_2$ inhibiting protein in rabbit neutrophils induced by glucocorticoids. *Proc. Natl. Acad. Sci. USA*, **77**, 2533–6

97. Wallner, B.P., Mattaliano, R.J., Hessian, C., Cate, R.L., Tizard, R., Sinclair, L.K., Foeller, C., Chow, E.P., Browning, J.L., Ramchandran, K.L. and Pepinsky, R.B. (1986). Cloning and expression of human lipocortin, a phospholipase $A_2$ inhibitor with potential anti-inflammatory activity. *Nature*, **320**, 72–5

98. Saris, C.J., Tack, B.F., Kristensen, T., Glenny, J.R. Jr. and Hunter, T. (1986). The cDNA sequence for the protein-tyrosine kinase substrate p36 (calpatin 1 heavy chain) reveals a multidomain protein with internal repeats. *Cell*, **46**, 201–12

99. Davidson, F.F., Dennis, E.A., Powell, M. and Glenney, J.R. Jr. (1987). Inhibition of phospholipase $A_2$ by 'lipocortins' and calpactins. An effect of binding to substrate phospholipids. *J. Biol. Chem.*, **262**, 1698–705

243

100. Snyder, D.S. and Unanue, E.R. (1982). Corticosteroids inhibit murine macrophage Ia expression and interleukin 1 production. *J. Immunol.*, **129**, 1803–5
101. Brinckerhoff, C.E., Plecinska, I.M., Sheldon, L.A. and O'Connor, G.T. (1986). Half life of synovial cell collagenase mRNA is modulated by phorbol myristate acetate but not by *all-trans*-retinoic acid or dexamethasone. *Biochemistry*, **25**, 6378–84
102. Leizer, T., Clarris, B.J., Ash, P.E., van Damme, J., Saklatvala, J. and Hamilton, J.A. (1987). Interleukin-1β and interleukin-1α stimulate synovial cells. *Arthr. Rheum.*, **30**, 562–6
103. Medcalf, R.L., Richards, R.I., Crawford, R.J. and Hamilton, J.A. (1986). Suppression of urokinase-type plasminogen activator mRNA levels in human fibrosarcoma cells and synovial fibroblasts by anti-inflammatory glucocorticoids. *EMBO J.*, **5**, 2217–22
104. Mitchell, M.D., Carr, B.R., Mason, J.I. and Simpson, G.R. (1982). Prostaglandin biosynthesis in the human fetal adrenal gland: regulation by glucocorticosteroids. *Proc. Natl. Acad. Sci. USA*, **79**, 7547–51
105. Crutchley, D.J., Ryan, U.S. and Ryan, J.W. (1985). Glucocorticoid modulation of prostacyclin production in cultured bovine pulmonary endothelial cells. *J. Rheum. Exp. Ther.*, **233**, 650–5
106. Hill, M.R., Smith, R.D. and McCallum, R.E. (1986). Interleukin 1: a regulatory role in glucocorticoid-regulated hepatic metabolism. *J. Immunol.*, **137**, 858–62
107. Mulkins, M. and Allison, A.C. (1987). Recombinant human interleukin-1 inhibits the induction by dexamethasone of alkaline phosphatase activity in murine capillary endothelial cells. *J. Cell Physiol.* (In press)
108. Bradley, L.M. and Mishell, R.I. (1982). Differential effects of glucocorticosteroids on the functions of subpopulations of helper T lymphocytes. *Eur. J. Immunol.*, **12**, 91–4
109. Paavonen, T. (1985). Glucocorticoids enhance the *in vitro* Ig synthesis of pokeweed mitogen-stimulated human B-cells by inhibiting the suppressive effect of T8$^+$ T cells. *Scand. J. Immunol.*, **21**, 63–71
110. Cockayne, D., Sterling, K.M. Jr., Shull, S., Mintz, K.P., Illeyne, S. and Cutroneo, K.R. (1986). Glucocorticoids decrease the synthesis of type 1 procollagen RNAs. *Biochemistry*, **25**, 3202–9
111. Forestier, J. (1922). The treatment of rheumatoid arthritis with gold salts injection. *Lancet*, **1**, 2235–7
112. Empire Rheumatism Council (1961). Gold therapy in rheumatoid arthritis: final report of a multicenter controlled trial. *Ann. Rheum. Dis.*, **21**, 315–33
113. Lipsky, P. and Ziff, M. (1977). Inhibition of antigen- and mitogen-induced human lymphocyte proliferation by gold compounds. *J. Clin. Invest.*, **59**, 455–66
114. Lipsky, P.E. (1981). Modulation of human antibody production *in vitro* by D-pencillamine and CuSO₄: inhibition of helper T-cell function. *J. Rheumatol.*, **9**, (Suppl. 7), 69–73
115. Hunneyball, I.M., Crossley, M.J. and Spowage, M. (1986). Pharmacological studies of antigen-induced arthritis in Balb/c mice. II. The effects of second-line antirheumatic drugs and cytotoxic agents on the histopathological changes. *Agents Actions*, **18**, 394–400
116. Paska, W., McDonald, K.J. and Croft, M. (1986). Studies on type II collagen induced arthritis in mice. *Agents Actions*, **18**, 413–20
117. Vernon-Roberts, B., Dore, J.L., Jessop, J.D. and Henderson, W.J. (1976). Selective concentration and localization of gold in macrophages of synovial and other tissues during and after chrysotherapy in rheumatoid patients. *Ann. Rheum. Dis.*, **35**, 477–86
118. Vernon-Roberts, B. (1979). Action of gold salts on the inflammatory response and inflammatory cell function. *J. Rheumatol.*, **6** (suppl. 5), 120–9
119. Hamilton, J.A. and Williams, N. (1985). *In vitro* inhibition of myelopoiesis by gold salts and D-penicillamine. *J. Rhematol.*, **12**, 892–6
120. Hamilton, J.A. and Williams, N. (1987). Effects of auranofin and other antirheumatic drugs on human myelopoiesis *in vitro*. *J. Rheumatol.*, **14**, 216–20
121. Waters, R.V. and Allison, A.C. (1987). Gold salts inhibit proliferation of promonocytic cells and accelerate their differentiation. *J. Rheumatol.* (Submitted)
122. Vaughan, J.H., Fosi, R.I., Abresch, R.J., Tsoukas, C.D., Curd, J.G. and Carson, P.A. (1984). Thoracic duct drainage in rheumatoid arthritis. *Clin. Exp. Immunol.*, **58**, 645–53
123. Ueo, T., Tanaka, S., Tominasa, Y., Osawa, H. and Sakurami, T. (1979). The effect of thoracic duct drainage on lymphocyte dynamics and clinical symptoms in patients with rheumatoid arthritis. *Arthr. Rheum.*, **22**, 1405–12

124. Bucy, R.P. (1986). Alloantigen-specific suppressor T-cells are not inhibited by cyclosporin A but do require IL-2 for activation. *J. Immunol.*, **137**, 809–13
125. Damle, N.K., Childs, A.L. and Doyle, L.V. (1987). Immunoregulatory T lymphocytes in man. Soluble antigen-specific suppressor-inducer T lymphocytes are derived from the CD4$^+$ CD45$^-$ P80$^+$ subpopulation. *J. Immunol.*, **139**, 1501–8
126. Harris, E.D. (1986). Recent insights into the pathogenesis of the proliferative lesion in rheumatoid arthritis. *Arthr. Rheum.*, **19**, 68–72
127. Mitchell, R.L., Zakas, L., Schreiber, R.D. and Verna, I. (1985). Rapid induction of the expression of the proto-oncogene *fos* during human monocytic differentiation. *Cell*, **40**, 209–17

# Index

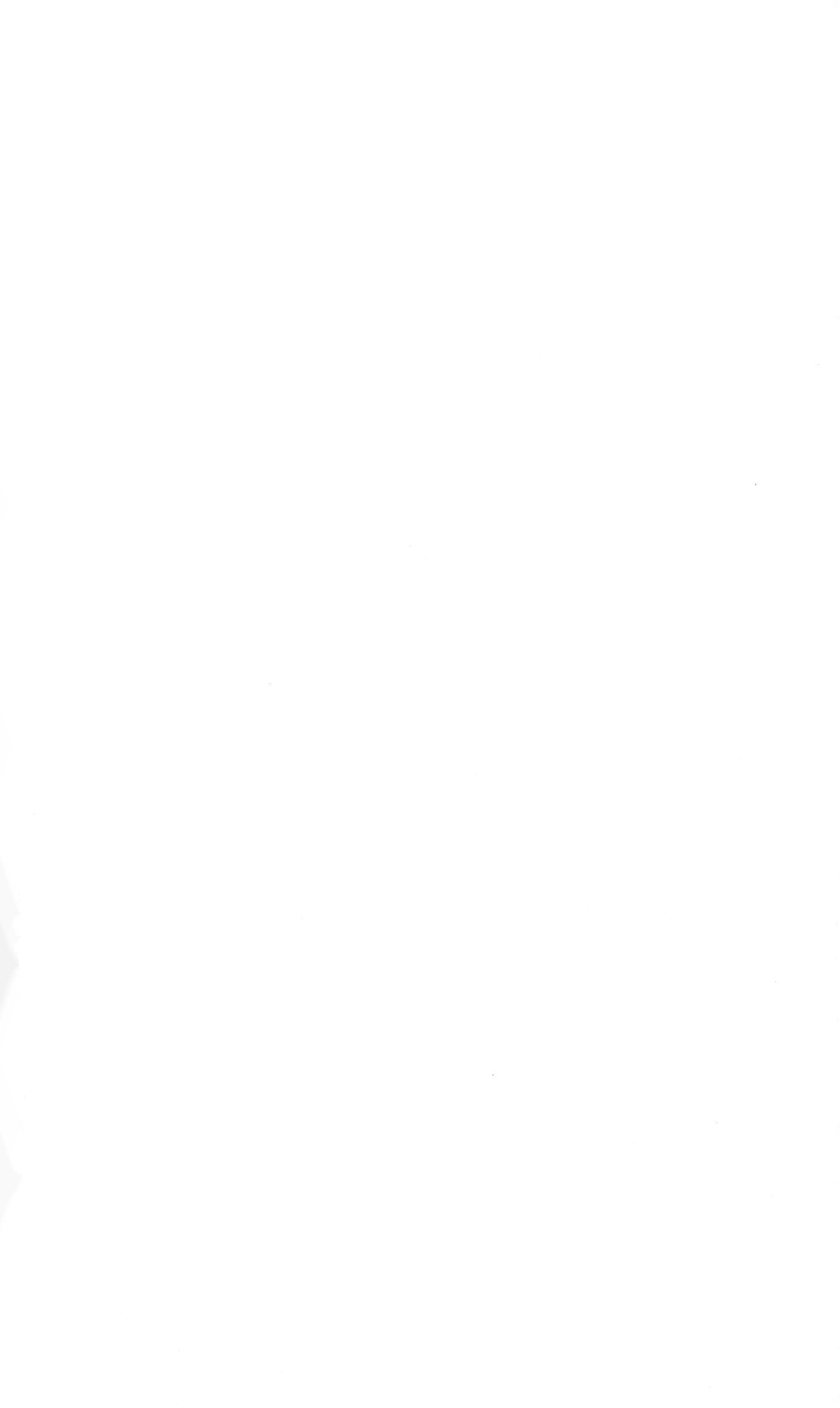

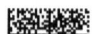